THE WORLD'S FITTEST BOOK

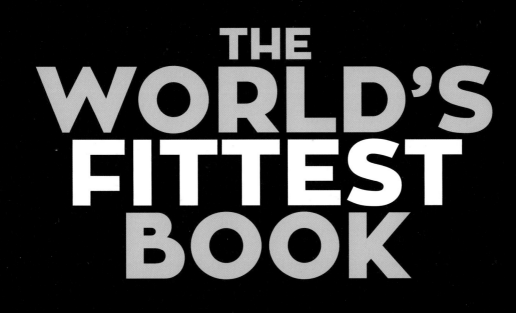

SPHERE

First Published in Great Britain in 2018 by Sphere

Copyright © Ross Edgley 2018

Every effort has been made by the author to ensure that all the information in this book is as precise and up-to-date as possible at the time of publication. It is recommended that before changing their diet or fitness regimes, readers always consult a qualified medical specialist for individual advice and to ensure any conditions specific to the reader are addressed. The author and publishers cannot be held responsible for any errors and omissions that may be found in the text, or for any actions that may be taken by the reader or any injury or illness caused as a result of any information contained in the text.

Photography: Allthingsgym.com (pp.244, 246); James Appleton (pp.10, 30, 53, 64, 66, 68, 69, 70, 71, 132, 269, 271, 274, 296, 320); Chris Bailey (pp.83, 105, 108, 109, 122, 123, 124, 192, 193, 194, 195, 239, 242); Anthony Barwell/BBC Photo Library (p.16); Rupert Bonington (p.136 (top)); Tani Devaux (Contents); Harvey Gibson (pp.32, 39, 43, 46, 54, 59, 95, 96, 107, 111, 120, 160, 186, 200, 216, 217, 228, 231, 233, 236, 255, 264, 283, 285, 287, 294, 295); Simon Howard (pp.21, 26, 88, 90, 134, 136 (lower 3 images), 151, 152, 161, 173, 177, 205, 206, 212, 254, 281); Richard Hunter (cover, pp. 13, 93, 125, 165, 180, 183, 201); Annie Mayne (pp.61, 155, 159, 174, 175, 176, 178, 179, 221, 223); Mike Poz (p.196); Phil Rowley Photography p.22; Hester Sabery (pp.98, 102, 103, 222); Hiroo Saso/BBC Photo Library (p.298); Tim Shieff/Bart Pronk (pp.72, 75, 77, 78); Shutterstock pp.4 (map), 14, 20, 33, 42, 76, 86, 97, 214, 236, 258, 268, 298 (globe); Adam Wiseman (pp.15, 19, 33, 34, 259, 299); Christie Wright (p.224)

Book Design: Sian Rance at D.R. ink

Illustrations: Emil Dacanay at D.R. ink

5 7 9 10 8 6

All rights reserved.
No part of this publication may be reproduced, stored in a retrieval system, or transmitted, in any form, or by any means, without the prior permission in writing of the publisher, nor be otherwise circulated in any form of binding or cover other than that in which it is published and without a similar condition including this condition being imposed on the subsequent purchaser.

The moral right of the author has been asserted.

A CIP catalogue record for this book is available from the British Library.

ISBN 978-0-7515-7254-4

Printed and bound in Italy by L.E.G.O. S.p.A.

Papers used by Sphere are from well-managed forests and other responsible sources.

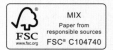

Sphere
An imprint of
Little, Brown Book Group
Carmelite House
50 Victoria Embankment
London EC4Y 0DZ

An Hachette UK Company
www.hachette.co.uk

www.littlebrown.co.uk

THE WORLD'S FITTEST BOOK: HOW TO TRAIN FOR ANYTHING AND EVERYTHING, ANYWHERE AND EVERYWHERE

ROSS EDGLEY

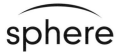

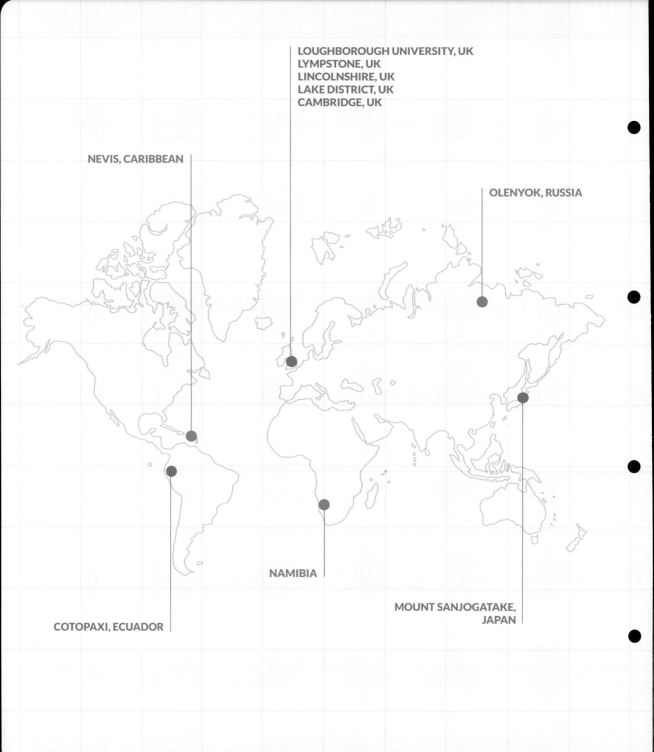

LOUGHBOROUGH UNIVERSITY, UK
LYMPSTONE, UK
LINCOLNSHIRE, UK
LAKE DISTRICT, UK
CAMBRIDGE, UK

NEVIS, CARIBBEAN

OLENYOK, RUSSIA

NAMIBIA

MOUNT SANJOGATAKE,
JAPAN

COTOPAXI, ECUADOR

Thank you to my mum and dad. You not only encouraged me to dance to the beat of my own drum, but you provided the drum and taught me how to play it.

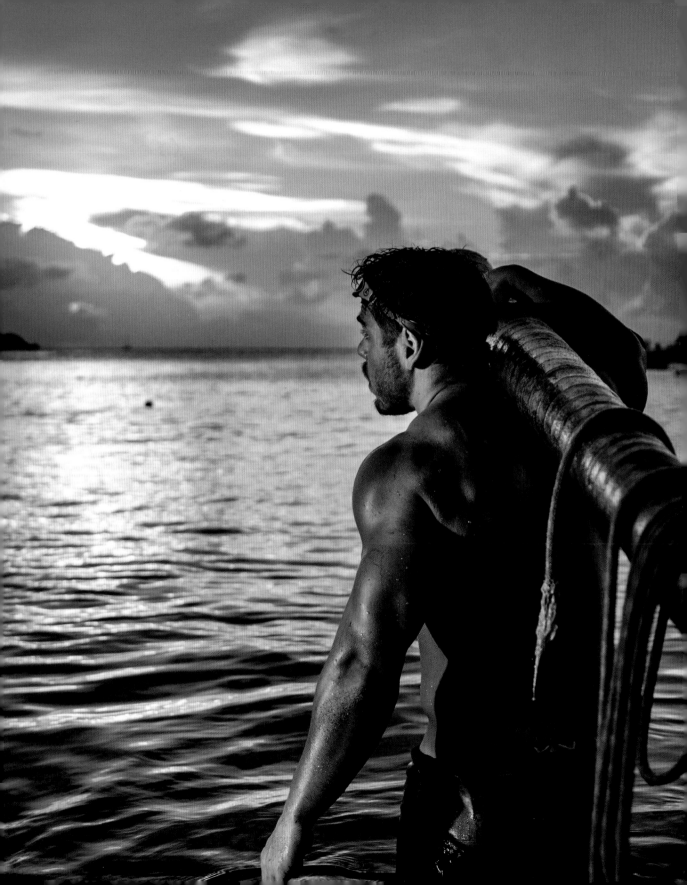

CONTENTS

FOREWORD

THIS IS NOT A FITNESS BOOK

This book is (unapologetically) different to most.

It's void of quick fixes, empty promises and magic pills. It doesn't present you with a training plan or diet guide and say: just blindly follow this. Instead, these 320 pages empower you to understand the principles of losing fat, building strength and improving endurance, so you can create your own fitness methods.

This approach is based on the work of American-born essayist Ralph Waldo Emerson. A pioneer in self-empowerment, he delivered more than 1500 public lectures on individualism and the importance of independence and self-reliance across the United States during the mid-19th century.

Empowering millions, he also shaped this entire book.

This is because in 1888 he wrote an essay aptly titled 'Self Reliance'. In it, he chose to ignore strict, insular **methods** in favour of more holistic, enduring **principles**. My favourite quote is:

'As to methods, there may be a million and then some, but principles a few. The man who grasps principles can successfully select his own methods.'
RALPH WALDO EMERSON

Which is especially relevant to our food and fitness.

Too many people are naively following 'methods' in the form of overpriced diet plans and training guides without actually understanding the 'principles' that govern them.

But this book was written to change all that...

MORE THAN A BOOK | A LITERARY REBELLION

Which is why, in many ways, this is not just a book. It's more like an empowering literary rebellion!

Based on the work of Brazilian educational theorist Paulo Freire and his concept of 'conscientization'[1], it promotes a critical way of thinking that teaches us to achieve an in-depth understanding of a subject – in this case food and fitness – so we can take action against limiting elements. By embracing this philosophy it's my hope we create an army of experts, not followers, because in reality no one knows your body better than you do.

You are your very best personal trainer.

You are your very best nutritionist.

Stop idolising gurus and looking for answers elsewhere.

'No one saves us but ourselves. No one can and no one may.
We ourselves must walk the path.'
BUDDHA

Instead, blaze **your own trail** and add strings to **your own bow**. Your best expert is you!

10-YEAR TOUR WITH THE WORLD'S FITTEST HUMANS

'I'm no prophet. My job is making windows where there were once walls.'
MICHEL FOUCAULT

This book is created from a melting pot of geniuses.

It cross-pollinates ideas and concepts from some extraordinary people who broke moulds, made waves and ruffled feathers in their chosen fields of strength, speed, endurance and food. From Olympic Champions and World Record Holders to remote tribes and celebrated members of the military.

Get to know them and you get to know fitness better than 99.99% of the population.

Now I acknowledge – and must state – that I'm not one of these fitness and food geniuses. Many times when writing this book I sat opposite them in awe. Eyes wide, mouth open and with most of their knowledge going over my head. Instead, my role has been to live and learn from each one.

With a notepad in one hand and a protein bar in the other, I travelled the world like a pen-wielding nomad to compile their teachings into the most eclectic and holistic fitness guide ever written. All so that you can become the strongest, leanest and fastest possible version of yourself.

WHY THE WORLD TOUR?

Learning should not be the study of one domain, but the combination of many.

This is an idea inspired by the brilliant book, *Mastery* by Robert Greene that I (randomly) read (many times over) during a lengthy boat ride down the Amazon river. It emphasises the importance of studying the work of other artists when trying to master a topic. Greene claims this is essential in the pursuit of mastery and uses Mozart as an example:

'Mozart never asserted any particular opinions about music. Instead, he absorbed the styles he heard around himself and incorporated them into his own voice. Late in his career, he encountered the music of Johann Sebastian Bach – a kind of music very different from his own. Most artists would grow defensive and dismissive of something that challenged their own principles. Instead, Mozart opened his mind up to new possibilities, studying Bach's use of counterpoint for nearly a year and absorbing it into his own vocabulary. This gave his music a new and surprising quality.'[2]

Which is why – inspired by Mr Mozart – I set off on my 10-year-long world tour, tracking down the world's fittest and most nutritionally advanced men and women.

It was from their collective teachings and inspiring stories that this book was born.

Ross Edgley

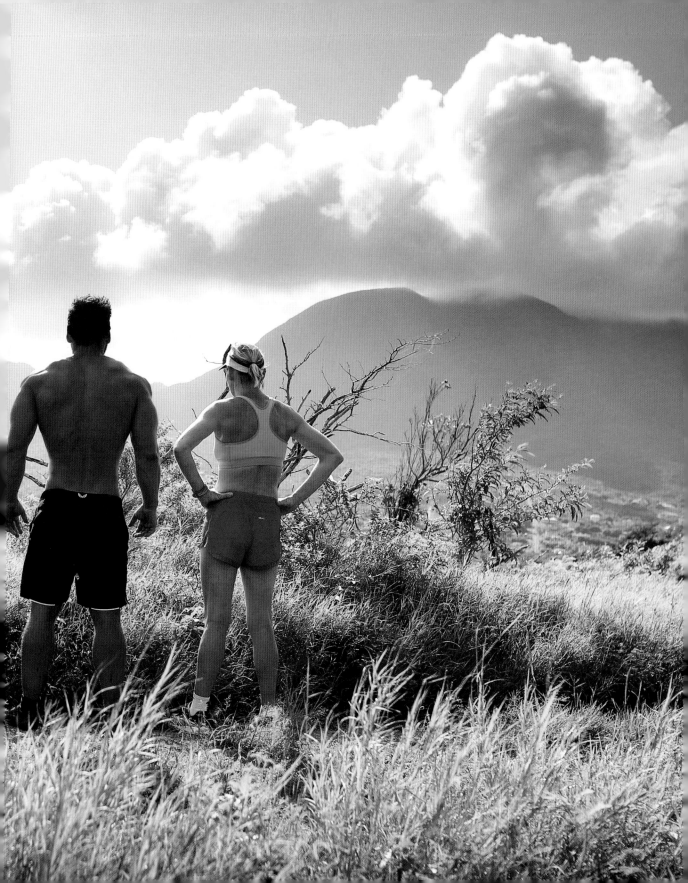

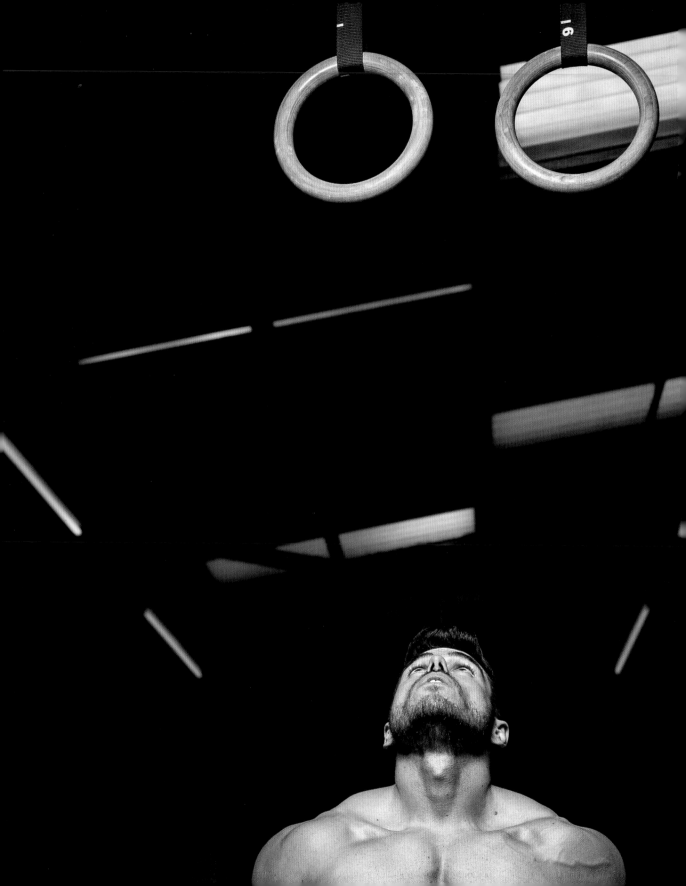

"WE MAY NEVER FULLY UNDERSTAND THE
MYSTERIES OF THE HUMAN BODY... BUT
SPENDING A LIFETIME TRYING IS ONE WELL
SPENT."

ROSS EDGLEY

PART I:
MY BEGINNING

WHEN THE BOOK STARTED | Andes Mountains, Ecuador (2008)

GRAB THE BULL BY THE HORNS

It's 11 March 2008 and I'm on a busy flight somewhere over South America.

I'm gripped by a strange blend of jetlag and adrenaline; sleep is a distant memory. Instead, I substitute hard-boiled sweets and caffeine for rest and recuperation as I research my next assignment.

See, graduation was a year earlier. Most of my friends left Loughborough University's School of Sport and Exercise Science and were immediately recruited by the English Institute of Sport. Taking up important roles as coaches, physicians and nutritionists, they'd later orchestrate the meteoric success of British sport at the London 2012 Olympics.

But life decided to deal me a different hand.

Equipped with pen, paper and a rucksack full of protein shakes I'd become this odd travel-writer-athlete hybrid. Developing a reputation for accepting even the weirdest of assignments, I'd spent a year flying, driving and sailing my way around the world, visiting the most remote and hostile places on earth.

It was far from conventional, but it was also far from dull.

Learning and living from men and women who were pushing the boundaries of human potential on a daily basis, my days consisted of everything from wrestling sharks in the Bahamas to charming poisonous cobras in Bangladesh. It basically made your typical extreme holiday look like a trip to Disneyland.

Now I'd like to say this was because of some noble quest. But if I can be honest, it was largely down to my complete aversion to boredom, child-like curiosity and inability to say 'no'. Still, to quote the early theologian St Augustine:

'The world is a book and those who do not travel read only one page.'
ST AUGUSTINE

So here I was, on yet another long-haul flight, reading a few more 'pages'. Heading to Ecuador in the hope that I would be accepted into a celebrated group of mountain cowboys known as Chagra as they prepared for this year's rodeo.

Duties would include wrestling, lassoing and branding wild bulls. Enduring hours of bum-numbing horseback riding. Finally, surviving all of this for 14 hours a day, at high altitude

(4000 metres above sea level), on a diet of soup and alcohol and void of anything that resembled a 'rest day'.

Was I excited? Yes.

Was I nervous? Very.

Was I completely out of my depth? Definitely.

But it was miles away from any treadmill or dumbbell – and on the muddy fields of this hacienda – that I learnt one of my most valuable lessons in fitness: to truly understand it, you have to live it.

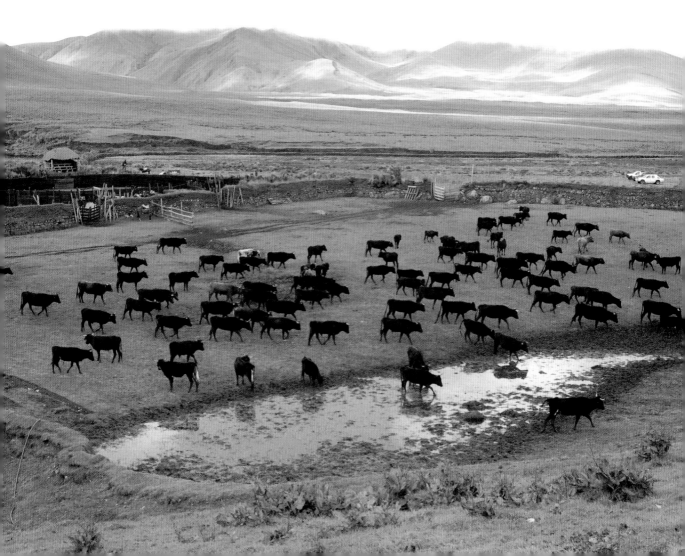

'STAY STILL!'

Two long hours had passed and the bull collapsed.

The rope around the horns was tight. My knee on his neck was firm. But the fight was far from over. That's because in an Ecuadorian rodeo the cavalry is never too far away and, unfortunately for me, that cavalry was this bull's bigger, angrier brother.

At around 900 kg (2000 lb), he was jet-black, foaming at the mouth and completely untamed. The battle scars on his face showed many had tried – but his unbranded hide showed that none had succeeded. Add to this a pair of deformed, jagged horns that were forever pointing in my direction and consider its aura of menace complete.

But it gets worse. This is Cotopaxi.

Over 5000 metres above sea level on the Andes Mountains, it's aptly named the Avenue of the Volcanoes. This is in reference to the fact that it sits on top of a collection of active ones. A place where altitude sickness taunts the lungs and plagues the muscles, and the threat of a potential volcanic eruption is always present.

However, these were way down my list of worries right now. At the top of that list was still the aforementioned bull that was now circling me, making his intentions quite clear. He had no regard for the medicine in my hand that I was trying to give to his smaller brother.

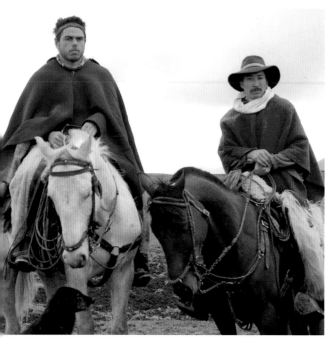

Me and Haraldo, a little hungover from the rodeo festivities the night before

He just saw a target that was my now tightly clenched buttocks.

So there I was. Unable to adjust my position in case the pinned bull sensed freedom and got up for round two. I looked to my mentor for guidance.

His name was Haraldo.

Chief Chagra, he stood 170 cm (5 ft 8 in) tall, had hardened leather-like skin and was the proud owner of the thickest and most impressive moustache I'd ever seen, like something out of a Hollywood movie. He'd also been lassoing bulls long before I was born. Which probably explains why, amid the mayhem, he casually sat on the fence of the hacienda – out of harm's way and carefully rolling a cigarette – and gave the following advice.

'Stay still! But if he charges don't stay still.'

Not quite the thorough plan I'd hoped for.

But then again this is South America's Wild West. There are no rules out here. If a bull chases you, be quick. If a bull catches you, be strong. But above all else, when the air is this thin, be fit. Basically agile, powerful and in the broadest sense of the word: just fit!

Inevitably the bull charged...

I ran...

Haraldo laughed...

A lot!

In that moment the sight of me leaping the 2-metre fence, headfirst and holding my buttocks, became cemented in Ecuadorian mountain folklore. That's because in the absence of TVs and books, Chagra stories become profoundly important. And the story of the terrified, airborne English sports graduate was practically Pulitzer worthy.

Needless to say, I returned to camp body intact, but ego heavily bruised.

But it didn't need to be. At around 11pm that night there was a knock at the door of the derelict garden shed I called home. It was Haraldo. It seemed my rodeo antics had earned me a 10-oz steak and a seat around the fire with some of the most respected Chagras in all of Cotopaxi. I of course eagerly accepted.

This was because I love steak and the Ecuadorian kind was known for being among the best in South America. But I also knew that to be semi-accepted despite not being entirely successful on the rodeo was a huge honour. So I grabbed my poncho and headed to this kind of 'cowboy gentlemen's club'. The festivities of which, I'd quickly learn, were more dangerous than the bull.

Among the steak, potatoes and open flames there was also an abundant supply of a specially home-brewed 70% alcoholic drink called *puntas*. Made from sugarcane, it can be mulled with cinnamon and fruit juices to make a cocktail, but whatever the serving suggestions, locals drink it like water, claiming it has medicinal properties.

This explains why, in the evenings, a sober Chagra is a rare phenomenon.

GET FIT OR GET DRUNK TRYING

No sooner had I arrived than my induction began.

A space was made for me to sit next to Manuel. The oldest and most respected of all the cowboys in Cotopaxi. How old? It was hard to tell. His wrinkled and weathered face told the story of a thousand rodeos. But his perfect posture, mischievous smile and constant playful taunting of the other Chagra led me to believe otherwise.

How respected? Very! All based on his battle scars and ability to drink like a fish: two valued qualities in this part of Ecuador. The latter I quickly learnt as my bum hit the seat and I was handed a hollowed-out bull's horn, filled to the brim with *puntas*, to serve as a shot glass.

I was, of course, keen to redeem myself from the day's failed bull wrestling. So we toasted. I drank. And everyone enjoyed my contorted face as it burnt my lips and hit the back of my throat. After waiting 10 seconds to be sure it wasn't going to come back up, I gestured with the bull's horn a second time to signal I was OK.

It was met with rapturous applause.

This format then continued long into the night. Songs were played on the guitar, stories were exchanged and my once-healthy and fully functioning liver slowly turned into pâté. But among the alcohol-induced merriment a special bond formed between Manuel and me.

This is because I don't mind admitting I'm not a hardened drinker. So it wasn't long before I was practically fermented. But Manuel was my rock. Sitting perfectly upright as I leaned against him to avoid falling in the fire, his body remained strong and sturdy as any concept of balance left mine.

With my head on his shoulder, I felt compelled to ask him something. How was it a man seemingly three times my age was able to outwork me in the day and outdrink me at night?

'Manuel, how old are you?' I asked.

This was met with more laughter around the fire. He put his hand on my head, took another shot and said, 'Who knows? Not me!'

Seeing my drunken confusion, Haraldo leant over and whispered 'Maybe 60. Maybe 70. But after his 50th birthday he stopped counting.'

I remember at the time thinking: this is genius. I was of course pretty drunk, but I thought that back home in England, society would tell him to retire. 'Experts' would tell him to take it easy. But (again) this is Cotopaxi. Void of restrictive ideals, Manuel was left to work, drink and party like he did when he was 21.

As a result, his body and mind seemed conditioned to completely defy Father Time.

'How old would you be if you didn't know how old you are?'
SATCHEL PAIGE, BASEBALL LEGEND

I slept that night very drunk, very tired and strangely inspired.

Morning came and I awoke on a wooden bench. My poncho offered some comfort as a temporary pillow, but my entire body ached from the night's alcohol-fuelled hospitality. Painfully hung over, I watched Haraldo – who'd already been awake for hours – as he chased horses across the mountains.

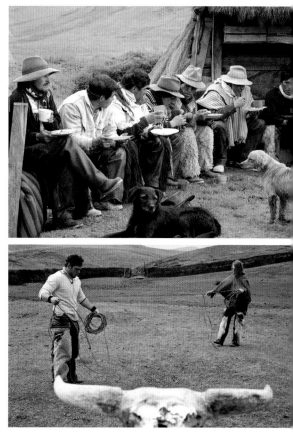

He'd drunk more than anyone last night! How was he still standing? In fact, how was he still conscious?

Another 14-hour day on the rodeo awaited me. I dragged myself off the bench and sobered up with some questionably served brown soup. In the cold light of day I was still utterly confused. Nothing made sense out here.

Four years of studying at Loughborough University's Olympic facility, and the physiology and nutrition of a Chagra baffled me. Everything from their crazy cardiovascular fitness, insane diet of steak and *puntas* and Manuel's complete lack of respect or concern for the ageing process.

All of which took place at sickeningly high altitude.

It was complete fitness ambiguity. It was in no book I'd ever read and no lecture I'd ever attended, but for some reason it worked. They had completely adapted to everything Cotopaxi could throw at them. I wrote the following *puntas*-induced epiphany in my notebook:

'We may never fully understand the mysteries of the human body...
But spending a lifetime trying is one well spent.'
ROSS EDGLEY

This signalled the end of my time in Ecuador, but the start of my fitness pilgrimage.

March 2008, and *The World's Fittest Book* had begun. Years would pass, pages would be written and I would come to understand the secrets of the Chagra and so much more.

WHY THE BOOK STARTED | Loughborough University (2006)

CHANGING THE RULES OF FITNESS

Returning to England, I realised the rules of fitness were about to change!

Why? Because they can! That's why.

Too many people see this idea of 'fitness' as a fixed doctrine. A set of infallible laws they must religiously follow. But this isn't true – just look at the Chagra. Instead, fitness is a vast, malleable and fluid concept. Within it are thousands of ideas you can learn, ignore, adopt or discard.

'It is often forgotten fitness is a complex state determined by several interacting components, each of which requires specialized training for optimal development.'
DR YURI VERKHOSHANSKY & MEL SIFF, Supertraining[1]

This is why the National Strength and Conditioning Association (NSCA)[2] and the American College of Sports Medicine[3] – both respected authorities in the area – were unable to define 'fitness' despite pages and pages of information published on it. Seriously, there's not one solid, agreed definition of fitness among all the gurus, magazines and organisations that each promise to help you improve yours.

But this isn't a bad thing.

We humans have a habit of always defining everything. Each stereotype, category and neatly organised pigeonhole helps us feel safe and secure. It makes us think we know how the world works. But by failing to define fitness in a general, broad context we can make it completely adaptive to our ever-changing and individual lives, bodies and goals.

That can only be good, right?

Everyone can interpret fitness differently! Yes, there are the often-quoted ten components of fitness (Cardiorespiratory Endurance, Muscular Endurance, Strength, Speed, Power, Flexibility, Coordination, Agility, Balance, Accuracy). But who's to say you can't train and eat for a triple-bodyweight deadlift (strength), a rapid marathon time (endurance) with rock-solid abs (body composition) and a side helping of protein pancakes?

Experts? Doctors? What about sports scientists?

What, the same people who told Roger Bannister it was physiologically impossible for the human body to run under a 4-minute mile? Well, that doesn't quite explain why the

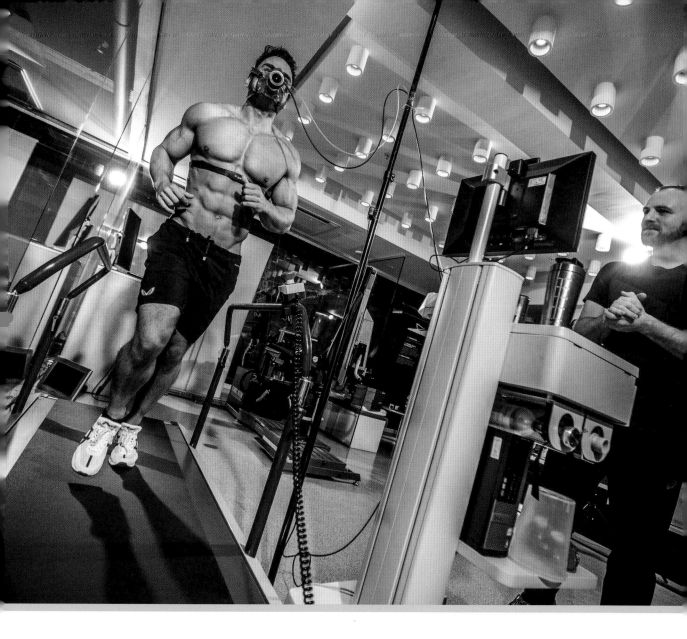

25-year-old former medical student took to Oxford's Iffley Road track on the evening of 6 May, 1954 to run a 3-minute-59.4-second mile time.

Which is exactly why this book was written.

Created with the help of some truly inspiring individuals who – like the Chagra of Cotopaxi – had no regard for rules, limitations or plateaus, it contains the teachings of champions, record holders, ancient tribes and sporting icons who broke the rules, crossed boundaries and pushed the limits of human potential.

All united by a desire to find their fitness.

They want to run faster, lift heavier and cycle further on their own terms. Refusing to be dictated to by others, they are masters of the Law of Biological Individuality. The only unequivocal law of human behaviour, it teaches us that, however alike we may be in many ways, our physiologies hold so many differences that each of us is truly biologically unique.

This is something I discovered on the floor of Loughborough University's library when I found that 51% of 'printed fitness' cannot be trusted. It's misleading, misinformed and wrongly mass-broadcasted as a solution to all.

A one-size-fits-all approach is an approach that fits no one.

50% OF FITNESS IS WRONG

'I can't bear art that you can walk round and admire. A book should be either a bandit or a rebel.'

D.H. LAWRENCE

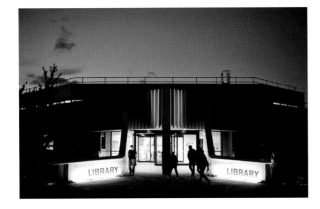

It's midnight on 25 July 2006 in a quiet corner of Loughborough University's library.

I'm two days away from handing in my dissertation proposal with no clue what it should be. Hence I'm sat on the floor among a diverse mix of sports science journals, fitness magazines and ancient philosophy. All the time desperately looking for inspiration and aimlessly making notes on a small notepad.

I wasn't hopeful either. Sleep was a distant memory, I hadn't showered or shaved for a week and the entire time I was semi-delirious from the heavily stimulated, home-made sports drink that I scientifically sipped on the hour to keep me awake.

I was like a medicated library-dwelling hobo.

But it was in my darkest, most unhygienic hour, while flicking through pages of Ralph Waldo Emerson and Plato, that I realised something. Those older books found in the corners of the library collecting cobwebs emphasised principles of enduring success. This is why they'd been there so long.

In contrast, the shiny, Photoshopped books from current authors were fixated on immediate results. They tended to become replaced as quickly as they'd arrived and were far less enduring.

So what was my caffeine-fuelled epiphany?

'Don't judge a book by its cover; judge it by its shelf life.'
ROSS EDGLEY (self-medicated and semi-delirious)

I quickly wrote down the above quote in big bold letters.

Then – with my senses now alive from the tyrosine and guarana cocktail – I began looking through pages and pages of books and magazines until eventually, somewhere between Socrates and *Sports Illustrated*, I noticed something: most commercial fitness magazines share a common 'literary formula'.

First, there's something I called a 'False Declarative' or 'Interrogative of False Intention'. These are terms I coined to describe bold statements or questions that almost promise results. They are then usually coupled with a superlative adjective or adverb, typically promising you'll be 'bigger', 'leaner' and/or 'stronger'. What's left is a collection of headlines like:

'Build Muscle in Five Easy Steps!'

'Want To Lose Fat Fast?'

'The Best Diet for Immediate Results!'

'Want Rock Solid Abs Fast?'

Sound familiar? I called them 'Fitness Fairytales'. The industry is riddled with them and on average they make up 51% of the headlines you'll find in fitness magazines[4]. I'm not the only one to think so either. The sports science genius Dr Mel Siff said it best:

'The public usually feels far more comfortable with cerebrally undemanding mantras and "fast food" solutions than with far more accurate, complex methods. This is a major reason why many fitness figures write as they do and market their catch phrases simplistically as they do – society has been processed by mass media to behave like that and they usually do not want to be forced to think too deeply or to have their convenient current beliefs questioned, because that entails a serious threat to their psychological safety.'
DR MEL SIFF

In summary, Fitness Fairytales sound great, but most over-promise and under-deliver. Bullet pointing short, snappy instructions for us to unquestionably obey, they fail to teach us even the most basic rules of food and fitness. Basically, thorough and in-depth education like in 'days of old' is all but forgotten.

Which is why, in that moment, I put pen to paper and my dissertation was written.

'I'm not interested in preserving the status quo; I want to overthrow it.'
NICCOLÒ MACHIAVELLI

TEACH A MAN TO FISH

'Give a man a fish and you feed him for a day; teach a man to fish and you feed him for a lifetime.'
ANNE ISABELLA THACKERAY RITCHIE

On a small side note, I don't blame modern writers for using Fitness Fairytales.

In a fast-paced, competitive capitalist society obsessed with quick fixes, the *Big Book of Hard Work, Patience & Fat Loss* probably wouldn't sell many copies. Granted, it would be more effective, but what good is that when your mum is the only one who turns up to your book signing?

Thankfully I love writing.

It's passion and not a profession and – at the risk of sounding like a Miss World speech – I always liked the idea of writing a book that would empower people even after I'm gone and training at the big gym in the sky.

In short, I want to teach people to fish.

That's why this book was written against the grain and without a commercial agenda. You won't be promised a perfect workout nor a magic diet plan that answers all your dietary prayers. Instead, the foundations are forged very differently from most.

If my mum is the only one at my book signing, so be it.

'The writer is fully aware that his message is not orthodox; but since our orthodox theories have not saved us we may have to readjust them.'
WEST A. PRINCE, Nutrition and Physical Degeneration

LIVE BEYOND REPS AND CALORIES

'You have to do stuff that average people don't understand because those are the only good things.'
ANDY WARHOL

Leaving university, I chose to ignore most modern magazines. Instead, I learnt about health, food and fitness through old books and barbells.

What did I find?

That human fitness is complex, powerful and infinite in its potential. In fact, it's fair to say we still don't fully know what the body is capable of and have barely scratched the surface in our understanding of it. So it stands to reason that we should not restrict our exploration of fitness with regimes, checklists and (false) glossy magazine headlines.

It was for this very reason that Bruce Lee – martial arts icon and one of the greatest pioneers of human physical excellence –famously once said:

'Use no way as way, use no limitation as limitation.'
BRUCE LEE

He was absolutely right, and not alone in his belief either...

Dr Yuri Verkhoshansky and Dr Mel Siff also knew this. Two of the greatest coaches ever to live, they pushed the boundaries of strength and conditioning, authored more than 500 scientific-methodological papers (each) and trained thousands of athletes to run faster, jump further and lift heavier than any before them.

How did they do this?

Well not through the age-old 'repetition/weight scheme' that most books and magazines broadcast, that's for sure. Instead, our strength and conditioning Yodas said:

'The summary of training approaches given in the table may be adequate for the average personal trainer or coach dealing with the average client or lower-level athlete, but it needs to be expanded upon to take into account the objectives stated.'
DR YURI VERKHOSHANSKY & DR MEL SIFF, Supertraining

Note the word **average**.

Variable	Strength	Power	Hypertrophy	Endurance
Load (% of one-rep maximum*)	80–100	70–100	60–80	40–60
Repetitions per set	2–5	1–5	6–15	25–60
Sets per exercise	4–7	3–5	4–8	2–4
Rest between sets (minutes)	2–6	2–6	2–5	1–2
Durations (seconds per set)	5–10	4–8	20–60	80–150
Speed per rep (% of max)	60–100	90–100	60–90	60–80
Training sessions per week	3–6	3–6	5–7	8–14

* 'One rep maximum' (1RM) is a term used to define the maximum amount of force that can be generated in one maximal contraction or lift.

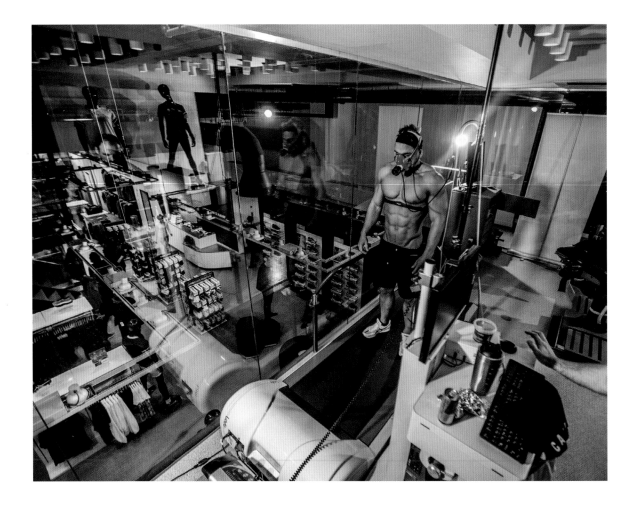

We've become regimented to the point of mediocrity. Wrapping our training in rules and formulaic tables to make us feel safe and assured. But it's not exactly progressive and pioneering. To quote a modern-day sports science legend (and friend), John Kiely: 'Such findings challenge the appropriateness of applying generic methodologies to the planning problems posed by inherently complex biological systems.'[5]

John was talking about the dangers of planning your training too much. Proposing that too many of us live within the parameters of sets and reps that were created to be tools, not limiting rules.

It's not just in fitness either. One of my favourite authors, Nassim Nicholas Taleb, claims – in his book *The Bed of Procrustes* – that we have this need for explanatory closure and aversion to uncertainty:

'We humans, facing limits of knowledge, and things we do not observe, the unseen and the unknown, resolve the tension by squeezing life and the world into crisp commoditized ideas, reductive categories, specific vocabularies, and prepackaged narratives.'

NASSIM NICHOLAS TALEB

This explains why your 'average personal trainer' can't think outside the repetition/weight scheme. Or why many runners seek solace in the treadmill, but fear the squat rack like the plague. Or even why so many strength athletes are capable of moving mountains, but mobility training and touching their toes seem alien. But we must think beyond 'pre-packaged' ideas if we want to progress. It's like learning to ride a bike and never taking the stabilisers off. And no one ever won the Tour de France with their stabilisers still on, did they?

'Uncertainty, in the presence of vivid hopes and fears, is painful, but must be endured if we wish to live without the support of comforting fairy tales.'

BERTRAND RUSSELL

Our nutrition is no more developed either.

According to the World Health Organization, 'More than 1.4 billion adults were overweight in 2008, and more than half a billion obese.'[6] Why?

Research published by the Cambridge University Press[7] believes 'Obesity and related diseases are problems not addressable through arithmetic dieting (i.e. calorie counting).' Basically, we're too mathematical and 'mechanical' in our approach to food.

'The meaning of life is that it is to be lived. It is not to be traded and conceptualized and squeezed into a pattern of systems.'

BRUCE LEE

Which is how this book came to be.

It starts with **Your Body's Five-point User Guide**, which teaches you how to train anything and everything, anywhere and everywhere, no matter what your goal, age or level of ability.

YOUR BODY'S FIVE-POINT USER GUIDE

The sum and substance of over ten years of research, I present... **Your Body's Five-point User Guide!**

A framework to achieve physical awesomeness, it's shaped into a **Pyramid of Priority** that I use in my university talks. Why a pyramid? Because it's the best-shaped graph to show how your attention should be organised when training your body, like a hierarchical (progressive) way to build your body from the ground up. Too many people are trying to lose fat or build muscle with no solid foundation.

But you can't build a castle on the sand, you can't shoot a cannon out of a canoe and you can't begin training without understanding the five laws of fitness that form the base of the Pyramid of Priority.

THE FIVE LAWS OF FITNESS

Everyone needs to read this section!

These laws govern 100% of all fitness goals. Whether you want to build a larger, more powerful physique or craft a leaner version of yourself, everything becomes easier when you understand these laws. If you're a beginner – or you've hit a plateau – read (or reread) this section because it will form the foundation of any fitness goal. These laws are covered in chapters 1–5.

ACHIEVE ANY FITNESS GOAL

This section is categorised by goals which are covered in chapters 6–9.

Each goal has a section devoted to it that comes packed with studies and secrets from all over the world. These are organised (again) into smaller Pyramids of Priority to show the hierarchical (progressive) way to focus your efforts on the things that will yield the biggest return.

- The lower parts of the pyramid make the biggest difference to that goal.
- The higher parts make a meaningful contribution to your goal, but only once you've laid the foundations.
- The top part of this (and every) pyramid is actually infinite and forever evolving. This is why they are all open-ended and may never have a peak, because our understanding and exploration of the body should never be 'capped' or concluded.

Pyramids of Priority

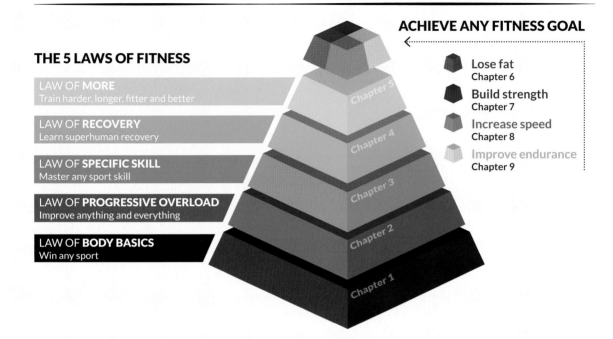

ACHIEVE ANY FITNESS GOAL

THE 5 LAWS OF FITNESS

LAW OF **MORE**
Train harder, longer, fitter and better

LAW OF **RECOVERY**
Learn superhuman recovery

LAW OF **SPECIFIC SKILL**
Master any sport skill

LAW OF **PROGRESSIVE OVERLOAD**
Improve anything and everything

LAW OF **BODY BASICS**
Win any sport

Chapter 5
Chapter 4
Chapter 3
Chapter 2
Chapter 1

Lose fat
Chapter 6

Build strength
Chapter 7

Increase speed
Chapter 8

Improve endurance
Chapter 9

HOW THE BODY AND BRAIN WORK

Your Body's Five-point User Guide is based on the work of leading psychologists. Believing this is how the human brain was designed to work, in 1936 the Swiss developmental psychologist Jean Piaget created a systematic way of studying mental development and found we learn through 'schemas'. These are building blocks of intelligent behaviour that we can again combine to deal with a task.

'Only education is capable of saving our societies from possible collapse, whether violent, or gradual.'

JEAN PIAGET

Fast forward to 1949 and enter the psychosocial pioneer Harry Harlow. He suggested that we humans – and other intelligent animals – notice patterns and shortcuts that make us more efficient learners. We not only learn, but we learn to learn, becoming faster at solving new problems as we gain experience solving older ones. This explains why if you learnt to become strong, learning to become fast should be easier. The process of tweaking and tailoring your training is very similar; it's just for another goal. To quote Mr Harlow, you have 'learnt to learn'.

> "THERE ARE MANY WAYS TO GET FITTER, STRONGER AND LEANER. YOU SHOULDN'T DISCRIMINATE AGAINST ANY OR STRICTLY FAVOUR ONE. AS SOON AS YOU DO, YOU CLOSE YOUR MIND AND LIMIT YOUR POTENTIAL."

ROSS EDGLEY

PART II:
THE FIVE LAWS OF FITNESS

CHAPTER 1
THE LAW OF BODY BASICS

"IF YOU HAVE BUILT CASTLES IN THE AIR, YOUR WORK NEED NOT BE LOST; THAT IS WHERE THEY SHOULD BE. NOW PUT THE FOUNDATIONS UNDER THEM."
HENRY DAVID THOREAU

THE LAW OF BODY BASICS | Olenyok, Russia

MASTER ANY SPORT

It's 21 April 2008, a month after I left the cowboys of Cotopaxi.

I remember this day well. It was the day I learnt the secret to mastering any and every sport.

This is because, having survived an alcohol-fuelled trip to Ecuador (my liver is still not sure what happened)… then having spent a month living with the Evenki reindeer herders of Siberia (my fingers and nose still defrosting)… I'm now en route to a derelict gym that's still standing from the days of the Soviet Union.

Why another random excursion?

Because I've always been fascinated by the strength and conditioning secrets of Eastern Europe. So when I was invited to train alongside a former soldier-turned-celebrated-wrestler I thought it was too good an opportunity to miss. Which is why, despite having never spoken a word of Russian and never wrestled a day in my life, I went in search of the man they called Nikolai.

At this moment I should point out I was completely out of my depth.

Yes, I had studied sports science from the comfort and confines of Loughborough University for the past four years of my life, but that was of little to no use out here. This was rural Russia after all. It was cold, it was harsh and it did not care about my degree.

A plane, train and taxi ride later I found myself standing before an entrance to a gym with my heart pounding in anticipation of what was to come. The damp, humid, sweat-

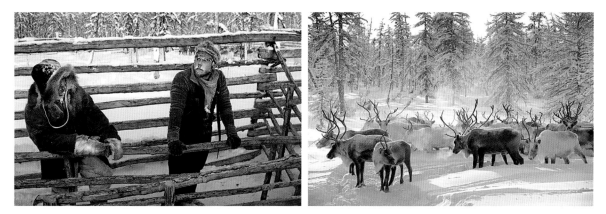

As you can tell from my beard, Olenyok is not warm

drenched walls and sound of grunting men and iron weights almost served as a warning to those brave enough to enter. But, determined, I pressed on and eventually found myself cautiously opening the doorway to the main hall.

Trying to remain inconspicuous, I failed miserably. The ancient hinges of the giant wooden door squeaked as it opened and instantly announced my arrival to the gym's (large) inhabitants. Now five of the biggest, scariest men I have ever seen are staring in my direction, one even pausing midway through a pull-up with what looked like 40 kg hanging from his waist to see what the strange Englishman was doing in their gym. If I'm honest, I don't blame them either. I must have looked so odd standing there, clutching my notepad with a few Russian phrases written on the first page.

I was like a tourist gone wrong.

Thankfully, salvation arrived in the form of a 65-year-old, locally celebrated, military-trained wrestling champion.

This was Nikolai.

After a few weeks of awkwardly translated emails (we both relied heavily on Google translate) it was great to finally meet the local hero. Words can't quite do Nikolai justice, but I will try.

Essentially, he was a lot like a man, only much bigger.

At 193 cm tall (6 ft 4 in) and over 104 kg (230 lb), he was built like most things in Russia: robust, hardwearing and utterly intimidating. Also, despite being three times my age he didn't have an ounce of fat on him, only lots of hair that sprouted from the holes in the old military T-shirt he was wearing and incredibly tight shorts that left very little to the imagination.

But questionable attire and ample body hair aside, as he greeted me with a vice-like grip and giant hands, I was grateful he was here. My association with him almost seemed to validate my presence to the other men mountains.

There was, however, a problem.

Without the aid of our mutual friend, Google translate, we had no way of communicating. Which, unfortunately for me, meant he would administer his lessons by throwing me around a wrestling mat until he got bored or broke me. Looking at his shovel-sized hands I feared it would be the latter.

'Wrestle,' he said as he walked over to the mats.

I got the sense this wasn't an invitation, but more a command, so hurriedly I fell in behind him. With the aid of the notes scribbled on my notepad and a pocket-sized Russian phrase book, I tried my best to explain I'd never wrestled before. He only looked confused and began stretching.

Clearly there was no turning back now and clearly this was not going to end well for me. So, preparing myself for the worst, I placed my bag on the floor and also began stretching, all in the vain hope that my sports background might help me in some small way.

It didn't. It was fair to say that on the day I came second.

Moments later, and despite my best efforts, my face was inevitably being squashed into the mat by the tree trunks he called legs. It was like wrestling a giant, sweaty bear. This continued for 50 minutes as a wrestling war veteran humped me up and down the mat, pinning me at his leisure.

What seemed like hours passed, and my body and ego were badly bruised. What's worse, news of my visit had reached the neighbouring school and now my entire demise was being witnessed by a group of children sitting on the perimeter of the gym to cheer on their local hero.

As they celebrated every painful 'body slam' and uncomfortable 'wedgie', I can safely say this was not my finest sporting moment. But weirdly it turned out to be one of my most valuable. That's because after another painful hour, Nikolai permitted me a short break from hitting the floor with my face. He offered me a cup of water from a defrosting block of ice and a seat beside him on the mat. I gratefully accepted and took the opportunity to 'talk' with him – by a combination of gesticulating, pointing and grunting – about all things training- and diet-related.

It was there – on a sweat-soaked wrestling mat in Russia – I learned to master any sport.

There was no denying Nikolai was an example of human physical excellence. He'd just absolutely embarrassed an athlete one-third of his age and barely looked out of breath doing it. But what baffled me that was he'd casually done it while claiming to have followed such a basic, generic training plan.

It was so simple it verged on the primitive.

With a shrug of his giant shoulders, he reached for his bag. Carefully unpacking the contents, he laid a collection of old training journals and military workouts he'd written onto the mat. He later told me he'd prepared them for my arrival but was waiting to deem me worthy before showing them to me.

I picked up the largest journal and scanned the pages. It was 500 pages thick. No preface, no contents page and no irrelevant literary foreplay. Just pure facts and sport/soldier-themed theory densely packed into every page. The workouts were no different: easy to understand with the repetitions and sets clearly detailed, they were regimented and well ordered, all with an emphasis on simple, often bodyweight, exercises.

Lots of push-ups – sometimes single-armed variations – dips, pull-ups, monkey bars, planks, lunges, split squats, single-leg balance drills, single-leg hops, L-sits, carries, single-arm overhead presses, single-arm overhead squats…

The list of illustrations was endless.

Seeing I was instantly and deeply engrossed in the contents, Nikolai stood up, patted me on the head with his huge palm, then walked to another corner of the gym to run some throwing and jumping drills with some of the younger athletes, leaving me to uncover Soviet training secrets on my own, one page at a time.

So what did I learn on the sweaty mat that day?

In short, I (painfully) understood Bodyweight Training and General Physical Preparedness.

Allow me to explain the latter first.

'Be general in your foundations so you can be specific in your goals.'
ROSS EDGLEY, Ego and body bruised

The Soviet Secret: General Physical Preparedness

This is a form of general training and conditioning used to improve strength, speed, endurance, flexibility and skill. It's completely non-specific. Instead, it encourages lots of big, functional movements that use universal motor recruitment patterns and improve work capacity – the amount of training you can complete (recover from) and adapt positively to.

It might sound complex, but as usual it's not. It's basically a training programme that encourages you to squat, lunge, jump, climb, press and throw as much as possible, as often as possible. All before you begin any specialist forms of training.

Simple? Yes.

Necessary? Absolutely.

By doing this, you improve your quality of movement, enhance your body's ability to handle greater workloads and prevent any imbalances. Nikolai was living proof of this. Having practised Russian General Physical Preparedness for years, he was still training and looked fresh as a daisy as I sat slumped on the floor reading. In many ways, this was the workout time forgot.

Today's commercial gyms are flooded with people trying to build strength, speed and stamina with no solid 'base' of basic fitness. They're running before they can walk, or rather curling before then can deadlift. The problem is that the foundations are weak. You can't build a castle on the sand and you can't create a fit, functional, good-looking physique solely with tricep kickbacks and calf raises.

When I returned to the UK to write up my notes, I discovered Nikolai wasn't alone in his training methodology. He was a child of the Russian training system known as the Process of Achieving Sports Mastery. Basically, a lifelong means of training and conditioning an athlete that was practised by all the great strength and conditioning coaches of the former Soviet Union. They believed General Physical Preparedness should make up a preparatory period of a training programme. This is usually a long period that takes place when there are no competitions or need for specific skills and game strategy. Or, in Nikolai's case, as a child growing up.

'The major emphasis of this period is establishing a base level of conditioning to increase the athlete's tolerance for more intense training. Conditioning activities begin at relatively low intensities and high volumes: long, slow distance running or swimming; low-intensity plyometrics; and high-repetition resistance training with light to moderate resistances.'

NSCA[1]

Even at five years old, Nikolai would have been performing some kind of General Physical Preparedness. Often it would involve running, climbing or throwing, and didn't really feel like exercise. On the odd occasion, he might have carried some kettlebells or weights, but generally it just seemed fun.

The theory underlying this system was that if an athlete develops a well-rounded athletic base their overall motor potential and just their ability to move will correspondingly improve. Over time, you can then specialise with this newly developed neurological efficiency and play any sport.Without it you will be forever training with the 'physiological handbrake' on.

The Soviet coaches believed the direct relationship between the central nervous system (CNS) and physical training played a paramount role in an athlete's adaptation to training. If they were neurologically efficient at a young age, they'd be able to mature and develop through the different stages of the Process of Achieving Sports Mastery framework – exactly how Nikolai had done with wrestling.

KNOW YOUR BODY

What I learnt on the sweaty mats that day is closely related to **kinaesthetic awareness**.

Don't be put off by the technical name. It's just a complex way of saying, 'know where your body is in space'. Developing this ability helps you in two ways:

1. Knowing when you're training right or wrong

Better kinaesthetic awareness means a better understanding of when the movements you're doing feel right or wrong. This kind of biological feedback helps you make adjustments to perform the movements better and more efficiently.

2. Better physiological intuition

It can also help with external coaching cues. These are verbal or visual prompts that focus you on the outcome of the movement. For instance, when getting people to engage their glutes during a deadlift, I might say 'Imagine squeezing a walnut between your butt cheeks'. Or if trying to get someone to bench press more powerfully, I might say 'Try to throw the bar to the ceiling'.

Basically, the better you understand how it feels for your body to move, the more sense external cues will make and the better you can apply them. You will have created a well-rounded, athletic base, rooted in general physical preparation, so that your overall motor potential – movement ability – will correspondingly improve when you want to specialise later.

All things considered, the formula is simple:

- Run, jump, push and pull first (Law of Body Basics).
- Learn to do more of these things (Law of Progressive Overload).
- Then you can specialise (and wrestle) later (Law of Specific Skill).

'This provides the base framework for the neurological construction of all subsequently developed motor skills.'
THE DEVELOPMENT OF THE RUSSIAN CONJUGATE SEQUENCE SYSTEM

CHAPTER 2
THE LAW OF PROGRESSIVE OVERLOAD

> " THOSE WHO HAVE NEVER BEEN TO THE EDGE AND LOOKED OVER WILL NEVER UNDERSTAND THAT IT IS BETTER TO LIVE ONE DAY AS A LION THAN A LIFETIME AS A SHEEP. THE ONES THAT HAVE BEEN TO THE EDGE KNOW THAT HARD TIMES DON'T LAST FOREVER, BUT HARD MEN DO! "
>
> ROYAL MARINES

YOU MUST ADAPT

All workouts ever created have one thing in common: **progressive overload**.

This is the gradual increase in weight, volume, intensity, frequency or time training in order to achieve a specific goal. Basically, the teeny tiny incremental improvements you make each time you step into the gym, lace up your trainers or enter the swimming pool.

Bicep curls, squats, marathon running, Olympic lifting and yoga are all designed to progressively adapt and improve something. This is because exercise, by its very nature, is an adaptive process. It's the whole reason we do it.

If you're not attempting to improve or progress in some way, it's probably not training.

Which is why a thorough understanding of progressive overload and the 'law of adaptation' is an absolute necessity. Too often people attack the weights rack or treadmill with no real comprehension of why they're doing it. It's like attending an art class with no paint or brush, but expecting to reproduce the Sistine Chapel.

Brief biology backstory

As long as we are alive, we will be adapting. But our understanding of this didn't fully develop until 1915, thanks to an American physiologist by the name of Walter Cannon and a French scientist called Charles Richet.

Cannon and Richet were instrumental in our understanding of something called **homeostasis**. This is the ability of the body to seek and maintain a stable internal state. Now this can get complicated, but like most things, there's no need for it to be.

So you know when your body temperature is good? Your immune system is OK? And millions of other internal mechanisms are running like clockwork to keep you healthy? All without you consciously having to lift a finger. This is homeostasis at work. It's that easy.

'The living being is stable. It must be so in order not to be destroyed, dissolved or disintegrated by the colossal forces, often adverse, which surround it. By an apparent contradiction, it maintains its stability only if it is excitable and capable of modifying itself according to external stimuli and adjusting its response to the stimulation. In a sense, it is stable because it is modifiable – the slight instability is the necessary condition for the true stability of the organism.'[1]

Fast forward to 1936...

An Austrian-Canadian endocrinologist by the name of Hans Selye used the work of Cannon and Richet to explain how certain 'stimuli' and 'stress' can impact our homeostasis and cause us to adapt and improve. To prove his theory, he took a lab full of rats and found that if he gradually subjected them to an increased dose of poison they began to develop a greater resistance to it, so much so that certain rats remained unharmed when later subjected to dosages that had previously killed them. 'By giving gradually increasing doses of various alarming stimuli, one may raise the resistance of animals... rats pre-treated with a certain agent will resist such doses of this agent, which would be fatal for not pre-treated controls.'

This became known as the 'General Adaptation Syndrome', and with his now-indestructible rates Selye discovered: 'It has been shown that when an organism is exposed to a stimulus to the quality or intensity of which it is not adapted, it responds with a reaction which has been termed the "general adaptation syndrome[2]".'

Basically, 'stress' and 'stimuli' (like exercise) cause us to adapt and improve.

Years later in his book, *The Stress of Life*, he added: 'Stress is the common denominator for all adaptive reactions of the body.'

OK, backstory over.

What does this mean for your training? At some point it's going to hurt.

Something the Royal Marines understand better than anyone.

THE LAW OF PROGRESSIVE OVERLOAD | Royal Marine Training Camp, UK

IMPROVE ANYTHING AND EVERYTHING

Tucked away in the south-west of England, the Commando Training Centre in Lympstone is the principal training centre for the Royal Marines. For over 75 years it's housed 3000 officers and men in 74 huts on 54 acres of prime East Devon countryside and has a proud heritage of recruitment, training and selection for the British military. Home to some of the fittest and most mentally resilient humans to ever live, it's a sacred place for many soldiers. Then you have me.

Arriving on base in my flip-flops – I'd been to the beach that morning – sweatpants and a hoodie, I looked like a Marine recruit gone (very) wrong. I checked in at the arrivals desk and made my way to the assault course on the bottom field.

It was March and very early in the morning and although the grass was relatively dry underfoot and the sun was shining, it was strangely and sporadically cold as the sea breeze changed from refreshing to chilling. I was jogging on the spot, flicking my feet out in front of me to force the blood (and feeling) back into my toes, for 20 minutes before my sporting saviours arrived.

Allow me to introduce Royal Marine Physical Training Instructor Alex 'Benny' Benstead and Royal Marine Captain Oliver 'Ollie' Mason.

Firstly, Benny is the pound-for-pound strongest Royal Marine–powerlifting hybrid I have ever met. Owner of the world's most dense shoulder and moustache combination, he bench presses 170 kg (375 lb), deadlifts 260 kg (573 lb) and squats 240 kg (529 lb), completed the Royal Marines Commando tests (twice) and will casually bust out 30-mile+ speed marches with 54 kg (120 lb) on his back.

Secondly, Ollie is without doubt the largest Marine I've ever met who casually smashes ultra-marathons on no notice. Standing at 193 cm (6 ft 4 in) and weighing 120 kg (264 lb), he plays rugby for the Royal Marines and owns a pair of legs and lungs that look like they should belong to a thoroughbred horse.

Needless to say, they were both experts in 'stress' and 'stimuli', and today both would administer some hard lessons on the subjects.

By 10am my flip-flops, sweatpants and hoodie had been traded for boots and military kit and I was (nervous and) ready to adapt and improve with whatever stress and stimuli they had for me.

THE PAINFUL TRUTH

'Never give in. Never give in. Never, never, never, never – in nothing, great or small, large or petty – never give in, except to convictions of honour and good sense. Never yield to force. Never yield to the apparently overwhelming might of the enemy.'
WINSTON CHURCHILL

10:30am on the rough moorland of Woodbury Common.

A short drive away from the base, this is home to the Royal Marines Endurance Course and has been used to administer stress and stimuli to new recruits for years. Thoroughly tried and tested as an effective training tool for physical adaptation and improvement, it consists of 2 miles of punishing hills, tunnels, pipes, wading pools and an underwater culvert known as the 'sheep dip'. All followed by a 4-mile run back to camp.

It's March, so the weather isn't warm, but it could also be a lot worse.

'How cold is the sheep dip?' I ask Ollie and Benny, trying to get an indication of how much 'stress' and 'stimuli' I need to prepare myself for.

'Not too bad today,' Ollie says casually. 'A few months back we had to break the ice before the recruits could get under it. That was fun. You had to run a little faster that day to keep warm,' he added, letting out the largest, deepest, Marine-themed laugh I have ever witnessed.

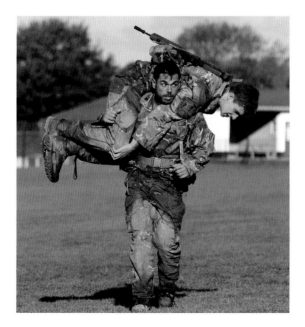

But what happens next surprises me.

This is because Benny is a physical training instructor who has comically muscular shoulders and shouts a lot. Ollie is a captain who has inexplicably large arms and legs and also shouts a lot. But beneath the moustaches, green berets and giant belt buckles lies a deep understanding of sports science.

Incredibly articulate Benny turns to me and says 'Yes, it's going to hurt. But for recruits to become fitter the body requires stress. You can't adapt to become stronger without experiencing some form of targeted stress. Your arms can't magically grow without lifting weight and your lungs won't be gifted with endurance without running to tax the body's cardio-respiratory system.'

Equally eloquent Ollie adds: 'This is why if you see any Physical Training Instructor making a recruit do extra burpees, or run another mile run or carry more weight in their backpack, they aren't doing it to be cruel. They're doing it to produce a physical adaptation so they improve.'

They were both absolutely right. It was an idea broadcast to the world of sport in September 1960 by Fred Wilt. He was the editor of *Track Technique* and published the article 'Stress and Training'.

It sounds so simple, but it's amazing how many people still fail to grasp this.

To reiterate: to improve, you must 'expose' your body to a specific 'stimulus to the quality or intensity of which it is not adapted'. There is no magic pill, quick fix or shortcut. You're going to have to sweat. You're going to have to work. And at times you might not like disrupting your comfy state of homeostasis.

Needless to say, over the next two miles my comfy state of homeostasis was disrupted.

ENDURANCE COURSE: MASTERCLASS IN STRESS AND STIMULI

Although my eyes were covered in mud and my senses numb from the cold, this is what I remember.

The course started with Benny guiding me through a warm-up. Within that warm-up was every bodyweight exercise ever invented and I was already breathing heavily before we started.

With little warning, he then took off like a shot.

Hurtling across the moorland at a rate of knots, I tried my best to keep up until we eventually arrived at an underground tunnel that was just big enough to crawl through.

'Get down and get in,' Benny yelled.

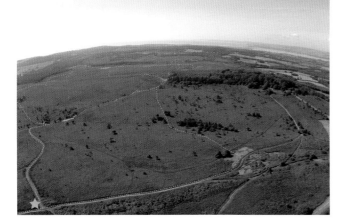

Diving into the entrance, I immediately regretted approaching it so fast as the sharpened rocks that lay across the floor ground into my knee-caps and – although I can't be sure because it was pitch black – I was pretty sure I left large chunks of skin in there.

Popping out the other side it was burpee o'clock and I owed Benny 50 before we continued running onto Obstacle 2, known as Peter's Pool, which Ollie told me contained 'Woodbury's freshest water'.

His smile led me to believe 'fresh' meant 'Baltic-like temperatures'.

I was right. Jumping in waist-deep I felt the blood leave my limbs as my legs and gentlemanly parts wondered what the hell was going on. With no time to think I was then told to dunk my entire body under and hold for 5 seconds. This was the longest 5 seconds in recent memory, but at least I was now clean (it wouldn't last).

'Good! You're now prepping the body for the sheep dip,' Ollie said.

Again, there is method to everything the Marines do, no matter how harsh it seems.

Now dripping wet, I felt like someone had put lead weights in my boots. Barely lifting my feet off the ground, I was made to race Benny to the next obstacle to keep the intensity (again more stress and stimuli) of the run. Despite being given a head-start, I came second.

With my lungs on fire, we reached the next obstacle (marked in red on the map). This applied the most severe amount of stress and stimuli to my shoulders, but was a short break for my sore and raw knees and suffering lungs. That's because I was made to crawl through bogs and marshes that were densely covered in thick mud, sludge and slime.

Again, I didn't mind this as much. The mud was almost soothing on my knees and because I was moving slower than a tectonic plate I didn't need to breathe as hard.

Next, we reached the infamous sheep dip (marked black on the map). It's a 1.5-metre underwater concrete tunnel that's too small to swim through. Instead, I had to hold my breath, become a human torpedo and trust that Ollie and Benny would push and pull me through it like large letterbox.

Delivered out the other side, we then immediately ran up another hill.

Cleaner but with boots now full of water, my legs and lungs began to complain (again). Reaching one of the highest points of Woodbury Common, I had no time to take in the view as I was made to bear crawl and duck walk in 200-metre circles until Benny granted me a small break by running down a long, downhill stretch.

Yes, the Marines class running downhill as a 'break'.

Heading to the woodland, the next obstacle applied the most severe amount of stress and stimuli my nose had ever experienced. I was crawling through what seemed like an endless streak of water and (I hoped just) mud, which was the consistency of yoghurt and seemed to change through black, brown and orange.

The smell was biblical and I now knew it definitely wasn't just mud I was coated in. After battling the course and my gag reflex, I arrived out the other side. I will be honest, at this point I had lost all my bearings and was just running, and/or crawling in whatever direction I was told to.

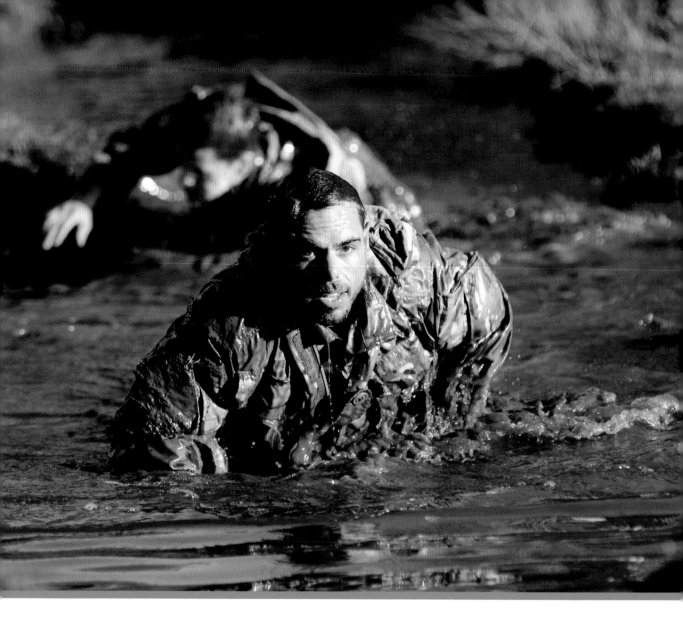

That direction was straight down the barrel of the next obstacle, the Smartie tubes.

Around 12 metres long, the tunnel is so narrow you have get on your belly, keep your hands and arms as tight and close to the body as possible, and basically inch-worm your way through. If you're claustrophobic this is your worst nightmare. Yes, there is light at the end of the tunnel, but it takes a lot of patience (and more skin from your elbows) to make it through.

'Watch out for the tunnel badger,' Ollie shouts, waiting until I'm halfway.

I didn't know if he was joking or not, but even if he wasn't I wouldn't have been able to do anything about it.

Fortunately, I encountered no badger. Emerging from the final Smartie tube I ran uphill towards the finish of the endurance course, only then to start my 4-mile run back to base. As I did (boots and kit still drenched and weighing me down) I reflected on what was a masterclass in stress and stimuli.

Every part of my body was in pain, which meant every part of my body would adapt.

DRINK, EAT AND GET DRY

Back at base I was told to drink, eat and get dry.

Note the word 'told' rather than invited. This is because the Marines understand recovery is critical. Yes, stress and stimuli are needed, but on the flipside there are those people who run, jump and lift as much as possible, as often as possible, every hour of every day. But this too – according to the work of Hans Selye – is destined to fail.

Why? In a word, **overtraining**.

You know those days when you just feel tired and flat? Your bench press has no power, your box jumps have no spring and your 40-metre-sprint time is too embarrassingly slow to even record. Well, chances are you've just pushed the stress and stimuli too far.

It's one run or one repetition too many.

It means your homeostasis is out of whack, your internal environment is a mess and your body is waving the white flag calling for you to surrender to the sofa. For this very reason, you, Royal Marine recruits and everyone who has ever set foot inside a gym must have at least some understanding of the three theoretical stages of Selye's General Adaptation Syndrome[3].

THE THEORY OF ALL TRAINING
ADAPTATION SYNDROME

Now this theoretical framework governs all training and all sports, but it's especially true at the Royal Marine Base. So, to use a military-inspired example, imagine you've just finished a 6-mile endurance course through lakes and swamps, 10 x 200-metre fireman carries and a (timed) 4-minute obstacle course. All while wearing 20 kg of armour.

You're now on the sofa. Your legs are tender, your back is fragile and your immune system has been taxed.

What happens now? Well, according to Selye's General Adaptation Syndrome there are three theoretical phases your body can go through.

1: Shock Phase

You're stiff and sore. This is the immediate response to stress caused by training. Often there's a reduction in performance that occurs at this phase and it's typically known that the fitter you are, the greater the stress and stimuli needed to induce shock. This explains why quite often the first session is always the hardest.

How your body reacts will determine which phase you visit next.

2: Adaptation Phase

Your body is able to tolerate the stress and now you're home with your feet up, resting. But inside there's a plethora of biological reactions going on. Hormonal adaptations, nervous system adaptations and muscle tissue building are just a few that will make you a stronger, fitter and better version of yourself the next day.

Worth noting is these adaptations are unique to each individual. It's (again) Biological Individuality, and some people bounce back better than others.

3: Exhaustion Phase

You're fatigued and ill. This occurs when the stimulus and stress used in training were too much for the body to handle. Maybe the distance was too long, the pace too fast to sustain or the weight of the backpack too heavy to carry. Whatever the reason, you feel beat up and your body is waving the white flag.

This is a phase you should never visit if you can help it.

In summary, the perfect adaptation is when you train to maximise the time spent in the Adaptation Phase, while avoiding any time spent in the Exhaustion Phase.

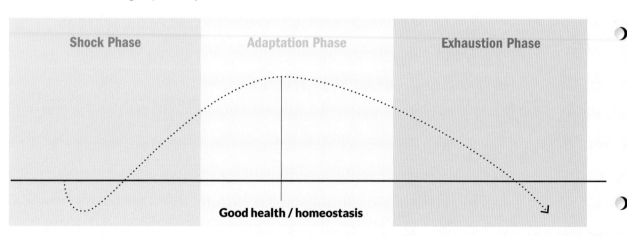

Whatever doesn't kill me...

Sports scientists later discovered training is not as simple as chucking loads of stress and stimuli at the body in the hope that you improve and break personal bests every week. Instead, they agreed we must expand on the work of Hans Selye. Why? Because, put simply, the General Adaptation Syndrome is general. It doesn't take into account all the different training programmes ('external conditioning') or the way individuals respond to those programmes differently ('internal conditioning').

This is why in September 1961, in an article entitled 'The Athlete and Adaptation to Stress', an Australian swim coach called Forbes Carlile stressed that General Adaptation Syndrome could serve as a theoretical framework for coaching.[4] But to truly master the law of adaptation we must master training stress and stimuli.

MASTERING TRAINING 'STRESS'

Introducing the Arndt–Schulz rule.

Hugo Paul Friedrich Schulz (1853–1932) was a German pharmacologist who discovered – through his work with yeast cells – that small doses of toxins have the opposite effect to large doses. Rudolf Arndt (1835–1900) was a German psychiatrist who – through his work with animals – found that low doses of certain toxins stimulated growth and fertility.

Combining their work, it was found:

'For every substance, small doses stimulate, moderate doses inhibit, large doses kill.'
ARNDT-SCHULZ RULE, 1888

But let's put toxins to one side and instead use a training example we can relate to.

Marathon | 'Small doses stimulate'

Imagine you're a beginner training for a marathon. Generally speaking, if you stood on your doorstep, laced up your trainers and completed a 5-mile run you'd probably make good progress, right? That's because it's a relatively low-level stress and stimuli, so adaptation would be stimulated and you'd become fitter.

Marathon | 'Moderate doses inhibit'

But what if instead of running 5 miles you decided to tackle a half marathon for your first day's training? Straight out of the blocks you just took off and clocked 13.1 miles! A bit ambitious I know, and you might find the adaptation would be inhibited and progress would be slow, if non-existent, due to the moderate dose of stress.

Marathon | 'Large doses kill'

But what if you decided you just wanted to dominate a marathon on your very first day. Ambitious? Yes. Successful? I'd say probably not. That's because that's one large dose of stress and although you wouldn't die, I think it's safe to say based on the Arndt–Schulz Rule, you probably wouldn't feel like training the next day.

So how do we train for a marathon?

We must identify our body's 'adaptation energy', that's how.

This is closely related to the current status of the body's defence/immune system. If we're feeling fit and full of beans it's likely our body's adaptation energy is good and we will respond well to training, stress and stimuli. If we're dragging our feet to the gym and feel a little under the weather it's likely our body's adaptation energy is bad and we won't respond well.

'The loss of acquired adaptation during the stage of exhaustion is difficult to explain but as a working hypothesis, it was assumed that every organism possesses a certain limited amount of 'adaptation energy' and once this is consumed, the performance of adaptive processes is no longer possible.'

HANS SELYE

Of course, 'adaptation energy' can be accurately measured with a few simple tests to monitor white blood cells, hormones and the body's immune system. But many involve needles and I personally hate them. Also relying on people in white coats to tell you how to train every day isn't practical for most people.

So instead, become your own expert and listen to your own body.

Although your programme might specify a 10-mile run, don't feel you have to if you honestly believe your 'adaptation energy' is low. Instead, work on mobility. Drill some technique and light active recovery. Or just go home, avoid the Exhaustion Phase and live to fight another day within the Adaptation Phase.

THE SECRET TO THE PERFECT WORKOUT |
0% FAILURE

YOU MUST ADAPT

Now we know that (in theory) the perfect adaptation is easy. You just have to understand that Progressive Overload is the gradual increase of stress placed upon the body during training and was pioneered by military physicians during World War II to aid rehabilitation. Now it can get complicated, but really there are three things to remember:

- **The Law of Progressive Overload must be constant.**
- **The Law of Progressive Overload is not linear.**
- **The Law of Progressive Overload must be specific** (see the Law of Specific Skill in the next chapter).

To explain, here's a story of a famous Greek wrestler and his pet bull.

THE LAW OF PROGRESSIVE OVERLOAD MUST BE CONSTANT

The story of Milo is famous in strength circles.

A celebrated 6th-century BC wrestler, Milo was born in the city of Croton and – like most successful athletes of that period – became the subject of some epic tales of strength, skill and power. Personal favourites of mine include his daily diet of 9 kg (20 lb) of meat, 9 kg of bread and 10 litres (18 pints) of wine, and how he could burst a band about his brow by simply inflating the veins of his temples.

But these aside, Milo was best known for epitomising the idea of progressive overload. All because the Greek fitness-themed fable details how Milo picked up a small baby cow and carried it on his shoulders every single day. As the cow grew, so did Milo's strength.

Days, months and years of progressive overload later and Milo was able to hoist a full-size, half-tonne bull onto his shoulders and stroll into town to pick up his weekly groceries. How? All through the gradual increase of stress (weight in this case) placed upon the body during training. It's the single most important component of anyone's training programme.

Without it you don't improve!

Unfortunately I'm not sure there's much science to back up the cow part. So don't spend next month's gym membership money on a baby cow. Instead, just understand the idea that Milo's story embodies. Always aim for a 'bigger bull'.

Of course, this is a concept that's been around for centuries, but it was only really developed by army physicians like Thomas Delorme, MD, who used it to rehabilitate soldiers after World War II.

'DeLorme's new protocol consisted of multiple sets of resistance exercises in which patients lifted their 10-repetition maximum. DeLorme refined the system by 1948 to include 3 progressively heavier sets of 10 repetitions, and he referred to the program as Progressive Resistance Exercise.'

NSCA[5]

Years later, Natalia Verkhoshansky expanded on this.

In an article entitled 'General Adaptation Syndrome and its Applications in Sport Training' she said: 'The athlete's progress in physical performance, during the training process, is assured by repetitive training workouts, which activate the specific mechanisms of the body's adaptation to the physical hyper function. These mechanisms assure the growth of specific proteins' contents in working organs, which leads to the increasing their functional capacity.'[6]

Put simply, continually subject your body to more than you did before. Cycle quicker on the bike than you did last session. Swim further in the pool than you did last week. Put more weight on the bar than you did last workout. (Again) it's that easy (in theory).

This is how you adapt and improve.

'Training may then be described as the process whereby the body is systemically exposed to a given set of stressors to enable it to efficiently manage future exposure to those stressors.'

DR MEL SIFF, Supertraining

THE LAW OF PROGRESSIVE OVERLOAD IS NOT LINEAR

So why is every strength athlete not able to lift a bull above their head?

Well, this is because when it comes to the human body no improvement – be that in strength, speed, fat loss or muscle – will ever be perfectly linear. It's impossible to add 1 kg to your squat every day in the hope you'll be lifting 365 kg (804 lb) more in a year.

The biology of our bodies doesn't work that way. Instead, think of it as occurring in waves.

In some training sessions you'll make these vast improvements. Strength might just inexplicably shoot through the roof and muscle will miraculously materialise. Then the following week you'll be lapped on the athletics track or fail to string together a collection of semi-decent lifts in the weights room.

Just know that in the long run you will reach the mountain peak if you keep walking. But due to our biological complexity the path is winding and inevitably gets rough in places.

'The gradual overload principle should be understood to be a fluctuating overload system.'

DR MEL SIFF, Supertraining

CHAPTER 3
THE LAW OF SPECIFIC SKILL

> "THE DIFFERENCES BETWEEN EXPERT PERFORMERS AND NORMAL ADULTS ARE NOT IMMUTABLE, THAT IS, DUE TO GENETICALLY PRESCRIBED TALENT. INSTEAD, THESE DIFFERENCES REFLECT A LIFE-LONG PERIOD OF DELIBERATE EFFORT TO IMPROVE PERFORMANCE."
>
> ANDERS ERICSSON

TIME TO GET SPECIFIC

There are a lot of similarities between Loughborough and Lympstone.

Great training facilities. Brilliant coaching. Years of tried-and-tested research on all things fitness and food. Finally, years of experience pushing the boundaries of human physical excellence. But there is one key difference between the elite Royal Marines of Lympstone and the world-class athletes of Loughborough University.

At Loughborough, you train to become a good athlete.

At Lympstone, you train to be a good Royal Marine.

Yes, you can be both and there are many incredible human beings who are.

But (generally speaking) the reason I make this distinction is because every day there's only a certain amount of stress, stimuli and adaptation energy you can successfully squeeze into 24 hours before you overtrain and visit the Exhaustion Phase.

If you're a Royal Marine, you use all that adaptation energy to throw stress and stimuli at the Law of Progressive Overload to adapt to everything and anything. What this means is you train to become a complete, well-rounded soldier who can run for miles, lift heavy loads and jump over a 180-cm (6-ft) wall if needed.

Royal Marines basically embrace the Law of Progressive Overload in all its forms.

But if you're an athlete, you use all that adaptation energy to adapt to a specific sport. What this means is you train to become a finely tuned, sports-specific specimen capable of running fast, lifting heavy or cycling far.

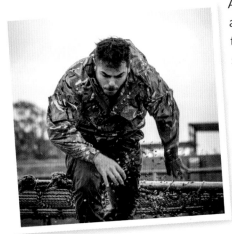

Athletes basically take the Law of Progressive Overload and make it incredibly specific by performing more targeted and specialised training to become good at one single task, rather than being competent in them all.

This, ladies and gentlemen, is The Law of Specific Skill.

The Law of Progressive Overload must be specific

The Law of Specific Skill is simply the Law of Progressive Overload made specific.

It's what happens when you take the theories of Selye, Cannon and Richet and focus them all into a very precise training programme and plan. In the world of sports science this is called the SAID principle.

Don't be fooled by the impressive-sounding acronym – as usual it's not complicated. It stands for **Specific Adaptation to Imposed Demands** and it just means you adapt specifically to the demands you place on your body. It's basically what happens when you make the Law of Progressive Overload specific.

▶ **Do you want to improve endurance?**

Do an activity that applies stress and stimuli to your cardiorespiratory system (heart and lungs).

▶ **Do you want to get stronger?**

Do an activity that applies stress and stimuli to your musculoskeletal system.

▶ **Do you want to get better at tennis?**

Buy a racquet and swing it.

It's that simple: you become more efficient at the things you repeatedly practise. And it's something I put into practice in 2016 in a full year of Specific Progressive Overload over five completely different events.

2016 | MY YEAR OF SPECIFIC PROGRESSIVE OVERLOAD

ADAPTING TO SPECIFIC STRESS

I finished 2016 bruised, battered and 20 kg lighter. That's because I had spent 365 days adapting to specific stress. I became a guinea pig of sports science. Practising what I called 'physiological puppetry' I bulked up and stripped down my 178-cm (5-ft-10) frame so it was tailored to each athletic adventure. As a result, my laboratory tests were completely different during each visit.

My weight 'bounced' from 104 kg+ to 84 kg depending on where I needed it to be. My **power to endurance ratio** was 'tweaked' on a monthly basis. Finally, my training and nutrition were manipulated to 'overrule' any limiting (inconvenient) genetic factors that came my way.

The result was an unforgettable year.

JANUARY	APRIL	AUGUST	OCTOBER	NOVEMBER
Ran a marathon (26.2 miles) around Silverstone race circuit pulling a 1400-kg car. I weighed 104 kg.	Climbed a 20-metre rope (repeatedly) for 19 hours until I'd scaled the height of Everest (8848 metres).	Covered 1000 miles (barefoot) in one month carrying a 50-kg Marine backpack.	Trained non-stop in 24 Olympic sports in 24 hours at Loughborough University.	Completed the Nevis Caribbean triathlon carrying a 45-kg tree. I weighed 84 kg (129 kg with the tree).

I won't lie: most of the training was brutal and I wouldn't recommend it to anyone.

But every blister, bruise and rope burn brought me one step closer to understanding The Law of Specific Skill and the infinite power of the human body. Which all culminated in one of the biggest (and strangest) training adaptations in my athletic career to date...

The World's First Tree-athlon.

THE LAW OF SPECIFIC SKILL | Island of Nevis, Caribbean

THE WORLD'S FIRST TREE-ATHLON

THE IDEA

12pm, 20 August 2016, and I raise my fork victorious!

Sitting in a small restaurant nestled among the secret streets of London's West End, I have just eaten four burgers in 40 minutes. Of course, onlookers had no idea of the calorie deficit I was nursing from that month, having just completed a strength-based session of epic proportions.

Instead, they just saw four empty plates, a man with food in and around his mouth and a giant cheesecake en route to my table that didn't stand a chance. But before I could attack the restaurant's supply of sweets I was joined by my good friend – and training partner – Jane Hansom.

Renowned in endurance-based sports, she takes the form of a petite, slender blonde woman who's rarely seen not smiling. But don't be fooled. Jane's appetite for competition is ferocious. She swims oceans for starters and has mountains for main courses. She's also an Ironman Kona Age Group World Champion and literally knows everyone in the world of triathlon.

This is because when she's not competing in them, she's managing them. As director of a London-based sports marketing agency it's almost inevitable that when we catch up, ideas of epic proportions are planned. Today was no different.

'Have you ever heard of the Caribbean island of Nevis?' she immediately asks as she takes a seat.

I shake my head, now unable to speak with a mouthful of cheesecake.

'It's a small island that wants to become 100% carbon neutral in the next ten years. It's also home to the most beautiful triathlon in the world, and I'm in charge of doing the PR for it.'

I pause for a moment.

An island that's carbon neutral! This is historic! How did more people not know about this? A potential turning point as we look to mend our fragile relationship with Mother Nature!

Jane agreed. I ate. We brainstormed…

'Why don't you do the triathlon carrying something heavy so more media cover it?' she asked.

We both sat there in silence for a moment. I even stopped eating to give my brain time to function…

'What about a tree?' I replied. 'Symbolic of the eco-friendly technology of the island.' Jane smiled. We nodded. Notepads were closed. More cheesecake was ordered.

At this moment in time I should mention that Jane is as blindly optimistic as me. Rightly or wrongly she put her faith – and the reputation of her company – in my hands. Over the coming weeks phone calls were made, emails sent and even the Minister of Foreign Affairs for Nevis was informed of our plan. This was either brilliant or stupid. Maybe it was both.

'To raise new questions, new possibilities, to regard old problems from a new angle, requires creative imagination and marks real advance in science.'
ALBERT EINSTEIN

But I had a plan and set sail for Lympstone to ask the Royal Marines about the best way to carry a tree.

THE TRAINING

So, how do you attach a tree to a bike?

You visit Lympstone to ask the Royal Marines, that's how. Which is exactly what I did when, at 6am on 25 August 2016, I arrived back at the Commando Training Centre in Devon. Only this time I had a 45-kg (100-lb) log, roughly 30 cm (12 in) in diameter and over 2 metres (6 ft) long, on my back. Thankfully, security had been informed of my (unusual and usual) visit, so my tree and me weren't a complete surprise to the large, heavily armoured gentlemen standing at the gate. Instead, I was wished 'the best of luck' and then told to report to the Officer's Mess (HQ) where my coach was waiting for me.

Now I know what you're thinking: what coach would be crazy enough to say yes to this?

The answer? Aled Jones.

A Welsh-born, military-trained fitness phenomenon, he was the Royal Navy Triathlon Captain and has served as a Royal Marine Commando for over a decade. What this means is he's become very good at running, swimming and cycling very long distances, but was also very good at carrying very heavy things very far.

Basically, he was a great coach, but a better friend.

Which is why I found myself gently placing the tree (and bike) on the floor next to his feet as I looked up at him in hope and desperation.

It was dawning on me that I had massively underestimated the cycling part of my newly invented sport. See, the log would float so the swim should be (semi-) safe. And the run can be done with it on one shoulder. (Again) I hope without too much trouble.

But the bike was proving tricky.

Yes, 45 kg of weight bearing down on my back wasn't pleasant, but it was manageable. Also I could make peace with the fact the bark was threatening to take a chunk out of the skin when resting on my shoulder. But if I lost my balance travelling 20 mph downhill I would most likely be found at the roadside wearing both the tree and the bike.

'How do carry it on the bike?' I asked desperately.

Seeing the panic on my face, Aled was unable to answer since he was laughing so much. Instead, he just signalled to the other Marines on camp to come and enjoy the spectacle. New recruits, physical training instructors and even the odd officer arrived to see what was so funny. I didn't disappoint.

Officers would later tell me that watching a civilian try to put a tree down his trousers while mounting a bike was one of the funniest things they'd seen in the Commando Training Centre's 75-year history.

'Cheerfulness in the face of adversity.'
ONE OF FOUR ELEMENTS OF THE COMMANDO SPIRIT

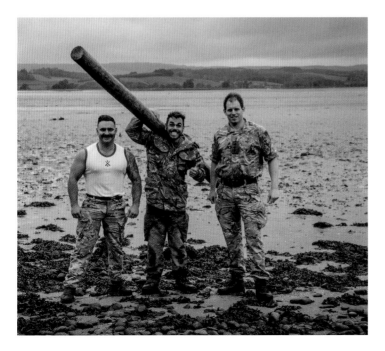

Within minutes everyone on the base was enjoying my sports-based idiocy.

If I wasn't the weird tree-athlete who'd agreed to swim 1.5 km, bike 40 km and run 10 km with a log on my back, then I think I would probably find it funny too. But I was. So there's still no smile on my face, only more panic.

Thankfully dinnertime arrived, which meant the crowd of commandos disbanded.

'OK, I'll help,' Aled said, now composing himself and assessing the best way to carry the tree.

'Have you thought about top-flatting it?'

I had no idea what 'top-flatting it' meant, so the answer was no.

'We carry our anti-tank missiles like that and they're a similar size and weight,' he said. 'You basically lay the log horizontal on top of the Bergen (Marine backpack) and then close the top flap over it and do the straps up.' It made sense.

We tried it. It worked. I did a mile on the bike and while it was far from stable, at least I was moving. Now I had to learn how to fuel an entire triathlon, through 10,000 calories and one all-natural raw energy ball at a time.

'If you wish to succeed in life, make perseverance your bosom friend.'
JOSEPH ADDISON

THE DIET

Whether running, cycling or swimming, as soon as you add weight you burn more calories.

That's according to scientists from the Chaim Sheba Medical Center[1] who found that additional weight alters your locomotion biomechanics – basically your technique – which leads to a 'significant increase in energy (calorie) cost over time'.

So how much will I burn during my tree-athlon?

At the time, the exact answer was hard to give. Now it's believed that if you complete an Olympic triathlon in the average 3 hours and 9 minutes you might burn between 1960 and 3000 calories total. Smaller athletes tipping the scales at 54 kg (120 lb) will burn a lot less while larger, muscular athletes who weigh 82 kg (180 lb) and more will burn towards the higher end.

Then there's my tree and me.

If you add the 45-kg (100-lb) log to my 84-kg (185-pound) frame, that means I will be attempting to drag 139 kg (285 lb) around the course, which includes two laps around the island on my bike, with each lap requiring me to tackle the infamous 5-km 'Anaconda' 12% hill gradient climb.

Couple this with the fact I could take anywhere between 4 to 6 hours to complete the triathlon, and what this means is my final caloric expenditure could be anywhere between 6000 and 10,000. What was clear was that I needed help. Help, chia seeds, nut butters and nutrient-rich fats and carbohydrates.

RAW ENERGY BALLS
by Annie Mayne

'One of the most efficient ways to get calories, carbohydrates and fats into the diet to fuel periods of intense training. Easy to make and even easier to eat, these energy balls are like small balls of performance-enhancing pudding.'

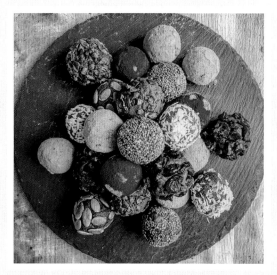

Ingredients

Serves 14

100g walnuts

100g almonds

75g cocoa powder

¼ tsp sea salt

390g pitted dates*

2 tbsp organic roasted cacao nibs from THE PROTEIN WORKS™

Various toppings to roll them in

*Preferably Medjool dates, but for a cheaper option, just soak the dates overnight so they're easier to work with.

Method

1. Put the walnuts and almonds in a blender and process until you get a fine meal. Add the cocoa powder and sea salt. Pulse to combine.

2. Put some dates in the food processor. It will probably hate this so put in only a handful at a time. Painful, I know, but better than having to buy a new food processor.

3. Once the dates have turned into a thick, sticky paste, add the nut and cocoa mix back in. You might prefer to do this in a bowl and get your hands involved.

4. Add the cacao nibs and any remaining walnuts you have. You can really play around with things you want to add: goji berries, dried fruit, nuts, seeds, all sorts. I like to grate the zest of an orange in the mixture, too, to give it that extra oomph!

5. Combine and form bite-sized balls (or bigger ones).

I get the most fun out of choosing what to roll the balls in. Cocoa powder, moringa, matcha, beetroot powder, coconut flakes, cacao nibs and chia seeds all work brilliantly, but don't be afraid to get creative.

	Calories	Carbs	Fat	Protein
Total	2589	332g	138g	57g
Per serving	185	24g	10g	4g

THE TRAINING PLAN

There are many workouts in this book I'd recommend.

My 12-week Tree-athlon Plan is not one of them. For most people, the sheer number of hours you have to commit to running, swimming and cycling with a tree makes it completely unrealistic. I only did it to raise money for charity and to illustrate an extreme example of The Law of Specific Skill. So, I'd suggest you:

- Read the following.
- Take lessons and inspiration from it.
- But don't take it as a viable training programme.

Unless (of course) you're like me and crazy enough to do a triathlon carrying a tree on your back. In summary, would I recommend the workout? No. Does it highlight an important point? Absolutely.

The theory

An Olympic-distance triathlon consists of a 1.5-km swim, 40-km bike ride and 10-km run.

While every athlete's training is different – researchers from the Department of Sport, Health and Exercise Science at the University of Hull stated there is no universally agreed consensus on the best way to train for endurance sports – generally speaking, the average athlete spends about 20% of the total race time swimming, 50% cycling and about 30% running, which is why most coaches would recommend that your training matches these splits.

What this means is you do an equal number of swim, bike and run workouts, but your swimming workouts should be shorter than runs and your runs shorter than your bikes.

To put this into an example: if you train 6 times per week, you will swim, bike and run twice but your longest bike ride might be one hour, whereas your swims last 30 minutes each and your runs 40 minutes. You then increase this 'workload' incrementally throughout the time you have available before your race, making sure you allow yourself enough time to recover.

And voila! This is the theory that governed the 12-week plan, all of which was done carrying a 45-kg tree to ensure I was conditioning my body to successfully complete a Tree-athlon and not a triathlon. All based on the SAID principle (see page 55) and inspired by the Bulgarian Olympic Lifting team's incredible ability to specialise in specialising.

Train like a Bulgarian

Bulgarian Olympic Lifting methods are world-renowned.

Why? Because despite limited resources and a poor economic conditions this small, south-eastern European country – with a population only slightly bigger than New York's – produced a team of weightlifters whose strength would become legendary. Under the tutelage of Ivan Abadjiev, who took over as head coach in 1968, Bulgarian athletes achieved things that were previously thought to be impossible.

How? Well, it's comprehensive, amazing and needs more than a paragraph to do it justice. But in brief, the gruelling Bulgarian Training System involved lifting close to your maximum weight, in a select number of exercises, every single day, 365 days of the year, for up to 8 hours a day.

Crazy?

Well, 12 Olympic Gold medallists and 57 world champions say otherwise.

So, what was the key to their success?

One reason was that Abadjiev placed such emphasis on the SAID principle in all his athletes' training. Essentially, Olympic Lifting consists of two moves: the clean and jerk, and the snatch. So why practise much else?

As Abadjiev said: 'Our athletes do not do any supportive exercises; they stay with full clean and jerk, snatch, and front squat. We have found that taking back squat out is more effective for the healthy lifter. Sticking with the three lifts named above as the only training for the advanced and healthy lifter. If the athlete is injured they will do back squat or parts of the lift (ie. high pulls, push press, etc). You must be extremely careful with the stresses you put on your athletes. You must have direct benefits from each exercise because the athlete has limited recovery capacity.'

Basically, if Abadjiev caught one of his athletes cheekily doing some bicep curls on the side or maybe running a marathon on the weekend there would be hell to pay.

Specialising in specificity was key.

Now you don't have to live by the same strict rules as Abadjiev. But do understand that you need to be specific in your goal every time you set foot into the gym. Inspired by the Bulgarians, I knew that most of my training from this day onwards needed to be done with a tree on my back.

THE WORLD'S FIRST TREE-ATHLON |
THE 12-WEEK PLAN

	Monday	Tuesday	Wednesday	Thursday	Friday	Saturday	Sunday
Week 1	Swimming specific · 10 minutes warm-up - 10 x 25m drills with 20 seconds rest · 10 x 50m (25m hard/25m easy) with 20 seconds rest · 5 minutes cool-down	Running specific · 10 minutes warm-up · 6 x 20 seconds hill reps and jog down recovery · 15 minutes running at 80% max. heart rate · 5 minutes cool-down **Strength session** 30 minutes	Rest day	Cycling specific · Turbo 40 minutes (10 minutes warm-up. 10 x 60 seconds high cadence (low gear at <75% max. heart rate) and 60 seconds easy. 10 minutes cool-down.)	Swimming specific · 30–45 minutes technique work	Running specific · 40 minutes easy and off-road · Strength session 30 minutes	Cycling specific · 60 minutes steady pace
Week 2	Swimming specific · 10 minutes warm-up · 10 x 25m drills with 20 seconds rest · 15 x 50m (25m hard/25m easy) with 20 seconds rest · 5 minutes cool-down	Running specific · 10 minutes warm-up · 8 x 20 seconds hill reps and jog down recovery · 15 minutes running at 80% max. heart rate · 5 minutes cool-down **Strength session** 30 minutes	Rest day	Cycling specific · Turbo 45 minutes (10 minutes warm-up. 12 x 60 seconds high cadence (low gear at <75% max. heart rate) and 60 seconds easy. 10 minutes cool-down.)	Swimming specific · 30–45 minutes technique work	Running specific · 45 minutes easy and off-road **Strength session** · 30 minutes	Cycling specific · 70 minutes steady pace
Week 3	Swimming specific · 10 minutes warm-up · 10 x 25m drills with 20 seconds rest · 20 x 50m (25m hard/25m easy) with 20 seconds rest · 5 minutes cool-down	Running Specific · 10 minutes warm-up · 10 x 20 seconds hill reps with jog down recovery · 15 minutes running at 80% max. heartrate · 5 minutes cool-down **Strength session** 30 minutes	Rest day	Cycling specific · Turbo 40 minutes (10 seconds warm-up, 15 x 60 seconds high cadence (low gear at <75% max. heart rate) and 60 seconds easy. 10 minutes cool-down.)	Swimming specific · 30–45 minutes technique work	Running specific · 50 minutes easy and off-road **Strength session** · 30 minutes	Cycling specific · 80 minutes steady pace

	Monday	Tuesday	Wednesday	Thursday	Friday	Saturday	Sunday
Week 4	**Swimming specific** · Complete 50% of race distance non-stop	**Running specific** · 10 minutes warm-up · 15 x 20 seconds brisk strides at 5k pace and 40 seconds recovery · 5 minutes cool-down **Weights** · 30 minutes	Rest day	**Cycling specific** · Turbo 25 minutes (10 minutes warm-up. 10 x 30 seconds at high cadence (low gear <75% max. heart rate) and 30 seconds recovery. 5 minutes cool-down.)	**Swimming specific** · 30 minutes technique work	**Running specific** · 30 minutes easy and off-road **Strength session** · 30 minutes	**Cycling specific** · 45 minutes steady pace
Week 5	**Swimming specific** · 10 minutes warm-up · 10 x 25m drills with 20 seconds rest · 10 x 100m (50m hard/ 50m easy) with 20 seconds rest · 5 minute cool-down	**Running specific** · 10 minutes warm-up · 6 x 30 seconds hill reps with jog down recovery · 15 seconds running at 80-85% max. heart rate · 5 minutes cool-down **Strength session** · 30 minutes	Rest day	**Cycling specific** · Turbo 40 minutes (10 minutes warm-up. 10 x 30 seconds at max intensity. 90 seconds easy. 10 minutes cool-down.)	**Swimming specific** · 45–60 minutes technique and endurance work	**Running specific** · 45 minutes easy and off-road. Find a hilly route to build leg strength	**Cycling specific** · 70 minutes hilly at steady pace. Stay seated on hills to build leg strength
Week 6	**Swimming specific** · 10 minutes warm-up · 10 x 25m drills with 20 seconds rest · 15 x 50m (25m hard/25m easy) with 20 seconds rest · 5 minutes cool-down	**Running Specific** · 10 minutes warm-up · 8 x 20 seconds hill reps and jog down recovery · 15 minutes running at 80% max. heart rate · 5 minutes cool-down **Strength session** · 30 minutes	Rest day	**Cycling specific** · Turbo 45 minutes (10 minutes warm-up. 12 x 60 seconds high cadence (low gear at <75% max. heart rate) and 60 seconds easy. 10 minutes cool-down.)	**Swimming specific** · 30–45 minutes technique work	**Running specific** · 45 minutes easy and off-road **Strength session** · 30 minutes	**Cycling specific** · 70 minutes steady pace

	Monday	Tuesday	Wednesday	Thursday	Friday	Saturday	Sunday
Week 7	**Swimming specific** · 10 minutes warm-up · 10 x 25m drills with - 20 seconds rest · 20 x 50m (25m hard/25m easy) with 20 seconds rest · 5 minutes cool-down	**Running specific** · 10 minutes warm-up · 10 x 20 seconds hill reps with jog down recovery · 15 minutes running at 80% max. heart rate · 5 minutes cool-down **Strength session** · 30 minutes	Rest day	**Cycling specific** · Turbo 40 minutes. (10 seconds warm-up. 15 x 60 seconds high cadence (low gear at <75% max. heart rate) and 60 seconds easy. 10 minutes cool-down.)	**Swimming specific** · 30–45 minutes technique work	**Running specific** · 50 minutes easy and off-road **Strength session** · 30 minutes	**Cycling specific** · 80 minutes steady pace
Week 8	**Swimming specific** · Complete 50% of race distance non-stop	**Running specific** · 10 minutes warm-up · 15 x 20 seconds brisk strides at 5k pace and 40 seconds recovery · 5 minutes cool-down **Strength session** · 30 minutes	Rest day	**Cycling Specific** · 25 minutes turbo. (10 minutes warm-up. 10 x 30 seconds at high cadence (low gear <75% max. heart rate) and 30 seconds recovery. 5 minutes cool-down.)	**Swimming specific** · 30 minutes technique work	**Running specific** · 30 minutes easy and off-road · Strength session 30 minutes	**Cycling specific** · 45 minutes steady pace
Week 9	**Swimming specific** · 10 minutes warm-up · 10 x 25m drills with - 20 seconds rest · 6 x 100m hard with 30 seconds rest · 5 minutes cool-down	**Running specific** · 10 minutes warm-up · 6 x 30 seconds hill reps and jog down recovery · 2 x 5 minutes running at 85–90% max. heart rate + 2 minutes active recovery · 5 minutes cool-down **Strength session** · 30 minutes	Rest day	**Cycling specific** · Turbo 45 minutes (10 minutes warm-up. 8 x 2 minutes at 85-90% max. heart rate and 60 seconds easy spin with 10 minutes cool-down.) · 5 minutes run	**Swimming specific** · 45–60 minutes, open water if possible. If not, include open-water skills	**Running specific** · 55 minutes off-road and easy. Run on terrain similar to race route **Strength session** · 30 minutes	**Cycling specific** · 70 minutes including 10 minutes at goal race pace

	Monday	Tuesday	Wednesday	Thursday	Friday	Saturday	Sunday
Week 10	**Swimming specific** · 10 minutes warm-up · 10 x 25m drills with 20 seconds rest · 8 x 100m hard with 30 seconds rest after each 100m · 5 minutes cool-down	**Running specific** · 10 minutes warm-up · 8 x 30 seconds hill reps and jog down recovery · 2 x 8 minutes running at 85–90% max. heart rate with 2 minutes active recovery · 5 minutes cool-down **Strength session** · 30 minutes	Rest day	**Cycling specific** · Turbo 45 minutes (10 minutes warm-up. 5 x 3 minutes at 85–90% max. heart rate with 90 seconds easy spin and 10 minutes cool-down.) · 10 minutes run	**Swimming specific** · 45–60 minutes open water if possible. If not, include open-water skills	**Running specific** · 55 minutes off-road and easy. Run on terrain similar to race route **Strength session** · 30 minutes	**Cycling specific** · 80 minutes including 15 minutes at goal race pace
Week 11	**Swimming specific** · 10 minutes warm-up · 10 x 25m drills with 20 seconds rest · 10 x 100m hard + 30 seconds rest · 5 minutes cool-down	**Running specific** · 10 minutes warm-up · 10 x 30 seconds hill reps and jog down recovery · 15 minutes running at - 85–90% max. heart rate · 5 minutes cool-down **Strength session** · 30 minutes	Rest day	**Cycling specific** · Turbo 45 minutes (10 minutes warm-up. 3 x 5 minutes at 85–90% max. heart rate and 2 minutes easy spin. 10 minutes cool-down.) · 15 minutes run	**Swimming specific** · 45–60 minutes open water if possible. If not, include open-water skills	**Running specific** · 40 minutes off road. Run on terrain similar to race route **Strength session** · 30 minutes	**Cycling specific** · 90 minutes including middle 20 minutes at goal race pace
Week 12	**Swimming specific** · 10 minutes warm-up · 10 x 50m drills with 20 seconds rest · 6 x 50m sprints at goal race pace and 30 seconds rest · 5 minutes easy cool-down	Rest day	**Cycling specific** · 15 minutes warm-up · 15 minutes sustained effort at goal race pace **Running specific** · 5 minutes at goal race pace and 5 minutes easy jog to cool down	Rest day	**Swimming specific** · 15 minutes including 5 x 25-50m sprints	**Cycling specific** · 15 minutes including middle 5 minutes at goal race pace **Running specific** · 5 minutes easy pace off the bike	Race day

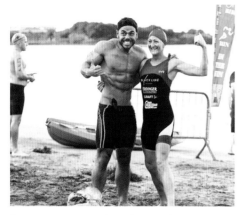

Jane Hansom, co-founder of the World's First Tree-athlon, and the reason I'm about to attach a tree to my trunks

TREE-ATHLON | DID IT WORK?

Before the race

It's 7am on 12 November 2016, the date of the Nevis Caribbean Tree-athlon.

Dubbed 'the world's most beautiful triathlon'. I could see why. The sun rose on the island and illuminated the different shades of green in the grass and trees. The pastel colours of the houses appeared to be custom-painted to complement the island's untouched natural beauty.

Even traffic – and therefore pollution – is almost non-existent as plants grow on every street corner.

But cycling to the start line I couldn't enjoy any of this.

Months of stress, stimuli and progressive overload were rushing through my head. Had I adapted? Was my 'bull' the right size? Had I become like Selye's indestructible rats? Did I visit the Adaptation Phase often enough? The honest answer to all of this is I didn't know.

But during a swim, cycle and run I would soon find out.

Moments later I was on the beach attaching a tree to my trunks. Spectators looked on in sheer bewilderment and Greg – friend and race director – had to assure them the strange Englishman knew what he was doing. I hoped he was right.

Athletes assembled on the start line. The gun was fired. My Tree-athlon had begun.

The swim | 1.5 km (0.93 miles)

I have to be honest: the swim was actually pleasant.

The water was warm and the tree floated. Also, although I started at the back to avoid hitting anyone with my 45 kg of wood, I managed to get up to speed and even overtook a few people. In fact, ever competitive, I quickly found myself locked in a back-and-forth battle with a local Nevisian who refused to be overtaken by a man dragging a log.

By 200 metres in I had abandoned the game plan to 'pace myself'.

Opening up a lead on my newly acquired swimming nemesis, I was ignoring my support team shouting from their kayaks and was determined to leave the water in a decent position. I would later regret this. The drag of the log and lack of swimming efficiency meant I was burning calories at a far greater rate than everyone else in the water.[2]

When I emerged from the water none of this mattered. The crowd cheered. I waved. My support team shook their heads.

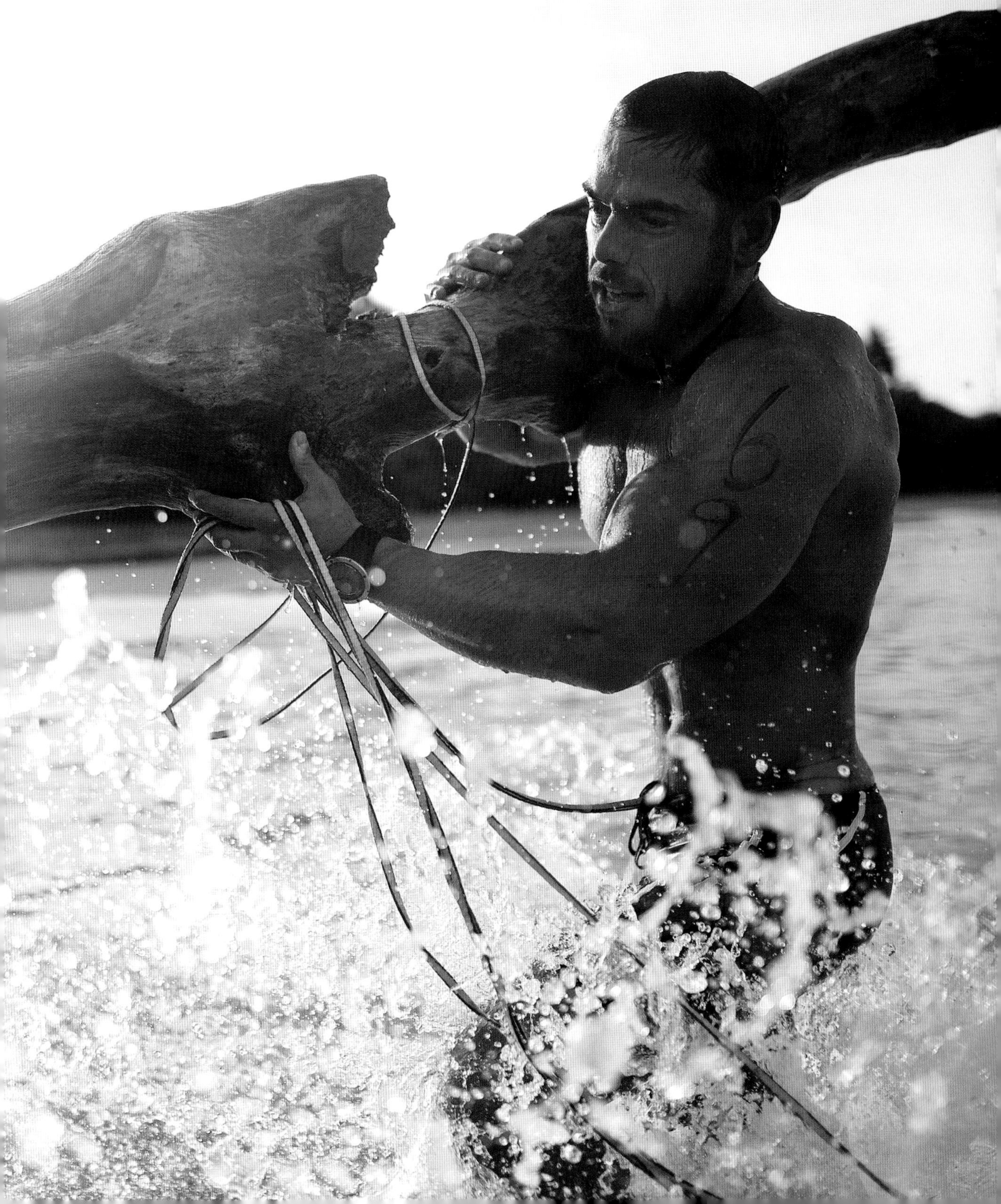

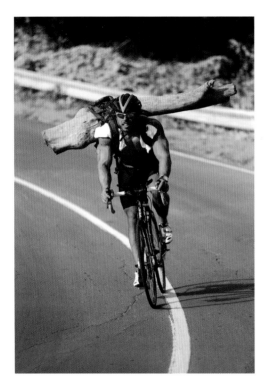

The bike | 40 km (24.8 miles)

The transition onto the bike was slow.

I had to untangle the tree from my swimming trunks and 'top flat' the log onto my Marine backpack as Aled had taught me. It's likely this was the slowest transition in triathlon's history and most of the athletes I'd overtaken on the swim were now cycling off into the distance.

But after 5 minutes the bike was mounted and I was moving.

Waving to the ever-supportive crowd, I left the town and began my slow ascent of the hill known as 'the Anaconda'. A 5-km incline with a 12% gradient, it winds into the volcanic mountains of the island with no end in sight and tests your mental fortitude as well as your legs and lungs.

It also proved to be the best ab workout I've ever endured.

All because during the next 30 minutes all the teachings of my core conditioning guide were put to use.

Like the research from the University of Jyväskylä in Finland that found stabilising exercises – like cycling with a tree – elicited a 'sufficient level of contraction of the trunk (core) muscles for the development of their endurance and strength characteristics'.[3]

Basically – and as weird as it sounds – the simple act of balancing a tree on a bike is a great way to get a six-pack.

Especially when you couple this with research from the Département de Mécanique Appliquée at the Université de Franche-Comté that set out to analyse muscular activity during two pedalling postures and found that 'the change of pedalling posture in uphill cycling had a significant effect on the muscle activity'.[4]

Specifically, they discovered the influence of the 'lateral sways' of the bike leads to greater activation in everything from the biceps, triceps, glutes to – most importantly – the rectus abdominis muscles that are responsible for your six-pack.

A few hours – and four punctures later – and I was lacing my trainers up for the 10-km run.

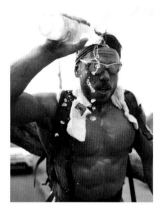

The run | 10 km (6.2 miles)

It was 10am and temperatures were approaching 30°C.

The sun, which I'd welcomed at the start of the swim, was now creating the strangest tree-shaped tan line on my back and I could feel the heat of the tarmac burning through the soles of my shoes. This meant each drinks station would also serve as a shower as I drank one bottle and poured a second over myself.

At this point I realised my time wasn't important, simply finishing was. Because as I passed the immaculately cut green grass of the island's golf course I was painfully aware this was the slowest 10 km I'd ever run.

One foot stepped in front of the other as I tried to remember research from the United States Army Research Institute of Environmental Medicine that examined the biomechanics of 16 males when carrying weighted backpacks of 6 kg, 20 kg, 33 kg and 46 kg.

What did they find?

That 'stride frequency increased and stride length decreased. All to improve stability and reduce stress on the musculoskeletal system'.[5]

Basically, I needed to take smaller steps, but more of them, to keep stable and keep moving.

After 6 km the sun was high, my stride was low and my run had turned into a shuffle. Looking at my Suunto watch and the cadence calculator confirmed that too.

Cadence is a term used to describe the total number of revolutions per minute (RPM) made by your feet. Experts generally recommend you aim for 180 steps per minute; any lower and you might begin to overstride, which can cause the knees to lock and the heels to slam into the ground. As well as putting undue stress on your joints, this is also much slower as every step serves as a 'brake' to your forward motion.

Thousands of steps and many miles later and the finish line was in sight. Speed increased and so did the number of photo opportunities with the people and press in attendance. Crossing the line, I knew I had adapted. Months of stress, stimuli and progressive overload had worked.

My 'bull' was the right size. I had become like Selye's indestructible rats and visited the Adaptation Phase just enough for the crazy idea forged at a burger bar in London and at the Royal Marine training centre in Lympstone to work.

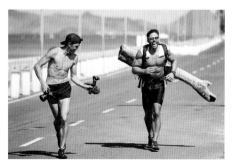

My friend James Appleton, a supremely talented runner; he is also an award-winning photographer, incredibly modest and much prefers being behind the camera

CHAPTER 4
THE LAW OF RECOVERY

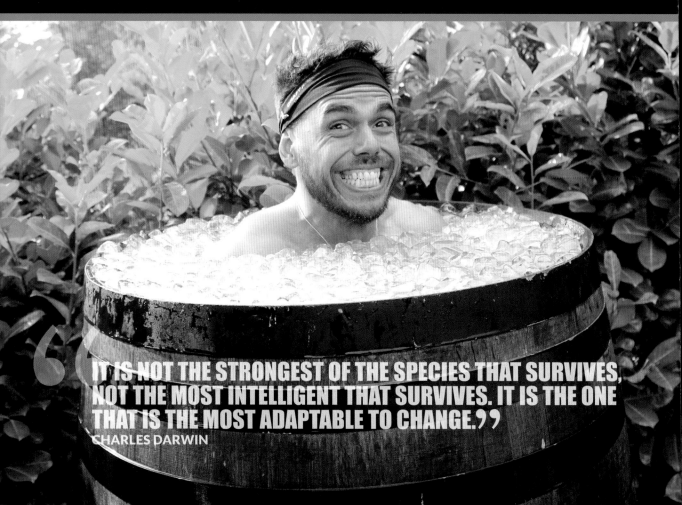

"IT IS NOT THE STRONGEST OF THE SPECIES THAT SURVIVES, NOT THE MOST INTELLIGENT THAT SURVIVES. IT IS THE ONE THAT IS THE MOST ADAPTABLE TO CHANGE."
CHARLES DARWIN

NEVER GET SICK, NEVER OVERTRAIN

In 2016 my charity fundraising schedule was ambitious.

Between the World's Strongest Marathon (pulling a 1.4 tonne car 26.2 miles) and the World's Longest Rope Climb (climbing 8848 m of rope) I discovered the mind was strong. The body was capable. But the immune system – and my resistance to overtraining and becoming ill – needed some tender loving care.

This is why, between the two events, I wrote in my GQ column:

'A powerful bench press is admired. A fast marathon time is impressive. But a strong immune system is essential. Why? Because all gym-based training goals, from losing fat to building muscle, become instantly more achievable when you're working with a healthy, fully functioning immune system.'
ROSS EDGLEY, British GQ

But there was a problem. From the thousands of medical journals I read – deep in the depths of Loughborough University's library – it appeared there weren't many studies that relate to strange men running car-weighted marathons or performing Everest-sized rope climbs in the middle of winter.[1]

'Exercise immunology has quite a short history relative to many branches of the exercise sciences, the modern era of careful epidemiological investigations and precise laboratory studies beginning in the mid-1980s.'[2]

So I formed a two-point plan…

First, I would lock myself in the library and learn from the 2200 peer-reviewed publications in exercise immunology (currently more than 2200 publications using search terms 'exercise' and 'immune') that have been published since the formation of the International Society of Exercise and Immunology (ISEI) in 1989. This took two months, lots of reading and very little sleep.

Next, I would contact Wim who had profoundly influenced the 2200 aforementioned publications by proving he was able to control his immune system. Then I would (wishfully and with fingers crossed) ask if he could teach me bulletproof immunity so I could complete a year of charity events and raise lots of money for some truly great causes. All thanks to the generosity of the Hof family, this took one week, less reading and lots of ice.

ONE PAGE | 2200 STUDIES | 20 YEARS OF SCIENCE

THE TWO-POINT PLAN, PART 1

The immune system is the body's defence against infectious organisms and other invaders. Through a series of steps called the **immune response**, the immune system attacks organisms and substances that invade body systems and cause disease.

Most athletes will have experienced an 'immune crash'.

It's simply the Exhaustion Phase that we've visited when – in an attempt to get stronger, quicker or more powerful – the periods of intense, heavy or high-volume training have been too much for our bodies to handle. As a result, we're left beaten up and slowing down as our immune systems wave the white flag, surrendering to any invading viruses or bacteria.

This has become known as Exercise-induced Immunodepression, and it will prevent even the world's fittest athletes training to their potential.

'Heavily exercising endurance athletes experience extreme physiologic stress, which is associated with temporary immunodepression and higher risk of infection.'[3]

So how's it possible to avoid getting ill while continuing to push the boundaries in training? The J-shaped theory[4], that's how.

In the 1990s, Dr Nieman formulated the 'J-shaped hypothesis' to describe the relationship between exercise intensity and the risk of acquiring upper respiratory tract infections (URTI). Very common in athletes, this is a form of illness that's caused by an infection of the upper respiratory tract (namely nose, pharynx, sinuses or larynx).

What was found?

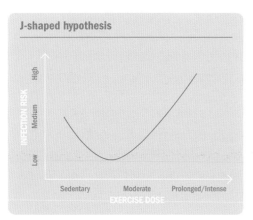

After looking up lots of noses and looking down lots of throats it was discovered that moderate exercise has the ability to improve immune function compared to sedentary people sitting on the sofa doing nothing. But high-intensity exercise depresses the immune system[5], which means our resistance to various viral and bacterial diseases[6] is weakened and we're doomed to enter the gym the next day as weak as a kitten due to overtraining.[7]

Represented on a graph it looks like a 'J', hence the name.

Putting graphs and science to one side…

All this means is a gentle jog on the beach could make us happy and healthy, but a fast-paced marathon has the potential to make us sad and sick. This is why many athletes are incredibly strong, fast and fit, but (should they train too hard) they could be equally unhealthy and have a poor resistance to illness.

Important to note is that evidence to support this isn't yet conclusive.[8]

It's also based on limited laboratory data[9] and (arguably) doesn't fully take into account the sheer complexity of the human immune system. The J-shaped theory was created when looking up athletes' noses for upper respiratory tract infections, not the thousands of other ailments and illnesses that often afflict athletes.

But it does make intuitive sense, which is why I decided to leave the library and check back in when science had more conclusive research for me:

'In the very near future, genomics, proteomics, and metabolomics may help exercise immunologists to better understand mechanisms related to exercise-induced modulation of the immune system and prevention (or reduced risk) of diseases by exercise training. In addition, these technologies might be used as a tool for optimizing individual training programmes. However, more rigorous standardization of procedures and further technological advances are required before practical application of these technologies becomes possible.'[10]

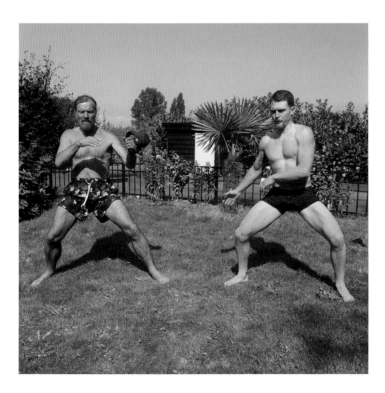

Instead I lived and learnt from Wim Hof, a man who had learnt to control his own immune system and body temperature and who held over 20 world records that range from the world's longest ice bath – 1 hour, 52 minutes and 42 seconds for those interested – to scaling Mount Everest wearing nothing but shorts, shoes and a smile. That's why they call him The Ice Man.

INTRODUCING THE ICE MAN | Amsterdam, The Netherlands

THE TWO-POINT PLAN, PART 2

'When we interact with nature, miraculous things can happen. Whenever you go against the rigid patterns of thinking, challenging yourself, you can receive a bounty of experience from hard nature.'

WIM HOF

10am, 10 February 2016 in Stroe, Amsterdam. I am naked in a barrel full of ice.

Now it's hard to explain what happens when you voluntarily jump into a thousand ice cubes, but as each minute passes you begin to become very aware of what's going on both inside and outside your barrel. Inside, your breathing becomes regulated, your body temperature stablises and your mental clarity heightens as your senses come alive with the cold.

Also – I won't lie – your severely shrivelled genitalia will begin to wonder what's going on.

Then, outside, you notice the sound of birdsong becomes louder, smells become more intense and there will be colours in the hedges that you have never noticed before.

Of course, all of this is new to me.

Equally, friend, fell runner and World Parkour Champion Tim Shieff didn't look all that comfortable in the barrel next to me. With barely any fat on his body, his lips had begun to go an odd colour and he had a quiver in his voice every time he tried to speak.

Needless to say, neither of us made a habit of plunging ourselves into a giant snow cone and this will easily be one of the most memorable training sessions. But for Wim Hof, our mentor, this was pretty standard. For him, this was just a Wednesday.

'How long have I been in?' I ask.

'Don't worry! You're doing great man. That's 20 minutes,' Wim replies.

I remember thinking '20 minutes is good, but I did that yesterday'. Ever competitive, I wanted to beat that (progressive overload) so I ask what the next goal should be.

I'd later learn this entire practice is not about forcing yourself to endure more. Instead, it's about listening to your body to reconnect with Mother Nature and reignite forgotten physiology. However, at this moment in time, Wim didn't want to tame my eagerness. So instead he smiled and said, 'If you really want to know...' he paused for effect. 'The next task is to get an erection in the ice. That's when you know you're really in control of your body.'

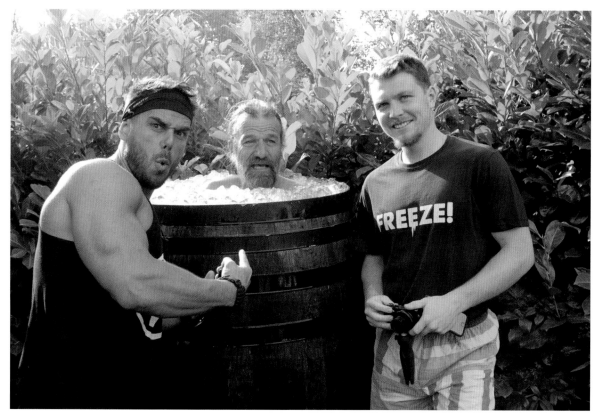

Me, Tim and Wim quite literally chilling in the garden at the Hof residence

We all burst out laughing.

Wim's sense of humour was almost as legendary as his ability to control his body temperature and immune system. But I saw his point and stopped trying to turn everything into a competition.

So what was I doing in Stroe that day (aside from attempting an 'ice erection')?

Well, despite a year of marathon car pulls, Everest rope climbs, 24-hour workouts and many miles wading through mud with Marines, I've not been ill once. Yes, my body has been tired and sore at times. But 24/7 for 365 days of the year my immune system was running at 100%.

I had become one of Selye's indestructible rats.

Destined never to visit the Exhaustion Phase, my weeks were spent testing my newfound bulletproof immunity with back-to-back marathons and 8-hour-long strength sessions.

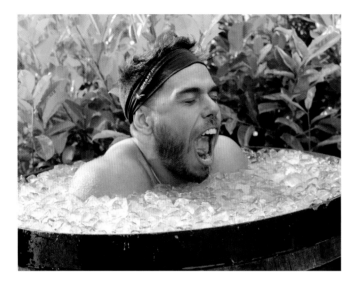

How? The honest answer is it has nothing to do with me, but everything to do with Wim.

He's one of the happiest and healthiest humans I've ever met. If you come to understand his story you will come to understand how never to become sick again. Your recovery from 'stress' and 'stimuli' will become almost instant and your adaptation from training perfect.

Interested? Me too. Which is how I came to be sitting naked in a barrel of ice in rural Amsterdam.

Hearing about my charity work earlier in the year, Wim, his son and team wanted to help and practically adopted me as their odd English son. Living at their house in Amsterdam I learnt more about my body and my immune system in a week than I did in two months of library-based research.

INTRODUCING THE WIM HOF METHOD

What Wim has achieved was thought to be scientifically impossible.

Before he was born it was believed that 'Both the autonomic nervous system and innate immune system were regarded as systems that cannot be voluntarily influenced.'[11]

Basically, during flu season you're at the mercy of the germs floating around. Yes, diet, rest and a good nutrition plan might help, but ultimately you just have to hope your immune system is healthy enough to fight should a virus strike.

But Wim claimed modern medicine was wrong and set out to prove this.

In 2007, the first scientific analysis was done at Feinstein Institute in New York. In 2011, the University Medical Center St Radboud in Nijmegen expanded on this research and after running several tests had to admit Wim – and those he taught – were able to voluntarily influence the autonomic nervous system.

Interested? Backed by years of research, here is an introduction to the Wim Hof Method.

THE WIM HOF METHOD

'The Wim Hof Method can be characterized by its simplicity, applicability and a strong scientific underpinning. It is a practical way to become happier, healthier and more powerful.'
WIM HOF

We humans have forgotten about our inner power. Over time, we've developed a different attitude towards nature and our body's ability to adapt to extreme temperature and survive within our natural environment. Because we wear clothes and artificially control the temperatures at home and at work, we've greatly reduced the natural stimulation of our bodies, atrophying the age-old mechanisms related to our survival and basic function.

Because these deeper physiological layers are no longer triggered, our bodies are no longer in touch with this inner power. The inner power is a powerful force that can be reawakened by stimulating these physiological processes through a system of practices: Cold Therapy, Breathing and Commitment.

'The present study demonstrates that, through practicing techniques learned in a short-term training program, the immune system can indeed be voluntarily influenced.'
Proceedings of the National Academy of Sciences of the United States of America

The Wim Hof method is based on two powerful pillars

Breathing	Cold Therapy
We're always breathing, yet we're mostly unaware of its tremendous potential. Heightened oxygen levels hold a treasure trove of benefits, and the specialised breathing technique of the Wim Hof Method unearths them all: more energy, reduced stress levels, and an augmented immune response to swiftly deal with pathogens.	The cold is your warm friend. Exposing your body to it in the right way starts a cascade of health benefits, including the build-up of brown adipose tissue and subsequent fat loss, reduced inflammation to facilitate a fortified immune system, balanced hormone levels, improved sleep quality and the production of endorphins – the feel-good chemicals in the brain that naturally elevate your mood.

'If you learn to control your mind anything is possible.'
WIM HOF

Step-by-step guide: Breathing exercise

Warning: important message, please read carefully.

The breathing exercise has a profound effect and should be practised in the way it is explained. Always do the breathing exercise in a safe environment (e.g. sitting on a couch/floor) and unforced. Never practise the exercises before or during diving, driving, swimming, taking a bath or in any other environment/place where, should you pass out, a serious injury could occur. Wim Hof breathing may cause tingling sensations and/or light-headedness. If you've fainted, it means that you went too far. Take a step back next time.

Do not practise the method during pregnancy or if you have epilepsy. Persons with cardiovascular health issues, or any other (serious) health conditions, should always consult
a medical doctor before starting with the Wim Hof Method.

1. Get comfortable

Sit in a meditation posture, whatever is most comfortable for you. Make sure you can expand your lungs freely without feeling any constriction. It is recommended to do this practice right after waking up, since your stomach is still empty, or before a meal.

2. 30 power breaths

Imagine you're blowing up a balloon. Inhale through the nose or mouth and exhale through the mouth in short but powerful bursts. Keep a steady pace and use your midriff fully. Close your eyes and do this around 30 times. Symptoms could include light-headedness and/or tingling sensations in the body.

3. The hold and retention after exhalation

After the 30 rapid successions of breath cycles, draw the breath in once more and fill the lungs to maximum capacity without using any force. Then let the air out and hold for as long as you can without force. Hold the breath until you experience the gasp reflex.

4. Recovery breath

Inhale to full capacity. Feel your chest expanding. When you are at full capacity, hold the breath for around 10 seconds and this will be round one. Steps 1–4 can be repeated three times in succession.

5. Meditative state

After having completed the breathing exercise take your time to enjoy the feeling. This feeling will be more and more like a meditation. When you start doing these exercises we recommend to take your time recovering from the breathing exercise. After doing the breathing exercise and when you feel good, you can start with taking the cold shower (page 81).

Breathe yourself healthy

When Wim was younger he did a lot of soul searching.

He says, 'I travelled the world studying everything from karate and kung fu to yoga and Buddhism. But nothing quite fulfilled me.' So with an understanding of Tummo meditation (a Tibetan Buddhist meditation practice) and pranayama yogic breathing, he created his own, more powerful, technique.

Perhaps the best way to describe this for anyone who's never seen it is a controlled form of hyperventilation. This sounds completely contradictory since hyperventilation happens involuntarily and is far from controlled. But imagine the sheer oxygenation of blood and cells without the panic or stress.

Wim says, 'You become charged. Carbon dioxide goes out. Oxygen comes in. The body becomes oxygenated. PH levels go up. At a certain point you're so fully charged, you change the chemistry in your body.'

Scientists from Radboud University Medical Centre would later call this change in chemistry 'intermittent respiratory alkalosis' and state, 'These results could have important implications for the treatment of diseases.'[12]

Step-by-step guide: Cold exposure

Warning: important message, please read carefully.

The cold is a powerful force. We strongly advise you gradually build up exposing yourself to the cold.

Always train without force and listen to your body carefully. If cold exposure is not practised responsibly, there is a risk of hypothermia. After the body scan of the previous exercise, you are ready to let your body embrace the cold. It is very important to try to relax as much as you can, really be with the cold, only then can your body process the signals and start thermogenesis. As Wim says, 'the cold is your warm friend!'

If you are new to cold exposure, just end your warm shower with 15–30 seconds of cold water. Begin with your feet and then follow with your legs, your stomach, shoulders, neck and back. Initial shock, shivering and hyperventilation is normal. Try to remain calm and breathe easily. Close your eyes and really try to embrace the cold.

Don't pour the cold water over your head if you are not comfortable with cold exposure. If you feel any strong physical discomfort, like heavy shivering, numbness or pain, get your body warm again as soon as possible. Cold exposure works like weight lifting: you get stronger over time.

There are little muscles around your veins that contract when they come into contact with the cold. After some time (only 1–2 weeks according to Wim) these become stronger, making your veins healthier and reducing the force that your heart has to use to pump blood around your body. You can increase exposure over time. At one point the cold will feel just as comfortable as wearing your favourite pyjamas and you can skip the warm shower completely.

Notice how you feel amazing after a cold shower and sluggish after a warm one.

Freeze yourself healthy

Ice therapy is basically free medicine!

No, seriously. Research published in *the European Journal of Applied Physiology and Occupational Physiology* wanted to test if our immune systems could be improved by a 'non-infectious stimulus'.[13]

The 'stimulus' used in the study was plunging people into cold water (14°C) for six minutes. What they found was that the cold signalled to the body to go into 'fight or flight' mode, which in turn triggered an immune response. After six weeks of cold plunges three times a week they recorded a 'small, but significant, increase in the proportions of lymphocytes'.

Lymphocytes are the body's cells that fight infection, so having more of these guys when you're feeling a little under the weather is a welcome physiological adaption of Jack Frost and the cold.

Get cold and get healthy!

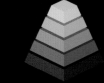

CHAPTER 5
THE LAW OF MORE

> "THE HIGHEST COMPLIMENT THAT YOU CAN PAY ME IS TO SAY THAT I WORK HARD EVERY DAY, THAT I NEVER DOG IT."
> WAYNE GRETZKY

YOU MUST DO MORE

'Patience, persistence and perspiration make an unbeatable combination for success.'
NAPOLEON HILL

Work capacity is the most underrated component of fitness. It's essentially the total amount of training you can perform (recover from) and adapt positively to. Remember the Law of Progressive Overload with Hans Selye's rats, Milo's bull and the importance of progressive overload? Well, a high work capacity means:

▶ You can train harder and for longer.

▶ You avoid the Exhaustion Phase and rarely overtrain.

▶ You're Hans Selye's indestructible rat and Milo carrying one massive bull.

▶ You're basically Geoff Capes (see page 86).

But here lies the problem. Too often the world of fitness places too much emphasis on minimalism, specificity and recovery. We seem to forget that eventually you just have to do more work. It's that simple. People seem surprised when they plateau doing the same training routine, with the same repetition/set scheme for several months. When this happens, work, work and work some more.

'Big jobs usually go to the men who prove their ability to outgrow small ones.'
RALPH WALDO EMERSON

Why? Because it increases the amount of training, stress, stimuli and progressive overload your body can tolerate and positively recover from so you visit the Adaptation Phase and avoid the Exhaustion Phase.

In short, greater work capacity means you can handle **more** training stress. which means you improve faster. Lower work capacity means you can only handle a **lower** amount of training stress, which means you improve, but at a slower rate.

Basically, don't be fooled. For all the tips, tricks and 'quick fixes' in the fitness industry, increasing your work capacity is the only way to constantly and continually improve. Athletes can only ever claim they've reached the 'genetic ceiling' of their physical awesomeness when they no longer have the ability to increase their work capacity.

'Work capacity refers to the general ability of the body as a machine to produce work of different intensity and duration using the appropriate energy systems of the body.'
DR MEL SIFF

Work capacity and recovery: The 'sink' analogy

'Talent is never enough. With few exceptions the best players are the hardest workers.'
MAGIC JOHNSON

Work capacity is: The amount of training you can complete (recover from) and adapt positively to.

'If you can't explain it to a six-year-old, you don't understand it yourself.'
ALBERT EINSTEIN

On that note, behold the 'Work Capacity Sink Analogy'.

Everyone (I hope) knows what a sink looks like. OK, imagine the water coming out of the tap is your training stress. Now imagine the plughole is your work capacity. When training with a low level of stress – like a steady 2 km run or a solid but manageable 30-minute weights routine – there's a slight trickle of water coming out of the tap (training stress) and it doesn't take a large plughole to drain it (work capacity and recovery).

But as you become stronger, quicker and fitter you will need more training stress to improve. That 2-km run and basic strength training routine is no longer enough. You need more water to come out of the tap, but equally you need a bigger plughole to drain it.

In short, a small plughole means you can only tolerate a small amount of water. The bigger your plughole, the more water you can put in your sink and the greater the improvements you'll see. All while making sure your sink doesn't overflow (overtraining).

'Let us rather run the risk of wearing out than rusting out.'
THEODORE ROOSEVELT

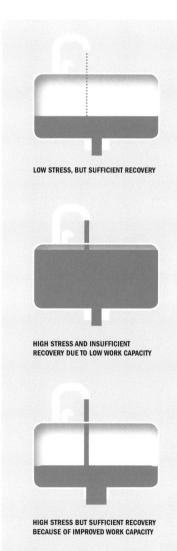

LOW STRESS, BUT SUFFICIENT RECOVERY

HIGH STRESS AND INSUFFICIENT RECOVERY DUE TO LOW WORK CAPACITY

HIGH STRESS BUT SUFFICIENT RECOVERY BECAUSE OF IMPROVED WORK CAPACITY

THE WORLD'S STRONGEST MAN |
Lincolnshire, UK

UNDERSTANDING WORK CAPACITY

11am, 14 February 2015, in the garden of one of the strongest men ever to live.

'Not a lot of people know I was a Churchill Scholar in 1974.'

I scribbled some notes. Sipped my freshly brewed tea. Then took another bite of home-made protein flapjack. This is a typical visit to Geoff Capes' house. Litres of tea are drunk, boxes of flapjacks are eaten and we talk about all things athletics and Strongman.

'I went to train and study in East Germany. In my own practical way I studied all the Communist Bloc and East German Bloc training systems. Then in turn they studied me. They basically wanted to know how I was throwing as much as them,' he added.

Despite the years between us, we both had a deep-rooted respect for all things Eastern European. Hours passed and I told him about my trip to Russia and my first (failed) foray into the world of wrestling with Nikolai. I revealed my pages of notes on General Physical Preparedness and the Process of Achieving Sports Mastery. All the time Geoff nodded politely.

He was there at the 1980 Moscow Olympics. He'd won the World's Strongest Man title. Twice! He represented Great Britain 67 times and completely dominated British shot putting for over a decade, remaining unbeaten in all that time. He even ventured to Scotland to add a string of Highland Games trophies to his mantelpiece.

Basically, none of this was new to him, but he happily sat there allowing me to discover it for myself.

Eventually I ran out of notes and flapjack.

I then asked Geoff what the East Germans never found out. How was it that a boy who grew up on the green fields of Lincolnshire in England was able to 'throw as much as them'?

We poured more tea and I discovered the following…

HOME-GROWN HERCULES

Geoff and I both call Lincolnshire home.

It's a county in the middle of England known for its agricultural history. In South Lincolnshire – where I'm told the soil is particularly rich – some of the most common crops include potatoes, cabbages, cauliflowers and onions. It's also famous for its Lincolnshire sausages, pork pies, gingerbread and my mum's home-made rice pudding! It's a beautiful part of the world. But I digress.

Putting Tourism PR to one side, the main difference between Geoff and me is that my name is not immortalised in our county's folklore. To this day, farmers recount the story of a young Mr Capes being 'Able to load 20 tonnes of potatoes in 20 minutes. Each day. Each week.' A feat I'm told no Lincolnshire farmer has even attempted since.

Talking about his farm-inspired physical strength, Geoff says, 'For a while, athletics lost its way; other sports, such as rugby, infiltrated the throwing talent that used to come from the industrial and farming heartlands. Compared with when I was growing up, partly because of increased mechanisation, few people work the land or work manually now.'

He adds, 'I try to instil that lost ethic into my group of athletes, but they are mostly students and think working for two hours is giving a lot. I worked eight hours a day on the land, then came home and worked three hours on my family's land and then went training for two hours.'

I remember at the time thinking: that's over 13 hours of hard labour. That's some serious work capacity!

Almost simultaneously a light bulb went on in my head. Turning to a page in my diary, I underlined the quote on General Physical Preparedness:

'The major emphasis is establishing a base level of conditioning to increase the athlete's tolerance for more intense training.'
NSCA[1]

Could hours of farm work be the reason Geoff's giant frame could tolerate so much training? Maybe…

THE WORLD'S CRAZIEST TRAINING PLAN

So how did Geoff use his inhuman work capacity?

Well, it seems he fused it with General Physical Preparedness. All to form this crazy, synergistic superhuman who dominated pretty much any sport he played.

'I loved competing,' he says. 'I played everything I could, from basketball to football. I'd throw the shot putt, javelin and discus. I even competed in track, running everything from 200m to cross-country. All at 23½ stone.'

It seemed he was the perfect Soviet specimen, groomed with General Physical Preparedness within the framework of the Process of Achieving Sports Mastery and sprinkled with unparalleled work capacity. It's just this all took place on the fields of Lincolnshire and not Eastern Europe.

'The real drug is to train like a madman, really like a madman.'

ALEKSANDR KARELIN, History's Greatest Greco-Roman Wrestler

Was he always destined for greatness? (By his own admission) it seems not.

'There was no coaching when I was a kid. I came second from last in the all-England schools (shot putt) because the boy who came last had three 'no throws'. The national coaches didn't look at me and say, "There's a national champion". They didn't even bother looking at me because I came 22nd out of 23.'

Tracking back through the history books, it seemed a year later he was undisputedly number one. How?

Training to become old-school strong

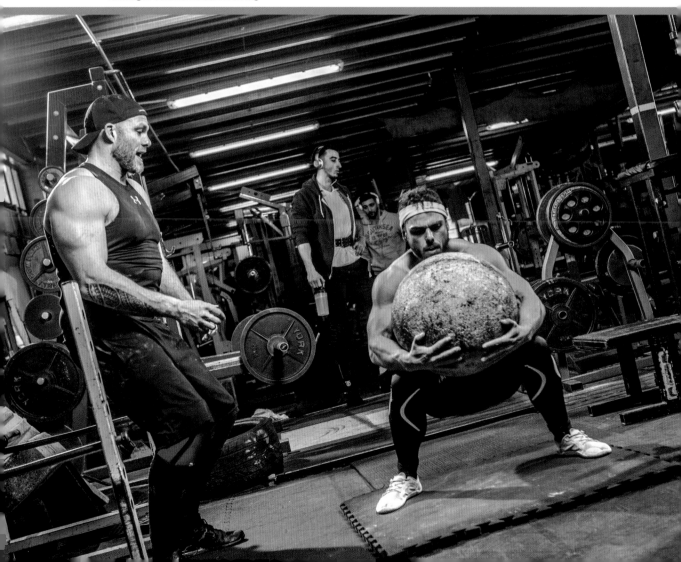

Just how did he condition himself to be a colossal one-man farming force, a one-man Olympics and a home-grown Hercules? All without the support of national coaches from a young age?

I asked. He replied. And the answer I got I could have never predicted.

'There was no sports science and theory back then. My heroes growing up were Alf Tupper, The Tough of the Track, and Wilson The Wonder Athlete from the British comic books of the 1960s.'

We both laughed. One of the strongest men to ever walk the earth credits his unrivalled athleticism and unbridled power to his childhood comic books. Geoff really did learn, make and break his own rules of fitness.

'And you won't find that in any sports journal. Nor could the East Germans in 1974,' he added.

He then sat back in his giant chair. Took in the picturesque view of his garden. Then recounted the early days of his training that involved running, climbing, carrying and throwing. All methods of training that most modern coaches have since reverted to.

'We're now going back to these old-school methods. We're leaving the comfort of these immaculate new gyms with all their shiny equipment and instead throwing tyres, logs and stones around. Why? Because that type of training has always and will always work. It did back then and it does now.'

Geoff then explained how his training had become a little more sophisticated throughout his career. Granted, it began with workouts inspired by Tough of the Track and Wilson The Wonder Athlete, but it quickly evolved into a four-stage training approach that he developed from Eastern European principles.

Sport's Four-point Training System

Unassociated	Partially associated	Semi-associated	Directly associated
Very general, often fun, multi-skill training. Examples include running, jumping, climbing and games.	Training that has some relevance to your sport. This could include medicine ball throws and tyre flips.	Training that directly aids your chosen sport. Examples include squatting, pressing and lifting variations.	Training that's specifically tailored to your sport and event.

Did it work?

Well, on this note I've never met anyone quite like Geoff.

He was a celebrated strength athlete in so many disciplines. He had a unique ability to adapt – and win – in so many different sports. Here's a quick look at his résumé.

- 2-time World's Strongest Man.
- 6-time Highland Games World Champion.
- Commonwealth shot putt champion.
- 2-time European shot putt champion.
- 3-time Olympian.
- Bench press: Unequipped 300 kg (661 lb).
- Squat: Unequipped 380 kg (836 lb).
- Deadlift: Unequipped from a deficit of 18 inches 454.5 kg (1000 lb).

His career was also sprinkled with other accolades.

Like marathons, fell-running victories and 200-metre exhibition races against celebrated Olympic, European and Commonwealth long-distance runner Brendan Foster, in which he (again) won.

This is why close friend – and rival – Bill Kazmaier famously once said, 'I'm the world's strongest man, but Geoff is the world's strongest athlete.'

Bill was a World Powerlifting Champion and three-time World's Strongest Man himself. But even he acknowledged Geoff's strength, power and unequalled athleticism.

All produced by a thorough understanding of work capacity.

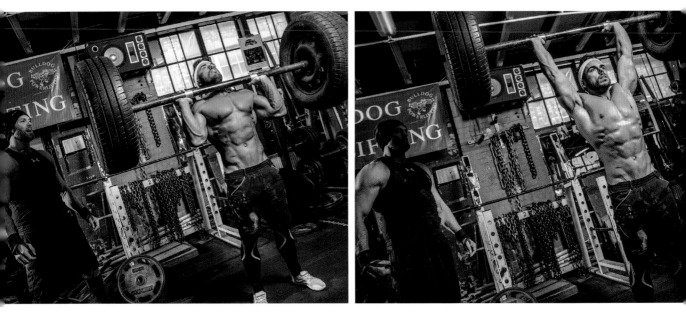

WORK CAPACITY | BEGINNERS
STARTING FROM THE SOFA

'In the beginner's mind there are many possibilities, in the expert's mind there are few.'
SHUNRYU SUZUKI

I would love to be a beginner again!

When starting out you set personal bests week in, week out. It's amazing!

This is because, as mentioned in the Law of Progressive Overload chapter, you only need a little stimuli or stress to load the body above what it's used to and therefore improve. It's true. If you've previously been sat on the sofa doing nothing, then you can improve strength with just a few press-ups a week. To improve your endurance the odd brisk walk would do. It's that easy!

You're basically Milo starting out with a tiny, baby cow.

This is why at Loughborough University, despite being at the very forefront of sports science and innovation, we used to have a saying:

'If you're strong, then train for speed.
If you're quick, then train for strength.
If you're neither, then just train!'
LOUGHBOROUGH UNIVERSITY GYM MAXIM

An idea echoed by Dave Castro. A decorated former US Navy Seal, Dave is now the Global Director of the CrossFit Games. What this means is it's likely he writes more programmes, for more people, than anyone else in the world. But despite his vast knowledge, expertise and experience he always has a way of cutting through the industry's often-unnecessary terminology. He told me when we spoke:

'There's no magic formula. Too many people get caught up in programming and formulas. It's the movements combined with intensity that's the secret. It's much simpler than people think.'

His advice if you're new to training?

'Get in the gym, try some stuff, make mistakes, take advice and learn yourself. You're not going to hurt yourself as long as you do the movements safely with the right technique. It's not going to kill you, that's the reality.'

So why are gym newbies not made aware of this basic law of fitness?

Because it's too simple! It won't sell and Fitness Fairytales sound much better. People like the sound of a band-resisted-vibrating-drop-set cable machine. It's perceived value. It's much more exciting than the tried-and-tested barbell.

Of course even the band-resisted-vibrating-drop-set cable machine offers some form of stimulus. This is better than nothing. But let's not be fooled by Fitness Fairytales.

It's far simpler than we're often led to believe.

'Everything should be made as simple as possible, but not simpler.'
ALBERT EINSTEIN

BEGINNERS | The simple science

Let's take away the illusion that 'fitness' is this hard, intricate thing few can achieve.

Too many people see getting fit as a complex activity that requires a gym, equipment and a personal trainer. It doesn't! Yes, when you're a highly tuned athlete going for the Olympics things become more complicated. But research conducted by the *British Journal of Sports Medicine* wanted to 'examine the effectiveness of brisk walking as a means of improving endurance fitness and influencing fat in previously sedentary women'.

After 12 weeks what did they find?

'The sum of four skinfolds body fat tests decreased with brisk walking and increased with detraining… These findings suggest that regular brisk walking can improve endurance fitness.'[2] Very similar results were found with inactive men too.

A study published in the *European Journal of Applied Physiology and Occupational Physiology* examined 'the influence of a 1-year brisk walking programme on endurance fitness and the amount and distribution of body fat in a group of formerly sedentary men'.

What they found was 'Heart rate and blood lactate concentration during submaximal treadmill walking were significantly reduced in the walkers… Skinfold body fat thicknesses tests on the anterior thigh decreased significantly for the walkers.'[3]

What if you don't like walking?

Then swim, cycle, crawl or hop! No, seriously. In a massive-scale study conducted at the University of Hull, England, scientists wanted to investigate 'whether there is currently sufficient scientific knowledge for scientists to be able to give valid training recommendations to long-distance runners and their coaches on how to most effectively enhance endurance'.[4]

Did they uncover a blueprint for success? No. They concluded there's no specific, set way to improve endurance.

The World's Easiest Kettlebell Workout!

I learnt this workout from friend and world-famous powerlifter Andy Bolton.

A strength and conditioning genius, he has seven WPC World Champion titles, two WPO Champion titles and a place cemented in history as the first human to ever deadlift 1000 pounds. But despite helping me personally squat, bench and deadlift more than I ever thought possible, it's this workout that he taught me under the leaking roof of Ralls' gym in Leeds in the North of England that I will never forget.

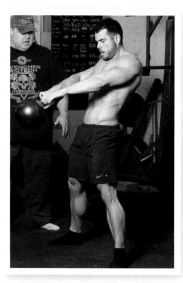

This is because despite all he's achieved Andy admits there's no secret formula for success.

He says too often we over-complicate our training. But this programme beautifully embodies the power of simplicity and it just requires one single piece of equipment and 10 minutes of your time. All to improve your work capacity.

Session 1: 5 repetitions of 5 sets. Performing the swings at the top of every minute.

This means you get just under a minute to rest between sets.

Add a rep each session...
Session 1: 5 reps x 5 sets
Session 2: 6 reps x 5 sets
Session 3: 7 reps x 5 sets
Session 4:: 8 reps x 5 sets
Session 5: 9 reps x 5 sets
Session 6: 10 reps x 5 sets (now you're doing 50 swings in 5 minutes)
Once you get to 10 reps for five sets start adding a set each session
Session 7: 10 reps x 6 sets
Session 8: 10 reps x 7 sets
Session 9: 10 reps x 8 sets
Session 10: 10 reps x 9 sets
Session 11: 10 reps x 10 sets (now you're doing 100 swings in 10 minutes)

Then, each workout, add an extra repetition to each set.

When you can do that with a 16-kg bell, switch to a heavier kettlebell and repeat until you can do this with the 48-kg bell — known as 'The Beast'. When you can do 100 crisp and powerful repetitions in 10 minutes – with The Beast – you will be strong and conditioned.

You'll also notice a weird and amazing carry-over to your barbell lifts, particularly the deadlift.

If you compete in sports that require strength, speed, power and/or endurance, you'll also find you are a much better athlete. And all that from 5–10 minutes of swings.

Again, learn to find power in simplicity.

Again, stressing the Law of Biological Individuality they said that, 'In the future, molecular biology may make an increasing contribution in identifying effective training methods, by identifying the genes that contribute to improved endurance.' But for now – and even when molecular biology does catch up – if you're a complete beginner, just get up and get active.

Someway and somehow, your body's endurance will improve since you only need the smallest 'training reaction' and 'activation reaction' to produce an Adaptation Phase'.

HORSEPOWER PROGRAMMING

Increasing work capacity for trained athletes

Problems occur when you're highly trained and have a high work capacity.

This is because you're already well adapted. You're like Milo with a fully grown bull: carrying a baby cow down the road once a week won't really bring about any training improvements since you need to subject your body to a greater degree of stress and stimuli for it to adapt.

So how do we increase work capacity? The honest answer is complex.

Since – again taking into consideration Biological Individuality – the right training programme will vary from person to person. But I recommend something I call **horsepower programming** which involves:

- Decreasing training intensity 5–15% and increasing training volume 20–50% over 2–4 months.
- Decreasing volume for heavy main lifts and increasing volume of bodybuilding-style lifts.
- Adding additional cardiovascular training.

Based on the above, here are some tried and tested strategies proven effective over time.

'Sheer effort enables those with nothing to surpass those with privilege and position.'
TOYOTOMI HIDEYOSHI

1. Add more sets

The first is also the most simple: add sets to your routines.

Let's say you can do three sets of three repetitions on a 140 kg squat. What would then be easier? Trying to complete three sets of three repetitions with 150 kg or just adding another 140 kg squat for one repetition at the end? I'd hope you'd say the extra repetition obviously.

Then, next session, add two repetitions with 140 kg, and three after that.

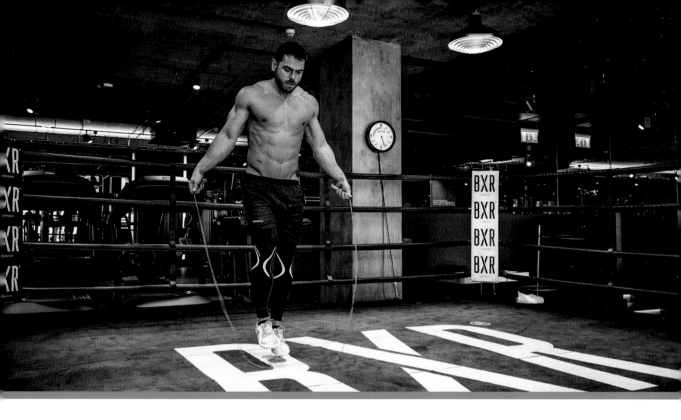

Once you're able to do five to eight sets of three repetitions your, work capacity has improved. Now it's time to drop back down to three sets with a bigger weight (maybe try that 150 kg).

The key is adding that one repetition per session. It's not that taxing on your body over your established baseline. Then when you drop back to just three sets, it's less volume than you've grown accustomed to, setting you up nicely for the subsequent re-ramping of the volume.

2. Add more reps

The second is equally simple: add reps to your routines.

Made famous by legendary Canadian strongman and weightlifter Doug Hepburn, you simply pick a weight you can do eight sets of one repetition with, then slowly add an extra rep to each set until you can do 8 x 2 repetitions, then increase the weight and start over with one repetition. This is simple yet very effective for many.

3. Add cardio

The third is to add additional cardio-based workouts around your strength training.

This could exist in the form of 20 minutes of cardio in the morning, like skipping. It has very little impact on the joints and isn't very taxing on the body, which would allow you to perform your usual strength-based training in the afternoon or evening. Or, depending on your circadian rhythm (i.e. your biological clock, which determines when your body 'peaks') and your work schedule, you could perform your strength training in the morning and your cardio in the evening.

Whatever method works best for you, know that adding cardio-specific workouts in and around your usual strength and conditioning routines remains one of the easiest ways to increase work capacity.

4. Add finishers

The final way is to add movement-specific 'finishers' to your strength training.

This is a favourite among strength athletes since many experts warn against the dangers of adding cardio to the end of your weight training. It's theorised that this floods the body with a cocktail of catabolic hormones that kills your body's natural anabolic response to training. Worth noting is that this is subject to debate and varies from person to person.

If you're in this camp, but want to increase your work capacity, 'finishers' are your answer. These are quick, intense, movement-specific exercises you can add to the end of your workouts:

- 5 x 20-metre sled sprints after a big leg session.
- 30 seconds x 10 battle ropes.
- 10 x 10-metre tyre flips after a colossal deadlift.

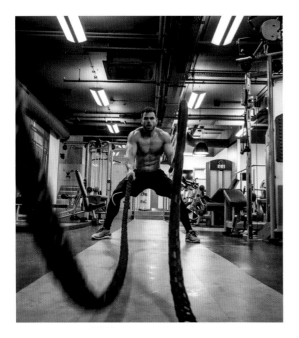

The list goes on and we're about to put them into a workout for you (page 106).

But know that, in summary, increasing work capacity is the 'secret' to fitness (if ever there was one), since throughout history the best athletes simply developed the ability to do more work than their competition.

This in turn allowed them to adapt, improve and ultimately win.

'Work capacity is the most important and most forgotten aspect of training.'
ROSS EDGLEY

THE WORLD'S LONGEST ROPE CLIMB |
Ashdown Forest, England

SCALING EVEREST ON A ROPE

'When the human body is put under exceptional strain, a range of dormant genes in the DNA are expressed and extraordinary physiological processes are activated.'

ANDERS ERICSSON

Chapter 7 details how I ran a marathon pulling a car to raise money for charity.

For whatever reason, it seemed that strange sporting events broadcast across my social media encouraged people to kindly donate to some amazing causes. But a few weeks after I'd finished the marathon I realised I was just short of my fundraising target. Visiting Alder Hey Children's Hospital in Liverpool, I learnt it costs £25,000 a year to pay for the ongoing maintenance and repairs of a specialist Teenage Cancer Trust Ward.

What this meant was although I had done well, I needed to do great. But I had a plan!

Toughest was Sweden's biggest obstacle race, boasting more mud and bigger obstacles than any other Nordic race. Its creators had won awards for their rope swings, ramps and giant mud slides, raised thousands for children's charities and built a business on electrocuting, catapulting and freezing competitors from all over Europe.

What's more, in April they would host their first-ever event on English soil. This was perfect!

If anyone would support another funny, fitness-based spectacle it was them.

A few emails and phone calls later and I met Adam and Per at their London HQ and immediately liked them. They were as kind as they were tall, Swedish and blond, which is why it only took one meeting, two cups of tea and three protein brownies for us to jointly dream up the idea for The World's Longest Rope Climb.

Our concept was simple…

1. I would commandeer the rig at the bottom of their course the day before their event.
2. We would attach a 10-metre rope to the top of it.
3. For 24 hours (or as long as it took) I would climb this rope (repeatedly).
4. I would finish once I'd scaled the height of Everest (8848 metres).

All the time Adam and Per would tell the health and safety marshals to ignore the strange Englishmen. My support team would sit around a campfire at the bottom of the rope and

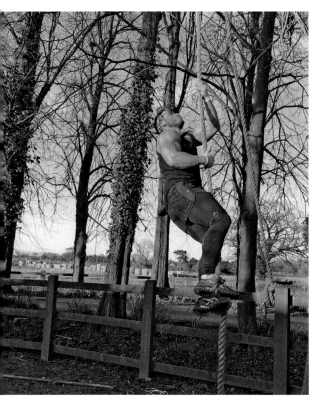

Over 400,000 ft of practice for The World's Longest Rope Climb

eat pizza and drink beer. Finally, 5000 confused spectators would arrive, watch and (hopefully) donate money. It was the perfect plan!

Money for charity would be raised… Ropes, for no reason, would be climbed…

And my 10 weeks of training began. It was an event the skin on my hands was not happy about, but it was also an event that taught me a lot about work capacity as we predicted it could take up to 24 hours to complete.

But first, I needed to build bulletproof biceps.

BULLETPROOF BICEPS

An efficient rope climb uses many muscle groups.

But it's an unavoidable truth that the biceps will take a battering. That's because, according to scientists from Duke University Medical Center, US,[5] who analysed muscle activation during climbing techniques, there is an 'abrupt peak in bicep and forearm muscle tension during the pull-up and lowering' phase of the climb.

This is why 'Upper-extremity muscle injuries from rock climbing are common' and 'a reduction in climbing-related muscle injuries may be achieved by a training program that emphasizes conditioning' of the relevant muscles.

Which is why I needed to find a way to train strength without the soreness.

STRONG, NOT SORE

Anyone who's ever set foot in the squat rack will experience the aches and pains that come with it.

You know the kind of DOMS (Delayed Onset Muscle Soreness) that makes climbing the stairs the day after seem like conquering Everest! But research published by the National Strength and Conditioning Association found that by mixing up the types of muscle contractions during training you can build strength and workout capacity without the soreness.

Interested? First, we need a quick Masterclass in Muscle Movement.

There are three basic ways the muscles contract:

- **Isometric contractions:** This is where the muscle contracts but does not shorten, giving no movement. The Plank is perhaps the best example of an isometric contraction.
- **Concentric contractions:** This is where the muscle contracts and shortens in length. The upward movement of a dumbbell in a bicep curl is a good example. Or imagine the spring back from a jump landing – as you extend your knees and jump back up in the air you'll notice the quadriceps (front of the legs) are shortening as they create force to push you off.
- **Eccentric contractions:** This is where the muscle is in tension while it lengthens. A good example of this is the downward movement of a dumbbell in a bicep curl. Or when you land on two feet from a jump and bend your knees you'll notice the quadriceps are in tension to cushion the impact, but are lengthening.

Why is this important? Because the NSCA scientists found, 'One critical differentiation is that higher levels of muscle tension can be generated during eccentric muscle actions.' Basically – if you imagine a squat, bench or deadlift – you can usually lower more weight than you can lift.

Researchers added 'Moreover, there is a significant amount of mechanical stress accrued during this part of the lift due to the lengthening of the muscle while cross bridge formation is occurring. Since mechanical stress is thought to be the chief factor stimulating muscular adaptation, researchers have concluded that the eccentric portion of a lift is that which induces many of the adaptations from resistance training. However, the damage produced by eccentric muscle action has the potential to cause a significant amount of soreness, fatigue, and inflammation.'

Let's put this in simple terms. Solely performing the concentric part of a lift and avoiding the eccentric phase means you could (in theory) avoid the 'soreness, fatigue and inflammation' usually associated with strength training. Which is why I spent hours flipping tyres, pulling weighted sleds across the gym with a rope, doing pull-ups and bicep curls with no downward (eccentric) phase. Or simply climbing a rope in my garden, but stepping on the fence to get back down.

No eccentric phase. No soreness.

Putting this knowledge into practice, I was able to:

- Train and condition my biceps and forearms seven days per week.
- Perform 1000+ repetitions per session.
- Spend hours a day battling gravity supported only by my hands and feet.

All while avoiding overtraining and muscle damage and dramatically improving work capacity as I spent less and less time on solid ground. Did it work? During 24 hours of climbing a rope in a field I would find out.

THE START

10am, 22 April 2016 and I'm standing in Ashdown Forest, England.

An ancient area of tranquil open heathland that occupies the highest sandy ridge-top of the High Weald Area of Outstanding Natural Beauty, Ashdown Forest is 30 miles south of London. The scenery is stunning as the hills seem to go on for miles, revealing every shade of green imaginable.

But this weekend this all changes. Recreational walkers and their dogs are to be replaced by 5000 mud-covered-thrill-seeking runners as Toughest host their first event on English soil, featuring miles of barbed wire from Stockholm and mountains of tyres from Malmö. Athletes from all over Europe have made the journey following a month-long social-media storm that promised this race would be the best of the year.

But my participation in the adrenaline-fuelled festivities will have to wait.

I have a rope to climb and money to raise.

The 'climb' before the storm

10:30am and I'm now standing underneath the scaffolding with my support team.

Looking up, the rope seemed to disappear into the clouds that were now menacingly circling Ashdown Forest. I wasn't sure if my hands were shaking from the nerves or the cold, but either way I firmly cupped the mug of coffee in the hope no one noticed.

But clearly not cupping it firmly enough, because my friend Matt did notice.

'You ready champ?' he asked, putting his hand on my shoulder.

The truth is, I wasn't. I don't think you can ever be ready to climb 8848m of rope.

But Matt's presence made me feel a little better. He was without doubt the best person I could have supporting me. A highly respected mountain leader, he practically lived outdoors and had set up the support team's base at the bottom the rope climb in just 20 minutes.

Breakfast was served over a stove, medical supplies were made ready and cameras were connected. We even had a giant whiteboard we could write on so that:

1. People could see how far up Everest we were.

2. We could record and I could strictly adhere to the 885 ascents of the 10-metre rope every 97 seconds to ensure I finished the 8848 metres in 24 hours.

Basically, it was only under Matt's supervision that the campsite was complete and running like clockwork.

From 10:35 to 10:45am porridge was eaten in silence. There was an eerie sense of anticipation in the camp.

We all knew this wouldn't be pretty and we all knew blisters, rope burns and blood were inevitable. The only question was how much of these would be needed to complete the climb. In 15 minutes I would finish my porridge. Begin the climb. Then collectively we would find out.

The technique

The clock struck 11am and I began my first ascent.

The team cheered, but I did my best to remain calm and remember the weeks of technique I had been drilling from a rope hung over a tree in my garden. I knew the success or failure of this event would largely depend on my climbing biomechanics.

Energy efficiency was key!

This is because all movements have what's known as a kinetic chain. Dr Arthur Steindler, one of the early pioneers of this theory, defines a kinetic chain as 'a combination of several successively arranged joints constituting a complex motor unit'.

Put simply, it's how all your joints and movements work together during certain movements. Needless to say, during a 24-hour rope climb you need one incredibly efficient kinetic chain. Without it, your legs and core fail to work in unison with your arms and your biceps are forced to battle gravity on their own.

This is one reason why the *Journal of Sports Medicine*[6] noted, 'Three-quarters of elite and recreational sport climbers will suffer upper-extremity injuries. Approximately 40% will be equally divided between the elbow and the shoulder.'

Now, worth noting is that there are many ways to climb a rope, from Navy Seal-inspired methods to CrossFit and Marine-taught techniques. During my 10 weeks of training I tested them all to find one that worked with my own individual physiology. For me this was the Marine-style brake technique:

- Single-wrap the rope around one of your legs and across the top of your foot.
- The foot of the unwrapped leg clamps down on the other foot, trapping the rope.
- You can now support your weight without using the power of your arms and hands.
- Reach up. Grab the rope as high as is comfortable (important not to overstretch).
- Then throw your feet up as high as possible, aiming to touch your hands.
- Single-wrap the rope around your foot (again). Trap it. Extend the body up the rope and climb.

I found this wasn't the quickest method…

But it was the most efficient in terms of energy expended, sustaining it for 24 hours and maintaining some sense of safety and stability when sleep deprivation kicked in.

As a result the first six hours were actually enjoyable.

Spirits were high in the camp. The porridge was finished and as I reached 2100m my support team's attention turned to celebratory quarter-way-mark pizza.

'Beef Bonanza or Ham Heaven?' Matt shouted. Halfway up the rope, my answer was, 'Both.'

PIZZA AND PATIENCE

Unfortunately, by 6pm both the pizza and skin on my hands were running thin.

Although my biceps and forearms were coping with the 'abrupt peak in muscle tension during the pull-up and lowering' phase of the climb, the rope was beginning to burn through the gloves and my skin. But they weren't like ordinary blisters: instead they were blistering where the skin had already torn. Basically, raw wounds were becoming even rawer.

It was unavoidable too, since I was gripping the rope in exactly the same spot each time. Turning to the support team for ideas produced no answers. We'd all had rope burns before, but these were making the ones I'd had before look like scratches.

'Try and climb gripping with your good fingers,' Matt suggested.

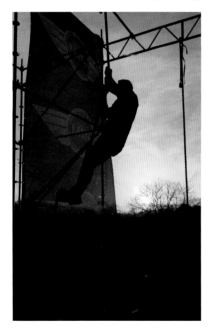

'I have no "good fingers" left,' I said, holding up each one individually to show they were all cut. 'What about your thumb on your right hand? That looks relatively healthy,' he said, laughing. I laughed too, since at this point that's all we could do.

We then taped them up as best we could, put on another pair of gloves and then headed into the night with my one good thumb leading the way as darkness descended on the forest…

THE DARKEST HOURS

10pm, and after 4000 metres climbed we were entering the night shift.

Temperatures had dropped, the support team were sleeping and all that remained was Matt, some very cold pizza and myself. This was figuratively and literally the darkest period of the climb and I was now the owner of unholy rope burns and blisters in places I didn't know you could get blisters.

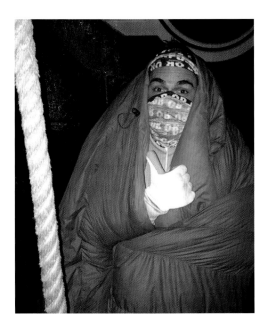

What's worse is that with limited lighting I would have to wait until the morning to see how bad they really were.

But despite the skin on my hands and the light in the sky failing me, Matt wouldn't.

Through the night he brewed litres of green tea, spoon-fed me porridge and between ascents – when I had roughly 60 seconds to rest – would wrap me in a blanket to keep my body warm and arms from seizing up. Hours passed and very few words were spoken.

Nothing needed to be said.

I have no doubt I would still be in that field now if it wasn't for Matt, and it was only because of him that I saw the sunrise with a glimmer of hope this might actually work.

MORNING AND MEDIA

6:30am, and morning arrived along with media crews.

After 7500 metres I was less than 1 km from my 'summit'. News had now spread across social media, and athletes racing that day had decided to arrive early to see the (not so) sprint finish of my rope climb. Tired and battered, I did my best to answer questions from journalists and smile for cameras.

But inside, my body was falling apart and my hands would no longer work like they were supposed to. Hours of pulling my body up and down a rope meant I could no longer fully extend or close my fingers. Holding a spoon was tricky. Tying my shoelaces was impossible. Every handshake was agony.

But do you know the worst part? I desperately needed the toilet. My diet of pizza and porridge had come back to haunt me and I now had a group of over 1000 spectators and a camera crew circling the rope, each expecting some heroic finish to the climb they'd heard so much about.

Eager to please, I managed 11 more ascents before my digestive system said no more.

Yes, finishing the event was important. But avoiding emptying my bowels when dangling 10 metres in the air above the English media was also quite high on my 'to do' list that day, which is why I politely excused myself and ran for the portable toilets, subtly grabbing the toilet paper en route.

BLISTERS, BANDAGES AND BATHROOM BREAKS

I will spare you most of the details.

Moments later I was lighter and relieved as I'd disposed of what seemed like kilograms of porridge and pizza that had been collecting in my stomach. But now I was painfully aware that I'd completely lost all dexterity in my blistered hands. What this meant was pulling my trousers up was proving tricky, but folding toilet paper so I could wipe things that needed to be wiped was proving impossible.

What seemed like hours passed as I fumbled and stumbled around. My trousers dropped back towards my ankles, the toilet paper fell to the floor and I collapsed into the cubicle wall. With so little room to manoeuvre and with no functionality left in my hands I began to worry this would be the end of The World's Longest Rope Climb. I even began thinking of the apology letter I would have to write to the Teenage Cancer Trust to tell them I couldn't finish the climb because I got trapped in a toilet.

That's not a letter anyone wants to write. I sat for a moment, considered my options and prayed for a toilet-based miracle. Then, somehow and someway, it worked. In the toilet next to me I heard a voice.

'Sounds like you're having some trouble in there?' the mystery voice asked, gently knocking on the wall. He had a strong Swedish accent, but spoke perfect English and sounded genuinely concerned. Also, although I didn't know for sure, he sounded quite old (maybe a grandad) and had an empathetic tone to his voice that lead me to believe he was one of the older competitors racing in the Toughest obstacle race that was due to start that day.

'Ermmmm...' I paused for a moment.

I needed help, but was unsure how much help you can ask from a complete stranger you've just met in a portable toilet in a field in the English countryside.

'Just experiencing a small technical difficulty,' I replied, trying my best to sound upbeat.

But my newly acquired toilet-dwelling friend could sense that my current plight was more than a 'small technical difficulty'. He then said he'd been obstacle racing all around the world and whatever predicament I was battling in my 1 x 1-metre cabin, he had probably been there at some point too.

He was my only hope. I decided there was no subtle way to broach the subject so asked, 'Have your hands ever been so blistered from rope climbing that you can't fold toilet paper to wipe your own bum?'

Silence now surrounded Ashdown Forest. This was officially the world's most awkward toilet break. Had I broken some European Toilet Treaty between England and Sweden where you don't confess you can't wipe your own bum?

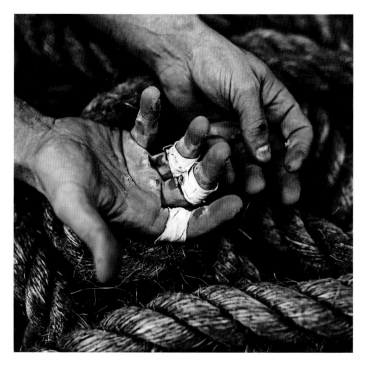

'Here we go my boy. The silence was broken. It seemed he'd only stopped talking so he could neatly and perfectly fold squares of tissue paper into a bundle and then pass them through the small gap at the bottom of the cubicle.

'Will this be enough?' he asked. 'Yes,' I said, a little emotional about the act of heroism I was witnessing.

Now (again) I will spare you the details, but the paper was folded with such precision it verged on origami art, which meant I was able to complete the task at hand by effortlessly cupping the loo roll without any need to grip. Whoever he was, my Swedish toilet-dwelling superhero had saved me, the rope climb and the charity donations. Emerging from the toilet I immediately looked for the man who had bravely liberated me from the confines of my potty prison, but he was gone and nowhere to be seen.

His cubicle was empty and to this day I have never had a chance to thank him. But needless to say, because of that man, Toughest obstacle race and the Toilet Treaty of Ashdown Forrest I will forever be indebted to the country of Sweden and the people of that great nation.

But with no time to waste, I had a rope to climb. Returning to the team, 'play resumed' and 1 hour later (at around 8:00am) I finished.

I had climbed 8848 metres and conquered Everest on a rope in a field in England, leaving most of my skin around the fields of Ashdown Forest. The World's Longest Rope Climb is essentially what happens when you fuse an increased work capacity with the unwavering support of a friend like Matt and the toilet-based heroism of a mysterious Swedish grandpa.

YOUR 12-WEEK WORLDWIDE BODYWEIGHT WORKOUT

THE WORKOUT EXPLAINED

Presenting the world's most travelled, tried-and-tested workout.

This routine has been around the world with me. I've hung from a tree on the beaches of the Bahamas, performed press-up variations in a backstreet gym in São Paulo and busted out weighted lunges through paddy fields in the village of Rahmatpur in Bangladesh.

It's bodyweight-based, requires very little equipment and perfectly embodies the Five Laws of Fitness so you can train anything and everything, anywhere and everywhere by combining:

- Nikolai's version of Soviet General Physical Preparedness.
- Geoff's four-point (multi-skill) training system.
- Bodyweight progressions inspired by the Royal Marines.
- The recovery methods of Wim Hof.
- The work capacity built from The World's Longest Rope Climb.

All so you can build a functional, well-rounded physique.

Essentially, it's a training programme that teaches you to 'know your body' – developing greater kinaesthetic awareness – so you can learn new movements, with greater proficiency, far faster. You then lose fat, build muscle, increase speed and improve endurance far more easily when you want to specialise later.

BODYWEIGHT TRAINING: A BRIEF HISTORY

Bodyweight training (also known as calisthenics) is as old as strength and conditioning itself.

In fact, you can trace its origins back to ancient Greece. Granted, not the complex, gravity-defying work of many of today's modern practitioners, but the humble press-up, lunge and chin-up have survived centuries of gimmicks and fads and have been used to forge some of the most elite[7] fighting forces in history[8].

And here's how...

As early as the reign of the Spartans between 600 and 400 BC young soldiers were conditioned through simple crunches, jumping jacks, lunges and squat variations. These were then coupled with skill-specific training like wrestling, boxing and javelin/spear work, all in an effort to create an ancient military super power.

Similarly, the superhuman fitness capabilities of the Shaolin Monks can be traced back to their mastery of calisthenics. According to research published in *The Oxford Handbook of Religion and Violence* (Mark Juergensmeyer et al, 2005) in 527 BC the monasteries were being robbed and looted and so in an effort to defend themselves and their land, the monks began training in physical combat and bodyweight training. Years later their enduring strength and lightning speed have become renowned around the world.

Finally, to use a more modern example, calisthenics has been used for years to assess the fitness of new recruits in the Royal Marines. To test strength, stamina and muscular endurance, soldiers must complete three events consisting of the push-up, sit-up and a two-mile run.

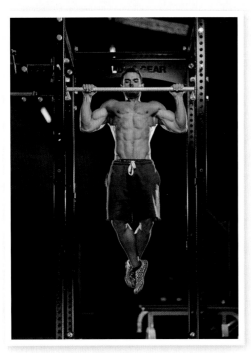

BODYWEIGHT TRAINING: HOW TO USE IT

You might be thinking, 'But I'm not a spear-wielding Spartan.'

Me neither. Nor can I do a Shaolin one-finger push-up. Well there's good news: you don't have to, and studies show that bodyweight training can still provide an array of benefits. Especially when you couple it with the principles of General Physical Preparedness and Conventional Strength Training.

Let me explain …

BODYWEIGHT TRAINING | Better mechanical energy

Who doesn't love bicep curls, right?

Also, few people would deny there's something satisfying about 'burning out' on a quad extension machine as your legs blow up twice the size from the volume. But neither of these exercises is particularly demanding on the body's mechanical energy and neither of them encourages the muscles and joints in the body to work cohesively.

In contrast, imagine a bar muscle-up, hanging leg raises or a handstand shoulder press. All the muscles in the body must work together to achieve the desired result. Now this isn't to say you should bid farewell to the preacher curl altogether. But to quote research published in the *Handbook of Sports Medicine and Science: Gymnastics*[9], 'An increase in skill difficulty corresponds to the demand for higher mechanical energy.'

For this exact reason, including some calisthenic work into your routine is ideal to build a strong, functional and aesthetically well-rounded physique.

BODYWEIGHT TRAINING | Greater muscle activation

Next, as well as improving your mechanical energy, it also seems swapping the machines in favour of 'free' exercises could also result in greater muscle activation. To test this theory, scientists from the College of Kinesiology at the University of Saskatchewan[10] in Canada took six healthy participants and monitored muscle activation during a Smith machine-assisted squat and a free weight squat.

Now it must be noted this wasn't strictly calisthenics; however, the principle of performing exercises unassisted by fixed equipment remains the same. After monitoring the electromyographic (EMG) activity of the legs, back and abs they found 'There were no significant differences between free weight and Smith machine squat for any of the other muscles; however, the EMG averaged over all muscles during the free weight squat was 43% higher when compared to the Smith machine squat.'

This led researchers to conclude 'The free weight squat may be more beneficial than the Smith machine squat for individuals who are looking to strengthen plantar flexors knee flexors, and knee extensors.'

Again this wasn't strictly calisthenics, but it would be interesting if the researchers took this one step further to monitor muscle activation during a unilateral, single-leg squat, which is exactly what research from *The Journal of Strength and Conditioning* did.

BODYWEIGHT TRAINING | Better core engagement

All bodyweight practitioners will tell you a strong core is absolutely key.

This is because you won't be able to perform certain exercises without engaging the entire core just because of the unstable, unilateral nature of calisthenics. Don't believe me? I bet you can perform a pretty heavy leg press while relaxing the core. But now try to do a single-leg pistol squat while relaxing the stomach.

I guarantee you will end up on the floor.

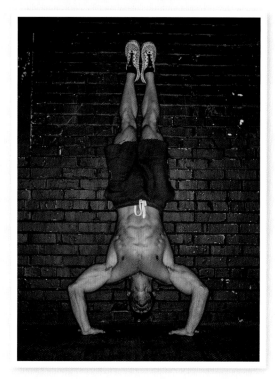

This idea is supported by research published in *The Journal of Strength and Conditioning*[11] that aimed to 'evaluate the effect of unstable and unilateral exercises on trunk muscle activation'. Using electromyography technology, they tested the activity of the muscles in the core and found 'The most effective means for trunk strengthening should involve back or abdominal exercises with unstable bases.'

Adding, 'Furthermore, trunk strengthening can also occur when performing resistance exercises, if the exercises are performed unilaterally.'

Training notes

- The sessions of this workout are biomechanically divided.
- This means your 'push', 'pull' and 'lower-body' movements are performed in different sessions.
- Every workout begins with a fast and explosive movement. The goal here is moving fast and efficiently to awaken the central nervous system, get the joints and muscles working cohesively and essentially prep the body for the rest of the workout and develop better mechanical energy and muscle activation.
- The number of workouts, sets, repetitions and volume increase from weeks 1 to 12 to increase work capacity.
- By weeks 9–12 you can begin to add sport-specific training (triathlon, football, basketball).
- The Full Body Centurion Workout is taken from the Primal 9 Training System. The most downloaded workout plan of 2017, it was a programme I co-created with *Men's Health Magazine* as a science-backed fitness test to mass monitor the physical ability of the millions that downloaded it.
- The Ab Routine is based on tried-and-tested movements shown to increase muscle activation in the core greater than the conventional sit-up/crunch alone.
- The entire 12-week programme is ideal if:
  - You are new to training.
  - You are off-season from your sport.
  - You want to rebuild your body, get back to basics and develop greater kinaesthetic awareness.
  - You have minimal equipment but want to train anything and everything, anywhere and everywhere.

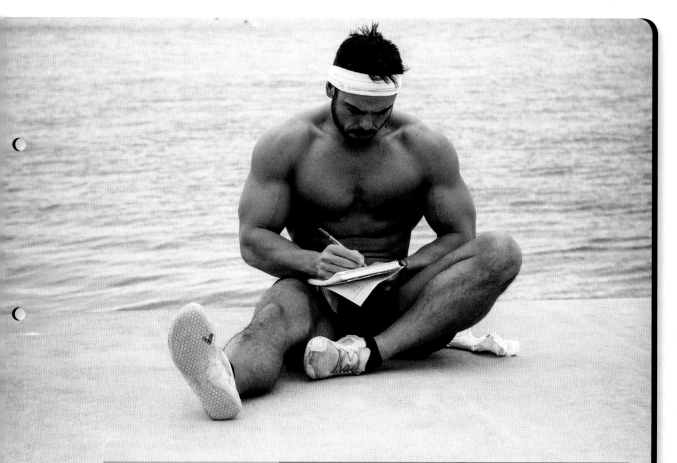

	4-DAY ROUTINE	5-DAY ROUTINE	6-DAY ROUTINE
	WEEKS 1–4	WEEKS 5–8	WEEKS 9–12
KEY FOCUS	Improve strength Refine technique Develop kinaesthetic awareness and better mechanical energy	Improve strength Refine technique Increase work capacity	Improve strength Refine technique Specialise
WORKOUT	Monday: 'Push' Training Tuesday: Lower-body Training Wednesday: REST Thursday: 'Pull' Training Friday: Full-body Centurion Workout Saturday: REST Sunday: REST	Monday: 'Push' Training Tuesday: Lower-body Training Wednesday: 'Pull' Training Thursday: REST Friday: Full-body Caveman Conditioning Saturday: Ab Workout Sunday: REST	Monday: 'Push' Training Tuesday: Lower-body Training Wednesday: 'Pull' Training Thursday: Ab Workout Friday: Full-body Caveman Conditioning Saturday: Sport Specific Sunday: REST
MAIN GOAL	Unlock the neurological potential of the body and develop kinaesthetic awareness.	Increase work capacity and therefore your body's ability to tolerate more training.	Use your improved neurological potential and work capacity to specialise 1 day per week.

4-DAY ROUTINE | WEEKS 1–4 | MONDAY: 'PUSH' TRAINING

Exercise	Reps	Sets	Rest	Coaching Cues	
Plyometric Push-up	5	3	90 secs	Get in a press-up position. Hands shoulder-width apart and back straight. Lower your chest to the floor, then push up explosively until your arms fully extend. Attempt to add claps into the movement while airborne if possible. (If you can't manage full press-ups, do them on your knees.)	
Spiderman Push-up	5 (each leg)	3	90 secs	Get into a traditional press-up position. Lower yourself toward the floor and bring your right knee to your right elbow, keeping it off the ground. Press back up and return your leg to the starting position. Repeat with the alternate leg. (If you can't manage full press-ups, do them with your hands on a bench.)	
Bench Dip	12	3	60 secs	Stand facing away from a bench. Grab it with both hands at shoulder width. Extend your legs out in front of you. Slowly lower your body by flexing at the elbows until your upper arms create a 90-degree angle. Use your triceps to lift yourself back to the starting position.	
Plate Press	20	3	60 secs	Lie on a flat bench holding a weight plate over your chest with your palms facing each other. Pinching and squeezing the plate, push up until your arms are straight, pause, then lower under control.	
Alternate Dumbbell Press	12 (each arm)	3	60 secs	Hold a dumbbell in each hand just above shoulder height with your palms facing forward and arms bent. Press one dumbbell up over your head without moving the other dumbbell. Return the weight to the starting position. Repeat for the opposite side, continuing to alternate between arms.	
Bear Crawl	10m forward then 10m backward	3	45 secs	Get down on all fours, with your hands directly under your shoulders and your knees under your hips. Bring your knees off the ground and travel forward. Keep your back flat at all times. Travel 10 m forward, then reverse.	

TUESDAY: LOWER-BODY TRAINING

Exercise	Reps	Sets	Rest	Coaching Cues	
Explosive Sprinter Step-up	5 (each leg)	3	90 secs	Place a bench or box in front of you and step onto it with one foot. As you plant your foot, aggressively drive through your other foot, bringing your knee as high as you can. Lower it back down to step back onto the floor. Repeat on the other side.	
Lateral Step-over with Weighted Plate	10 (each leg)	3	90 secs	Holding a weight plate at your chest, stand to the right side of the bench and place your left foot on top. Push from your left heel and raise your body onto the bench. Touch down on the bench with your right foot, then lower your left foot to the other side of the bench. Drive back up and repeat on the other side.	
Bulgarian Split Squat	12 (each leg)	3	60 secs	Stand facing away from the bench. Rest one leg on the bench behind you with the laces of your shoes facing down. Squat with your standing leg until the knee of your trailing leg almost touches the floor. Push up through the front foot to return to the start position.	
Paused Bodyweight Squat	20	5	60 secs	Stand with your feet shoulder-width apart. Bend the knees and sit back with your hips until your knees are at a 90-degree angle. Pause, then reverse the motion until you return to the starting position.	
Duck Walk	5m forward then 5m backward	4	60 secs	Lower into a squat so your thighs are parallel to the floor and place your hands behind your head. Slowly walk forward 5 m in a controlled manner, keeping your balance at all times, then reverse the movement back to the start position.	

4-DAY ROUTINE | WEEKS 1–4 | THURSDAY: 'PULL' TRAINING

Exercise	Reps	Sets	Rest	Coaching Cues	
Dumbbell Single Arm Sumo High Pull	5 (each arm)	3	90 secs	Stand with your legs wider than shoulder-width apart with a dumbbell in one hand. Lower your body into a squat position until your thighs are parallel to the floor. Push through your heels and raise the dumbbell to your chin, so your arm bends and the elbow is in line with the top of your head. Squat down and repeat.	
Pull-up	8	3	90 secs	Grip the bar with hands shoulder-width apart. Raise your feet off the floor and hang. Pull yourself up until your chin is over the bar and repeat.	
Incline Dumbbell Row	12	3	60 secs	Holding a dumbbell in each hand, lie face-down on an incline bench. Keep your core tight and back straight as you row the weights up to your chest. Lower and repeat.	
Reverse Incline Scaption	20	3	60 secs	Lie face-down on an incline bench holding 2 dumbbells by your sides. Arc the weights up to touch above your head, keeping your arms straight at all times. You should feel a strong stretch across your shoulders. Return slowly to the start position.	
Kneeling Drag Bicep Curl	10	4	60 secs	On your knees with your back straight, hold a dumbbell in each hand in front of your thighs with an underhand, shoulder-width grip. Curl the weights and, as your hands rise, drive the elbows back so the dumbbells stay as close to your torso as possible. Squeeze your biceps at the top and then lower the weight under control.	
Paused Seated Dumbbell Curl	12	4	60 secs	In a seated position, grab a pair of dumbbells with palms facing out. Raise the dumbbells on both sides so that the elbow is flexed at a 90-degree angle. Curl both dumbbells up to the nose. Pause for 1 second, then return to the 90-degree angle. The beauty of this exercise is the biceps are constantly in tension.	

FRIDAY: FULL-BODY CENTURION WORKOUT

This fitness test is simple enough. Created by myself and *Men's Health* to mass-test the fitness of millions who downloaded the Primal 9 training system, it gets you to do 25 reps of four moves – 100 reps – without a break. Then you rest. Then you do another round. And another. And another. You're aiming for 10 rounds – and 1000 reps in total – to complete the whole thing. I know. Sounds impossible and very few will be able to finish it without some large tactical rest breaks. But that's the point.

Get as far through The Centurion as you can now and – trust me – once you progress through the 12-week programme, you'll soon be storming through it since the improvements are both biomechanical (better movement) and physiological (enhanced endurance).

Exercise	Reps	Coaching Cues	
Bench Jump-over	25	Stand next to the bench and grasp it with both hands. Jump over with both feet while keeping hold of the bench, landing on the other side. Jump back over and continue hopping from side to side, landing lightly.	
Lateral Step-over	25	Stand to the right side of the bench and place your left foot on top. Push from your left heel and raise your body onto the bench. Touch down on the bench with your right foot, while at the same time lowering your left foot to the other side of the bench. Drive back up and repeat on the other side.	
Bear Crunch	25	Assume a press-up position. Crunching your core as you turn, bring your left knee towards your right hip. Repeat on the other side.	
Bench Toe Tap	25	Stand with one foot on a bench or high step. Jump and swap your feet over, tapping the bench lightly with your toe.	

That's one round.

Rest as long as you need, then do another.

Complete 10 rounds. Note down your time. That's your Centurion personal best.

5-DAY ROUTINE | WEEKS 5–8 | WEDNESDAY: PULL TRAINING

Exercise	Reps	Sets	Rest	Coaching Cues	
Paused Explosive Dumbbell Deadlift	10	3	90 secs	The paused deadlift is brutal. Essentially, it's a standard deadlift from the floor, but instead of pulling continuously until lockout, you pause below the knees around mid-shin level for a 2–3 second count. This increases strength and time under tension, which improves overall muscle growth.	
Pull-up	8	3	90 secs	Grip the bar with hands shoulder-width apart. Raise your feet off the floor and hang. Pull yourself up until your chin is over the bar and repeat.	
Renegade Row	10 (each arm)	3	60 secs	Get into a press-up position with your hands on the handles of 2 dumbbells. Keeping your core tensed, row the right dumbbell up to your abs and then return to the start position. Repeat with the left dumbbell to complete one repetition.	
Spider Dumbbell Curl	10	4	60 secs	Lie on an incline bench and hold a dumbbell in each hand. Let them hang underneath your shoulders. Use your biceps to curl the dumbbells towards your shoulders. Slowly return to the starting position.	
One-arm Plank Dumbbell Bicep Curl	12 (each arm)	4	60 secs	Place a dumbbell on the ground and set up in the up position of a press-up. Keep your feet shoulder-width apart. Grip the dumbbell in your right hand. Complete a bicep curl with your right hand by flexing at the elbow and curling upwards towards your shoulder. Lower your arm by fully extending it to the starting position. After 6 repetitions, repeat with the other arm. That's one set.	

5-DAY ROUTINE | WEEKS 5-8 | FRIDAY: FULL-BODY CAVEMAN CONDITIONING

Presenting The Mountain. The most popular full-body caveman conditioning circuit that was downloaded 1.2 million times, you might finish this quickly, or it might take a very long time indeed. Just make sure you complete the 10 rounds. Easier said than done. For your first session of Caveman Conditioning you're going to spend 20 seconds doing each Mountain Climber at varying angles. You can only rest after finishing your hands-elevated Mountain Climbers.

Repeat this process 10 times.

If you need more rest, you can take it. But you've got to make it through those 10 rounds.

Exercise	Reps	Sets	Rest	Coaching Cues	
Feet Elevated Mountain Climber	20 secs	10	n/a	Set up on the floor as though in a sprinter's blocks, with your feet resting on a bench. Explosively piston your knees in towards your chest. Repeat for 20 seconds. Go straight into the next move without rest.	
Mountain Climber	20 secs	10	n/a	Set up on the floor as though in a sprinter's blocks. Explosively piston your knees in towards your chest. Repeat for 20 seconds. Go straight into the next move without rest.	
Hands Elevated Mountain Climber	20 secs	10	60 secs	Set up on the floor as though in a sprinter's blocks with your hands resting on a bench. Explosively piston your knees in towards your chest. Repeat for 20 seconds. Then rest for 30 seconds (enjoy it) before starting another round of the three moves. Do 10 rounds.	

5-DAY ROUTINE | WEEKS 5–8 | SATURDAY: AB WORKOUT | TRAINING NOTES

This ab workout is very different to most.

Placing a greater emphasis on large, full-body movements that produce more muscle activation in the abdominal area, it's been designed to condition and create a strong, functional and aesthetic core. All tried, tested and based on the findings from years of research within the world of 'six-pack sports science', which is why instead of listing exercises for you to blindly follow, I will explain the theory behind this workout (and all others in this book) before we even roll out the yoga mat and pour out the pre-workout.

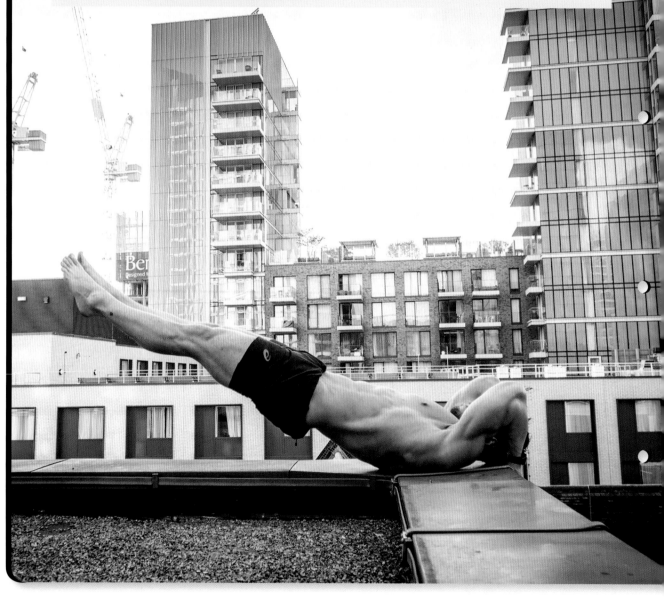

There's NO perfect six-pack guide...

There's no single best stomach exercise.

Why? Because research in *The Journal of Manipulative and Physiological Therapeutics* conducted a large-scale literary review of 87 core-related studies only to find 'Overall, the studies retrieved lacked consistency, which made it impossible to extract aggregate estimates' and find the best ab routine.

Enter the researchers from Department of Kinesiology at The Pennsylvania State University, USA. They wanted to specifically challenge the crunches dominance as the best 'six-pack' exercise and decided to monitor which techniques activated the muscles the best. Large, integration movements like the plank that require different parts of the body to work in harmony. Or smaller, isolation movements like the standard crunch that only target the muscles of the stomach.

The results were as follows...

Increase your 'ab activation' by 27%

Sports scientists took a group of athletes.

Each was made to complete a series of core exercises while they were connected to surface electromyography (EMG) electrodes to monitor muscle activation. What did they discover? Activation of the abdominal muscles was greatest during larger, compound, integration movements. Not even a little, but a lot greater!

The rectus abdominus (the muscles of the 'six-pack') and external obliques (the muscles found down the side of the stomach) showed 27% greater activation during the 'plank with reach' compared to a traditional crunch. Activity in the lumbar erector spinae (the muscles of the back and spine) was also two times greater during the 'plank with reach' compared to the crunch. The 'tripod stance' of Mountain Climbers 'results in a greater activity for all the muscles'. The examples go on.

Get strong, functional 'compound' abs

These basic principles have been echoed and practised in sports for years. (This is especially true in gymnastics.)

'This extreme difference is an illustration of how the integration exercises may be a superior choice for a training regimen as they target a wider range of muscles for a more comprehensive strengthening effect.

JOURNAL OF STRENGTH AND CONDITIONING RESEARCH

In summary, results from the Pennsylvania State University study clearly show there was greater activation in the stomach muscles during big and integrative movements. That's not to say isolation movements aren't without their benefits, but it does mean that a core routine that is heavily based around crunches and sit-up variations might need to be redesigned.

Enter The Four Key Principles of Ab Training that each get progressively harder...

Core Principle 1: Learn to balance

Simply balancing can build your core.

This is based on research from *The Journal of Human Kinetics* that showed something as simple as performing your push-ups (or planks) with your feet placed in gymnastic rings elicited a different kind of muscle activation in the stomach when compared to a traditional push-up on the floor. 'Therefore, suspension push-ups may be considered an advanced variation of a traditional push-up when a greater challenge is warranted.'[12]

They're not the only ones to think so either.

The Journal of Exercise Physiology states 'A suspension device elicited a greater activation of the stomach muscles.'[13] Again supporting this idea to take your planks and press-up variations off the floor and onto something less stable like an exercise Swiss ball.

It's worth noting that unstable surface training still divides the strength and conditioning community and research published by the NSCA stated its application is 'still very limited'. But it is acknowledged that 'unstable surface training has been shown to increase core muscle activity and alter neuromuscular recruitment patterns'.[14]

So, if your goal is to build a stronger core: learn to balance, alter your neuromuscular recruitment patterns, shock the abs into working over a different range of motion and add some variety to your push-ups.

How to perform 'T' push-ups

- Assume a standard push-up position, your body aligned from ankles to head.
- Lower your body until your chest nearly touches the floor.
- As you push yourself back up, rotate one side of your body up as you raise the same side arm your towards the ceiling.
- Pause, and return to the starting position and perform another push-up.
- Alternate sides with each rep.

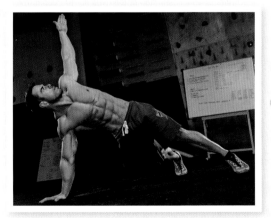

Core Principle 2: Learn to hold

Hold and do nothing. This is one of the best ways to strengthen your stomach. This is because most strength and conditioning coaches will agree that L-sit variations and all kinds of holds will tax your stomach far more than any crunch or sit-up. If you've ever attempted hanging from a bar with a weight between your legs you'll know exactly what I mean.

This is, again, supported by research published by the American Association for Health, Physical Education and Recreation that found 'The exercises found most effective in strengthening abdominal musculature as revealed by the high magnitude of action potential are: L-sits and V-sits.'[15]

How to L-sit

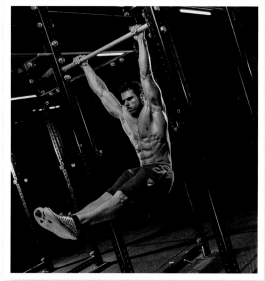

- Hang from a bar or rings.
- Place your hands around shoulder-width apart.
- Keep your legs straight and together.
- Using your lower abs and hip flexors, lift your legs.
- Once parallel to the floor, hold.
- Hold your legs at a 90° angle to your torso. This is the L-sit position.
- Once you've mastered this, try adding weight.

What if you can't L-sit? No problem.

Researchers from the University of Jyväskylä, in Finland, showed you don't have to in order to activate your core. They tested the effect isometric upper-body exercises had on the muscles of the stomach. Put more simply, they wanted to see if upper-body exercises where you hold a static position could engage the abdominal muscles.

What they found was that these exercises, like the Pallof Hold, elicited a, 'sufficient level of contraction of the trunk muscles for the development of their endurance and strength characteristics'.[16]

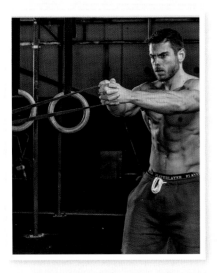

How to perform a Pallof Hold

This can be performed with a resistance band, cable or even a rope with training partner offering the tension.

- Take the rope/cable and hold it at your sternum (arms fully extended).
- Point your left shoulder towards the point to which the rope/cable is attached.
- Stand far away enough to feel the tension.
- Keep your shoulders and hips square.
- Hold the rope/cable straight out in front of your body.
- Resist the tendency to rotate and hold for 60 seconds.
- Keep your abs tight.

Core Principle 3: Learn to hang

Hanging is a lost art form and forgotten method to condition your core.

This is based on research published by the American Association for Health, Physical Education and Recreation that studied muscle activation in the stomach during 10 strenuous abdominal exercises. What they found was 'Intensity of contraction was greatest in the basket hang, followed by three variations of the hook sit-up.'

It beats the conventional sit-up in terms of muscle activation. Researchers added 'The apparently strenuous nature of the basket hang, which is primarily a movement of thigh rather than trunk flexion, implies that this exercise may be useful in the abdominal training of highly conditioned athletes.'[17]

How to perform a twisted hanging leg raise

This is a more difficult progression of the L-sit.

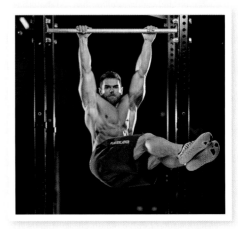

- Lift your legs towards one shoulder and go as high as you can.
- You'll need to tilt your pelvis slightly forward to complete the movement.
- Hold for a second at the top, then slowly lower your legs.
- Repeat on other side.

Core Principle 4: Learn to control

This core principle is linked to an ab exercise launched into the mainstream consciousness after featuring in the Rocky IV training montage set in rural Russia. Known as 'The Dragon Flag', this exercise – unlike most conventional core conditioning – forces the muscles of the stomach to eccentrically contract. They are in tension, but lengthening. This is much like the downward phase of a bicep curl.

Why is this important? Because research from *The Journal of Applied Physiology* concluded that 'eccentric exercise offers a promising training modality to enhance performance'.[18] Put more simply, forcing the muscles to contract and work during the downward phase is often forgotten. However, it can provide a valuable training stimulus to improve the strength and functionality of any muscle group.

In this instance, your newly chiselled, Rocky-inspired six-pack.

How to dragon-flag

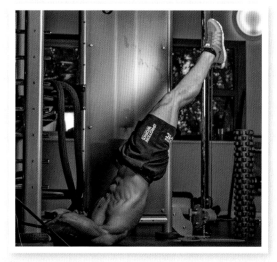

- Lie on the floor while holding onto something stable with your hands by your head.
- With only your head and shoulders in contact with the floor, raise the rest of your body off the floor.
- Keeping as straight as possible, lower yourself to the floor.
- Pause for one second when at the bottom of the exercise.
- Then return to the upright position, all the time ensuring only your head and shoulders are in contact with the floor.

5-DAY ROUTINE | WEEKS 5–8 | SATURDAY: BEGINNER AB WORKOUT

Exercise	Reps	Sets	Rest	Coaching Cues	
T-Plank	10 (each side)	3	90 secs	Start by getting into a conventional plank position. Bend the elbows. Rest your weight on your forearms. Your body should form a straight line, shoulders to ankles. Engage your glutes and abs. Rotate your body so your weight is on the side of one foot. Raise an arm and form a T shape with it. Hold this position, lower your arm and repeat on the other side.	
Suspended Side Crunch	10 (each side)	3	90 secs	Suspend your feet in TRX equipment or gymnastic rings. Draw your attention to your core and focus on maintaining a clean, straight plank, belly button locked in. Draw both knees towards the outside of one elbow, maintaining straight arms and a tight core. Maintain your focus on your tight core and return both legs to a straight start position. Repeat with both legs to the other elbow and return to a start position to complete 2 reps.	
Pallof Hold	60 seconds (each side)	3	60 secs	This can be performed with a resistance band, cable or even a rope with training partner offering the tension. Take the rope/cable and hold it at your sternum (arms fully extended). Point your left shoulder towards the fixed point. Stand far away enough to feel the tension. Keep your shoulders and hips square. Hold the rope/cable straight out in front of your body. Resist the tendency to rotate and hold for 60 seconds. Keep your abs tight.	
Basket Hang	10 (each side)	3	60 secs	Hang from a pull-up bar. Place the hands shoulder-width apart. Contract your lower abs. Bring your knees to your chest. Twist your hips to one side in a controlled manner, keeping your chest forward at all times. As you do crunch your ribs to your hips. Pause, then perform on the other side.	
Double-knee Tuck Dragon Flag	10	3	60 secs	Lie on the floor while holding onto something stable with your hands by your head. With only your head and shoulders in contact with the floor, raise your entire body from the floor. Keeping as straight as possible, but tucking the legs, lower yourself to the ground. Pause for 1 second when at the bottom of the exercise, then return to an upright position, all the time ensuring only your head and shoulders are in contact with the floor.	
Bear Crunch	60 secs	3	60 secs	From a plank position, bring your right knee under and across your body to meet your left elbow. That is one rep. Now repeat to the other side. When done correctly this move challenges your core stabilisers and your obliques simultaneously.	

6-DAY ROUTINE | WEEKS 9–12 | MONDAY: 'PUSH' TRAINING

Exercise	Reps	Sets	Rest	Coaching Cues	
Close-grip Plyometric Push-up	5	3	90 secs	Get in a press-up position, hands shoulder-width apart and back straight. Lower your chest to the floor, then push up explosively until your arms fully extend. Attempt to add claps into the movement while airborne if possible. (If you can't manage full press-ups, do them on your knees.)	
One-arm Push-up	10 (each arm)	3	90 secs	Get into push-up position, with one hand on the surface and spread your feet wide apart. Tense your entire body and hold your free hand tight against your lower back. Lower your body slowly until your chest nearly touches the floor, then explode up to the starting position. (If you can't manage full press-ups, do them on your knees.)	
Alternate Arnold Press	12 (each arm)	3	60 secs	Grab a set of dumbbells and bring them to shoulder height, with arms bent and palms facing the body. Gripping the dumbbells as tightly as possible, press one overhead (keeping the other dumbbell at shoulder height) rotating the dumbbells until the palms are facing forward at the top of the press. Pause, and then slowly lower the weight, reversing the rotating so that the palms end facing the body at the bottom of the press. Repeat on the over arm.	
Uchi Mata Push-up	6 (each leg)	3	60 secs	A push-up inspired by a judo throw that increases activation of your core, lower back and hamstrings and boosts demand on the shoulder muscles. Starting in a push-up position, lift your right foot so your leg is parallel to the floor. Lower your body until your chest nearly touches the floor. Raise your lifted leg higher into the air. Push back to the starting position. Switch legs and repeat.	
Incline Dumbbell Fly into Hex Press	12	3	60 secs	Lie flat on the bench holding 2 dumbbells above your chest with your palms facing each other. With a slight bend at your elbows, lower the dumbbells down to your sides until you feel your chest stretch. Bring the dumbbells into the centre of your chest and push them back up to the start position and repeat.	
Weighted Bear Crawl	10 m forward then 10 m backward	3	45 secs	A tough final test to finish the last pushing session of the 12-week programme, here we add weights to what is an already hard exercise in the bear crawl. Complete over 10 m forward and backward and (optional) on the final set, go until complete failure.	

6-DAY ROUTINE | WEEKS 9–12 | TUESDAY: LOWER-BODY TRAINING

Exercise	Reps	Sets	Rest	Coaching Cues	
Knee-to-feet Box Jump	5	3	90 secs	Knee jumps will develop the posterior chain (lower back, glutes and hamstrings) and by adding a box jump after it becomes a continuous movement where you are jumping twice in a row without any time to rest. To perform them, get down on your knees with the top of your feet flat on the ground behind you. Sit back on your feet, lean forward, and bring your arms behind you. Swing your arms forwards, while simultaneously extending your hips forwards. As you come up off the ground, raise your knees up and plant your feet on the ground to catch yourself. Try to land as softly as possible and immediately go into a box jump.	
Bulgarian Split Squat with Plate	12 (each leg)	3	60 secs	Stand facing away from the bench, holding a plate against your chest. Rest one leg on the bench behind you (the laces of your shoes facing down). Squat with your standing leg until the knee of your trailing leg almost touches the floor. Push up through the front foot to return to the start position.	
Paused Goblet Squat	12	3	60 secs	Standing tall with your feet shoulder-width apart, grab the head of a dumbbell with both hands and hold it vertically in front of your chest. Keeping your back straight, squat down until the crease of your hip drops below the knee and the tops of your thighs are at least parallel to the floor. Pause and hold for 3 seconds. Extend your hips and knees to return to the starting position.	
Plate Extended Squat	12	5	60 secs	A conventional squat while holding a weighted plate with your arms extended in front of your chest to increase activation of the core. Lower into a squat position and ensure your thighs reach slightly below parallel.	
Forward and Reverse Lunge into Forward and Reverse Duck Walk	10m (forward and back)	4	60 secs	A brutal way to finish any leg session, here we combine the finishing exercises of the previous lower-body workouts and perform them back-to-back in what will be a gruelling leg-specific fitness challenge.	

6-DAY ROUTINE | WEEKS 9–12 | **WEDNESDAY: 'PULL' TRAINING**

Exercise	Reps	Sets	Rest	Coaching Cues	
Alternate Dumbbell Sumo High Pull	6 (each arm)	3	90 secs	Stand with your legs wider than shoulder-width apart with a dumbbell in one hand. Lower your body into a squat position until your thighs are parallel to the floor. Push through your heels and raise the dumbbell to your chin, so your arm bends and the elbow is in line with the top of your head. Squat down, change hands and repeat.	
Dead-hang Pull-Up	5	3	90 secs	Raise your feet off the floor and hang so the arms are fully extended. Pull yourself up until your chin is over the bar and repeat, ensuring you go back to the hanging position with arms fully extended so the muscles have to work harder to overcome the loss of momentum.	
Incline Bench Dumbbell Reverse Fly	12	3	60 secs	To begin, lie down on an incline bench with the dumbbells in each hand, palms facing each other (neutral grip). Extend the arms in front of you, perpendicular to the angle of the bench. Keep your legs still and apply pressure with the ball of your toes. This is the starting position. Maintaining the slight bend of the elbows, move the weights out and away from each other (to the side) in an arc motion while exhaling. Tip: Try to squeeze your shoulder blades together to get the best results from this exercise. The arms should be elevated until they are parallel to the floor. Slowly lower the weights back down to the starting position while inhaling.	
Upright Row	20	3	60 secs	Hold a dumbbell in each hand, resting in front of your thighs. Lift the dumbbells vertically until they're in line with your collar bone with your elbows pointing out. Lower the dumbbells back down and repeat.	
Spider Zotterman Curl	10	4	60 secs	Lie down on an incline bench. Hold a dumbbell in each hand at arm's length, elbows close to the torso. and palms facing each other. This is the starting position. Holding the upper arm stationary, curl the weights while contracting the biceps as you breathe out. Only the forearms should move. Your wrist should rotate so that you have a supinated (palms-up) grip. Continue the movement until your biceps are fully contracted and the dumbbells are at shoulder level. Hold for a second as you squeeze the biceps. Now, rotate your wrist into a pronated (palms-down) grip with the thumb higher than the pinky. Slowly begin to bring the dumbbells back down. As you reach the lower part of the movement, start rotating the wrist back to a neutral (palms facing your body) grip. Repeat.	
Burpee into Pull-up	100	1	As much as you need to finish 100	The burpee is a four-point move. From standing, drop into a squat with your hands on the ground just in front of your feet. Then kick your feet back behind you, keeping your arms extended so you are in a raised plank position. Complete a push-up, then jump your feet back towards your hands. Squat, then jump into the air with your arms straight above you. Grab the bar and complete 1 pull-up. That's 1 repetition.	

6-DAY ROUTINE | WEEKS 9–12 | THURSDAY: ADVANCED AB WORKOUT

Exercise	Reps	Sets	Rest	Coaching Cues	
Full Dragon Flag	10	4	60 secs	Lie on the floor while holding onto something stable with your hands by your head. With only your head and shoulders in contact with the floor, raise your entire body from the floor. Keeping as straight as possible, lower yourself to the ground. Pause for 1 second when at the bottom of the exercise, then return to an upright position. All the time ensuring only your head and shoulders are in contact with the floor.	
Window Wiper				Essentially a basket hang but with straighter legs to add difficulty. Hang from a pull-up bar, hands shoulder-width apart. Contract your lower abs. Bring your knees to your chest. Twist your hips to one side in a controlled manner, keeping your chest forward at all times. As you do, crunch your ribs to your hips. Pause, then perform on the other side.	
Suspended Pike	12	3	90 secs	Get in push-up position. Rest the tops of your feet in the TRX equipment. Keeping your legs as straight as possible, bend your hips and pull your feet towards your chest. Pull your feet towards your hands. Hold at the top for three to four seconds, then slowly roll back to the starting position.	
L-sit	60 secs	3	60 secs	Hang from a bar or rings. Place your hands about shoulder-width apart. Keep your legs straight and together. Using your lower abs and hip flexors, lift your legs. Once parallel to the floor hold. Hold your legs at a 90° angle to your torso. This is the L-sit position. Once you've mastered this, try adding weight.	
Dumbbell Wood-chop into Bear Crunch	10 (each side) into 60 seconds of bear crunches	3	60 secs	Hold your dumbbell with both hands next to the outside of your right thigh. Twist your torso to the side and lift the weight up and across your body with straight arms. As you lift, turn your torso so you end up facing the dumbbell, which is above your left shoulder. You should be using your core muscles to control the movement. Return to the starting position, reversing the twist and bringing the weight down as if chopping wood.	

6-DAY ROUTINE | WEEKS 9–12 | FRIDAY: FULL-BODY CAVEMAN CONDITIONING

Congratulations you've made it to weeks 9–12.

Welcome to the bigger brother of The Mountain, which we call The Everest! This takes Caveman Conditioning to a new level as you aim to complete 44.24 seconds of mountain climbers at varying angles, resting for 44.24 seconds only after finishing your hands-elevated mountain climbers.

Repeat this process 10 times.

Why 44.24 seconds?

Because it's double the time you complete for The Mountain, plus 1 set (with rest) equals 176.96 seconds, symbolic of the height of Everest if you climbed up and down it (17,696 m).So your goal is to conquer this entire workout in 1769.6 seconds (or 29.49 minutes)

Exercise	Reps	Sets	Rest	Coaching Cues
Feet Elevated Mountain Climber	44.24 secs	10	44.24 secs after the last set	Set up on the floor as though in a sprinter's blocks, with your feet resting on a bench. Explosively piston your knees in towards your chest. Repeat for 44.24 seconds. Go straight into the next move without rest.
Mountain Climber	44.24 secs			Set up on the floor as though in a sprinter's blocks. Explosively piston your knees in towards your chest. Repeat for 44.24 seconds. Go straight into the next move without rest.
Hands Elevated Mountain Climber	44.24 secs			Set up on the floor as though in a sprinter's blocks with your hands resting on a bench. Explosively piston your knees in towards your chest. Repeat for 44.24 seconds. Then rest for 44.24 seconds (enjoy it) before starting another round of the three moves. Do 10 rounds.

6-DAY ROUTINE | WEEKS 9–12 | SATURDAY: SPORT SPECIFIC

Success! After nine weeks you can now begin to specialise…

You have built greater kinaesthetic awareness and unlocked your neurological potential through the Soviet Union sporting concept of General Physical Preparedness. Increased your work capacity inspired by the bodyweight exercise progressions of the Royal Marines. Now you are ready to perform Directly Associated training based on Geoff's four-point (multi-skill) training system.

Whether this is football, rugby, running or swimming — or in my case a Tree-athlon — you now 'know your body' better and will be able to learn new movements, with greater proficiency, far faster.

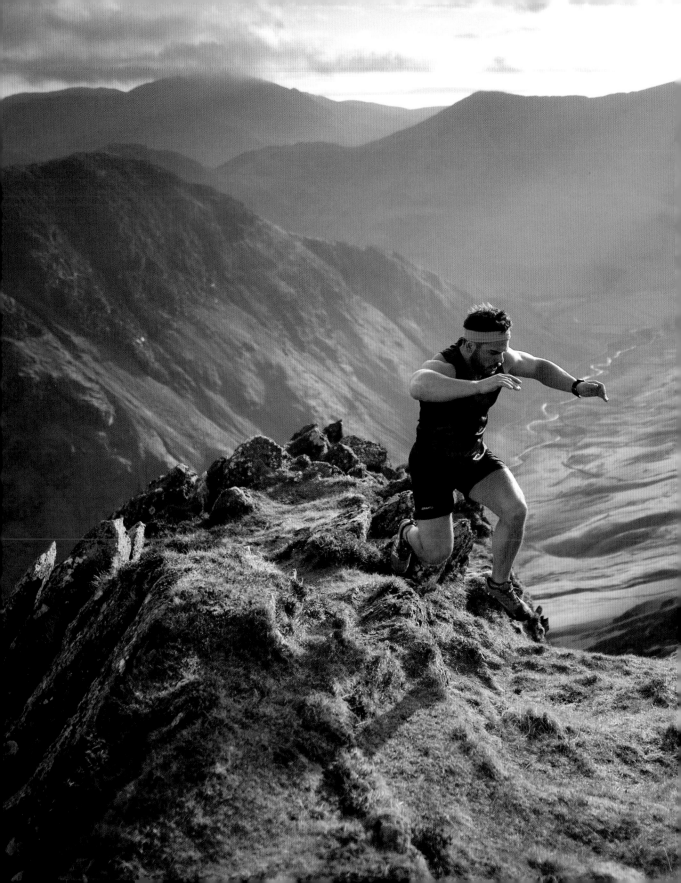

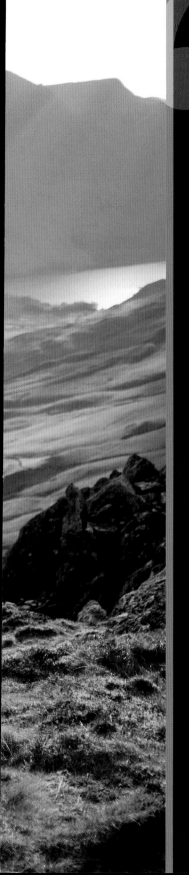

"THERE ARE NO LIMITS. THERE ARE PLATEAUS, BUT YOU MUST NOT STAY THERE, YOU MUST GO BEYOND THEM."

BRUCE LEE

PART III:
THE SECRETS OF RECORD-BREAKING FITNESS

CHAPTER 6
HOW TO LOSE FAT

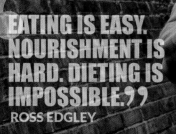

EATING IS EASY. NOURISHMENT IS HARD. DIETING IS IMPOSSIBLE.
ROSS EDGLEY

FOOD RULES (ARE THERE TO BE BROKEN)

During 2013, my approach to food and fitness was very different to most.

This is because I had returned from my global travels and settled back into life in England, forming part of the founding team at THE PROTEIN WORKS™. A sports nutrition brand later dubbed, 'The world's most innovative', we didn't eat and train like the rest of the industry.

We created the world's first protein popcorn, invented the Caramel Macchiato and Lemon Shortcake protein shake and even had ambitions to build Europe's biggest protein bakery.

'Here's to the crazy ones, the misfits, the rebels, the troublemakers, the round pegs in the square holes… the ones who see things differently – they're not fond of rules. You can quote them, disagree with them, glorify or vilify them, but the only thing you can't do is ignore them because they change things… they push the human race forward, and while some may see them as the crazy ones, we see genius, because the ones who are crazy enough to think that they can change the world, are the ones who do.'
STEVE JOBS

For me it felt like home.

Where the weird was welcomed and innovative invited in. I rarely wore shoes, attended meetings in shorts, trained on the roof in my lunch hour and would visit the Protein Popcorn room for breakfast, lunch and dinner. But to the team, this was normal and they accepted my feral jungle habits.

All because together we were raising (protein) bars, rewriting the rule (cook) book and baking outside the box.

THE CHEFS' ROUNDTABLE

This is where fitness meets fine dining.

All the recipes within this book have been created by these three culinary geniuses. I take no credit for any of them and only consider myself incredibly lucky to have sampled what came out of their pans, bowls and ovens. Now sharing their brilliance with you, allow me to introduce three of the most skilled people I know with a spoon…

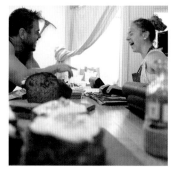

This is **Annie Mayne** and your taste buds will love her.

She lives in Keswick in the north of England and I can only describe her as the creator of the tastiest and healthiest home-made recipes that will ever cross your kitchen table. This is a bold statement, I know, but with each Acai Bowl and Keto Taco recipe contained within this book you will start to understand why.

Fuelling so much of my endurance training – which takes place in Keswick as you'll come to see in Chapter 9 – she is an amazing friend and an incredible cook.

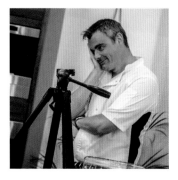

This is **Simon Partridge**, a wizard of the kitchen.

Simon and I first met during a BBQ photoshoot (yes, it was as awesome as it sounds) for Athleat Meat, a company that specialises in providing quality-sourced meat for elite athletes. I was there to talk about the nutritional science of their grass-fed produce and Simon was there to make it taste amazing.

The man's a genius and has led brigades in a fine-dining hotel kitchen, cooked all over the world and even baked for Hollywood royalty. Yes, he's that good.

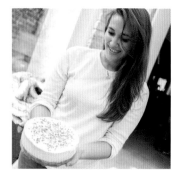

This is **Hester Sabery** and she was the Head Chef for The World's Longest Rope Climb, The World's First Tree-Athlon and The World's Strongest Marathon.

She's also my girlfriend.

But outside of those two roles she is also the commercial manager for one of Europe's largest cupcake manufacturers. What this means is she's very good at making food taste great, but also very good at mass producing it.

Considering I eat over 10,000 calories on a big training day, this basically makes her my perfect girlfriend.

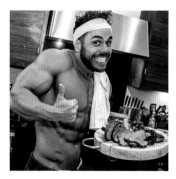

This is me and I'm better at eating than I am cooking.

But I have worked in sports nutrition for over a decade, which means there's not a snack, shake or protein bar I haven't taste-trialled. This is why my role at the chefs' roundtable is to eat, drink and show you how to use the nutrient-dense, flavour-packed recipes each one of these geniuses has created, all so you can stick a proverbial finger up to the diet industry, have your cake and eat it, too.

THE WORLD'S MOST INNOVATIVE SPORTS NUTRITION BRAND

It's 6pm, 2 December 2013 at the famous Christmas market in Manchester, northern England.

Without doubt the happiest place on earth for anyone who loves their food and drink. This is also without doubt the strangest place on earth to conduct the Research and Development for one of Europe's biggest sports nutrition brands. Yet miles away from our sports lab, that's exactly what we are doing.

I say 'we' because my evening of edible exploration was by no means a solo venture. I was standing arm-in-arm with the other founding members of THE PROTEIN WORKS™ singing Frank Sinatra's version of 'Jingle Bells' as the smell of mulled wine filled the air and pastries, pork sausages and festive merriment filled our bellies. So, what exactly was the method to our merriment?

We were flavour hunting.

See, for the past six months we had been taste-trialling every chocolate, sweet and pudding as part of our mission to help people's taste buds and tummies work in harmony. Our goal was simple: make healthy shakes and snacks so full of taste and texture that sticking to a 'diet' was no longer a chore because people would be unable to tell the difference between our nutrient-dense recipes and the unhealthy, calorie-dense counterparts.

A bold plan I know, but this was all based on a year-long study of this thing we call 'diets':

'Regardless of assigned diet, 12-month weight change was greater in the most adherent. These results suggest that strategies to increase adherence may deserve more emphasis than the specific diet.'
INTERNATIONAL JOURNAL OF OBESITY[1]

What does this mean?

Basically, the nutritional value of your food is of course important. We all need the right vitamins, minerals, fats, protein and carbohydrates to be happy and healthy. But equally significant to a successful eating strategy is your enjoyment and ability to stick to a meal plan – 'adherence'.

(Again) the best diet plan in the world is useless on paper if you can't follow it in real life.

That smoothie in your cupboard that tastes like pond water and the protein bars in your gym bag that provide a workout for your jaw instead are just two vital ingredients that produce a recipe for dieting disaster.

But we wanted to change all that. So, with a spoon in one hand and a giant, refillable, decorative mug in the other, we went to work!

Gareth headed for the barrels of German-styled wine that were being fused with every herb and spice imaginable. Karl and Mark were quizzing a man to see how he got his Portuguese pastries so soft. Nick was last seen among the carol singers because that was closest to the sweets and candyfloss.

Me? I had gone AWOL! No food stall is safe.

I had convinced the people on the cookie-dough stand to make me a cookie wrapped in a chocolate crêpe. I then asked for a serving of ice cream to be folded into the mix as the proverbial cherry on top of what was an already powerful pudding.

This went on for about 40 minutes. Tasting and testing every flavoured crêpe combination I could dream up, I was even having a fruit-based ice cream between servings to act as a sorbet palate cleanser.

But round six was interrupted by one of the strangest things I'd seen at a Christmas market. Gareth came bounding through the crowds, balancing an elf hat on his head and clutching two massive tankards with Bavarian symbols down the side in each hand.

Arriving short of breath having run through the crowds like a festive ninja, he thrust a tankard at me. I could tell whatever was in the giant mug was clearly more important than another crêpe, so I put down my fork and charged my taste buds.

"Taste this!" he commanded.

I nodded and raised the cup…

He smiled and raised his eyebrows…

All the time his eyes wide with anticipation as he studied my initial reaction closely…

As soon as the contents of the novelty-sized mug hit my lips I understood his excitement. It was a German-style mulled wine (called Glühwein) and it had the perfect apple and cinnamon blend we had been searching for to use in our protein shakes. After months and months our quest was over. We needed the recipe!

'Which barrel did it come out of?' I asked.

'That's the problem, I don't know! I was given these by one of the beer maids walking among the crowds of people and barrels of beer and wine. It could be any and there's an entire street filled with them.'

Looking at the never-ending line of wine, beer and alcohol, we knew what we had to do.

Not all heroes wear capes; some come bearing decorative tankards painted in Bavarian art. We both pressed the thumb-lever on our hinged pewter lid and got to work.

'You start at that end, I will start at this end… then let's meet in the middle.'

Gareth nodded and one-by-one we heroically set out to conquer each barrel.

During the first five our search was enthusiastic, but fruitless…

Numbers 5 to 9? Still no sign of apple or cinnamon…

By barrel 10 I won't lie, I was no longer completely sober (or walking in a straight line), but the taste buds were still functioning, so I decided to persevere.

Number 11? A spiced orange flavour that had bits floating in it.

Number 12? An odd elderberry concoction.

Number 13? I have absolutely no idea.

Then it happened. Lucky number 14. It was like an orchestra of flavours that was playing on my palate, but it smelt like comfort and tasted like Christmas as the sweetened cinnamon bathed in a barrel of white wine and apple juice with more freshly cut apples for taste, texture and effect.

Gareth had seen my face through the crowds of people.

Rushing over, he didn't need to speak a word. He knew. We both filled our cups and toasted. Our six-month journey of edible exploration was complete. We found the recipe and weeks later used it to create that year's best-selling whey protein shake.

Is this how product development works in sports nutrition? No.

Did we later win awards for our flavours? Yes (many).

Which is why ever since that day we have been challenging the status quo of the food industry, one recipe at a time, the best of which you'll find throughout the pages of this book. Each have been created, cooked and calculated by THE PROTEIN WORKS™ family of chefs and eaten by yours truly.

All to prove that sweets and a six-pack can co-exist.

The Fat-loss Pyramid of Priority

So, what did I learn from 2013 to 2014?

Why was I not sidestepping the Christmas food stalls in fear I'd catch a calorie like the plague? Why was I merrily sipping from a novelty-sized mug of spiced wine without a side serving of guilt? But above all else, how was I six crêpe creations in with my six-pack still intact?

Let me explain with **The Fat-loss Pyramid of Priority...**

'Individuals who engage in rigid dieting strategies reported symptoms of an eating disorder, mood disturbances and excessive concern with body size/shape. In contrast, flexible dieting strategies were not highly associated with BMI, eating disorder symptoms, mood disturbances or concerns with body size.'[2]

APPETITE, Behavioural Nutrition Journal

HOW TO USE IT

This is a hierarchical (progressive) illustration of how to focus your efforts when losing fat.

- The lower parts make the biggest difference to your fat loss.
- The higher parts make a meaningful contribution to your fat loss, but only once you've laid the foundations.
- The top part of this (and every pyramid) is infinite and forever evolving. This is why they are all open-ended and may never have a peak, because our understanding and exploration of the human body should never be 'capped' or concluded.

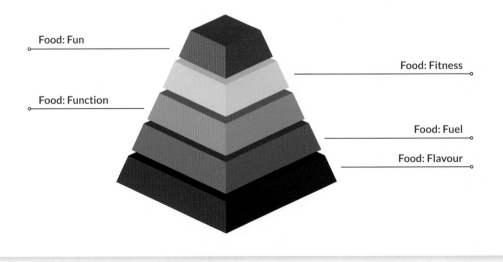

Food: Fun

Food: Fitness

Food: Function

Food: Fuel

Food: Flavour

FOOD: FLAVOUR

In your 'foodiverse' there are two groups of people:

- **Chefs:** These make food taste great. Our taste buds love these people.
- **Nutritionists:** These make food nutritious and keep calories in check. Our waistlines love these people.

Now the ideal nutrition plans are the ones created with input from both. You need something your taste buds love as much as your tummy.

FOOD: FUEL

Our primary (and primitive) use of food is to use it as fuel.

Our caveman ancestors would hunt and harvest food (fuel) in order to survive. But finding fuel (calories) is no longer an issue for modern man. Instead, rising obesity figures show our issue is that we're 'harvesting' and eating too much, which is why understanding a calorie deficit, calorie surplus and calorie balance is key to climbing The Fat-loss Pyramid of Priority.

FOOD: FUNCTION

We extract more than just calories from our food. We also eat food for function, using the protein to aid recovery and fats and carbohydrates (our energy-yielding macronutrients) to power our bodies, as well as an almost infinite list of vitamins, minerals, phytochemicals, enzymes and micronutrients that are involved in millions of functions within the body.

FOOD: FITNESS

The truth is, you can lose fat without exercise.

It's slower and boring, but it is possible, which is why Food: Fitness appears higher up The Fat-loss Pyramid of Priority. But once you master this part, shedding fat and building a leaner version of yourself becomes a whole lot easier.

FOOD: FUN

The moment you have all been waiting for...

Only once all other aspects of The Fat-loss Pyramid of Priority have been mastered are you able to introduce chocolate, wine and an extra hour in bed as a legitimate fat-loss aid. Yes, this is all completely different to what the more 'compliant' members of the fitness industry will tell you, but it ensures your fat loss is fun and sustainable.

So let's delve into Food: Fuel, which begins with a short history of the calorie.

1. Pick a number and stick to it

This is how most people set a deficit.

This is where you decide you want to lose a certain amount of fat per week. Typically, this is around 0.45kg (1 lb) per week and since 1 lb of fat has about 3500 calories, you'd need to be in a calorie deficit of 500 per day[6].

For most people this works since it's simple and achievable.

The problem is that this size deficit might be too aggressive for some and too slow for others. If you're already maintaining your weight at 2000 calories per day (your maintenance calorie number), cutting your food intake by 25% might be too drastic. In contrast, if you maintain your weight at 4000 calories per day, you might be able to achieve a faster rate of fat loss with a larger calorie deficit.

2. Pick a number based on a percentage

Take your maintenance calorie number and subtract 20%.

If your maintenance calorie number works out at 2000 per day and you cut this by 20%, it means you'll be slashing your calorie intake by 400 calories a day (giving you a calorie intake of 1600). Many believe this is a better approach since it scales your calorie intake to your energy needs, rather than assigning a set number that might not suit your biological individuality.

People with a higher maintenance calorie number will be able to eat more and lose fat. People with a lower maintenance calorie number will have a smaller deficit that's more appropriate for their calorie intake.

3. Pick a number based on a goal weight and timeframe

This is perhaps the most advanced method of the three; however, beginners need not shy away from it.

Now that we know 1 lb of fat is 3500 kcal we are able to do the maths of fat loss.

Say you want to lose 9.5 kg (21 lb). That equates to 21 lb x 3500 kcal = 73,500 kcal. Now let's say you are getting married or going on holiday in 14 weeks (98 days), which gives us the required deadline. We simply divide 73,500 by 98 to give us 750kcals. That is our deficit each day to achieve that fat-loss goal.

The reason this method is the most advanced is that we aren't taking anything personal into account other than our (potentially unrealistic) goal. However, contrary to popular belief, faster rates of weight loss have not been shown to cause worse 'rebound' weight gain. The key message with this point is that, whatever deficit you end up with, it must be something you can stick to.

CALORIE DEFICIT: FIVE FINAL 'FAT' THOUGHTS

To repeat: your calorie deficit is crucial to fat loss, therefore here are five final things to consider.

1. Fast vs slow fat loss

Larger calorie deficits will produce the highest rates of fat loss.

Therefore, severely cutting calories will mean you reach your body-fat goal quicker. But the problem is that people often cut too many calories, which according to the *American Journal of Clinical Nutrition* can reduce your metabolism,[7] down regulate your fat burning hormones[8] and become completely counter-productive. And it's certainly no fun.[9]

Therefore, ask yourself what suits your biological individuality for sustained fat loss.[10]

2. Long-term fat loss

Some people are better at sticking to small deficits and some people prefer large ones.

Smaller deficits are usually easier to maintain.[11] They're easier on the body, not as severe and you're better able to manager appetite and hunger.[12]

Larger deficits tend to be harder to stick to as they require more exercise and/or food restriction and are generally harder to achieve. But to offer a different perspective, because larger deficits help you lose weight faster, for some people they're more effective because of the more obvious and rapid results.[13]

Again (and honestly) ask yourself what suits your biological individuality as well as your psychological preferences.

3. Sports performance and fat loss

Large deficits make it harder to train[14] and recover from workouts.[15]

In some cases, the negative effects of a calorie deficit aren't worth the dip in performance. Also, even if you're not a performance athlete, maintaining the intensity of your strength workouts is essential for preserving your lean muscle mass while dieting, which is why it's important to see point 4.

4. Lean muscle mass

It makes sense that the larger the calorie deficit the more muscle you'll lose.[16] [17]

However, most of the people in these studies were not strength training or eating enough protein to prevent muscle loss. If you set up your diet correctly with adequate protein and strength training, then you can limit muscle loss to a very small amount. In fact, some male[18] and female[19] bodybuilders have been shown to limit it altogether.

If you're already fairly lean, larger deficits will generally make you lose some muscle, even with strength training and adequate protein. If you're overweight, however, then you can usually restrict your calorie intake more without losing as much, or any, muscle. Your body has thousands of extra calories to burn from fat, so it's less likely to break down your muscle for energy.

5. Metabolism and moving less

When you cut calories you burn fewer calories.

This is for a variety of reasons, not least because you weigh less, therefore you use less energy. You also move less [20] [21] when on a larger caloric deficit due to something called 'Non-Exercise Activity Thermogenesis', which essentially means the activity outside your formal training sessions going down. Likewise, there is also a small but significant drop in metabolic rate. This can make tracking your activity a good option, for example tracking step counts and keeping this consistent for the duration of your diet.

MIX UP YOUR CALORIE DEFICIT

You don't need to use the same deficit for your entire diet, or even each day. I never do. Depending on what I'm training for I'll jump between a low, moderate and high calorie deficit and might:

- Start with a larger deficit and move towards a smaller deficit.
- Start with a smaller deficit and move towards a larger deficit.
- Have some days where I'm in a much larger deficit and other days with less severe deficits.

Basically, I use whatever size deficit suits my lifestyle at the time.

FOOD | FUNCTION

HOW WE USE FOOD

We extract more than just calories from food.

This is based on research published in *The Journal of the International Society of Nutrition* that states 'Biologically speaking, a calorie is certainly not a calorie.'[22]

This led scientists from the Albert Einstein College of Medicine in the US to publish a great paper entitled 'How calorie-focused thinking about obesity and related diseases may mislead and harm public health.'[23] In it they say 'In particular, the authors consider how calorie-focused thinking is inherently biased against high-fat foods, many of which may be protective against obesity.'

In essence, they are campaigning to stop the vilification of all dietary fats.

Perhaps for good reason too, it seems.

Since while it's true that fat contains nine calories per gram – carbohydrates and protein contain four – research conducted at Vanderbilt University, USA, discovered the fat known as medium-chain triglycerides found in coconut oil 'stimulates thermogenesis'.[24]

Thermogenesis is a fancy way of saying 'the burning of energy'.

They also say that 'This increased energy expenditure provides evidence that excess energy derived from medium-chain triglycerides is stored with a lesser efficiency.' Basically, the fat content of medium-chain triglycerides can help increase the rate at which we burn it.

This idea is supported by scientists from the School of Dietetics and Human Nutrition at McGill University, Quebec, Canada, who even proposed medium-chain triglycerides could be a 'potential agent in the prevention of obesity', concluding: 'Medium-chain triglycerides increase energy expenditure and may result in faster satiety and facilitate weight control.'[25]

Now it must be noted that coconut oil is just one food source. There are thousands more with impressive nutritional benefits. But hopefully it shows why we should stop vilifying certain healthy food sources within our current calorie-controlled framework.

'Each food has a story to tell that's far more interesting than its calorie content. It's our job to discover those stories.
ROSS EDGLEY

Basically, the previously mentioned Professor Nicolas Clément-Desormes and Wilbur O. Atwater were pioneers.

Their calorie-counting approach to nutrition was revolutionary, and we should be forever grateful to those who laid the foundations. But now we must build upon these if we want to advance our understanding of food and fat loss.

Why? Because we don't just use food for fuel (calories), we also use food for function (protein, fats and carbohydrates).

An idea echoed by research from the State University of New York Downstate Medical Center which states 'Attacking the obesity epidemic will involve giving up many old ideas that have not been productive. "A calorie is a calorie" might be a good place to start.'[26]

So let's move up The Fat-loss Pyramid of Priority.

MACRONUTRIENTS

'Don't study nutrients in isolation. Each one impacts the other in more ways than we will ever know.'

ROSS EDGLEY

All nutrients are interdependent within the body.

What this means is that fats, proteins, carbohydrates, vitamins and minerals will all impact each other in more ways than we will probably ever know. They operate in a complex system of interrelationships where inevitably Monday's choice of breakfast will impact Friday night's choice of dinner.

The problem is, too often science fails to acknowledge this.

Food is studied in complete isolation and nutritionists compartmentalise nutrients that are never compartmentalised in nature. We are unfortunately – yet again – failing to take into account the complexity of the human body and all its different variables.

What's the end result? Our kitchens and bodies are a mess and riddled with nutritional imbalances. How do we tidy them up? We consider our diets in their entirety, that's how. This begins with your body's macronutrients: protein, fats and carbohydrates.

PROTEIN

Protein is often associated with building muscle.

On its most basic level this is true. But dig a little deeper and you'll find protein can also help control hunger better than fats or carbohydrates.[27] You'll actually burn more calories at the dinner table eating certain forms of it.[28] Finally, it's also pretty important to our immune system and overall health.

It's safe to say protein is pretty important.

Protein: The best choices

For 90% of people meat, eggs, fish and protein shakes represent practical sources of protein.

But, as always, don't be confined to lists. That's one of the downfalls of modern diets. Most have this restrictive list of foods you can and can't eat. Follow them and you're destined to eat through charts and checklists for the rest of your life.

But it's wrong. We're biologically wired to seek variety. According to *The American Journal of Clinical Nutrition,* 'There would have been no single universal diet consumed by all extinct hominin species. Rather, diets would have varied by geographic locale, climate, and specific ecologic niche.'[29]

So experiment! Put things in your mouth and enjoy the wide spectrum of foods available on Mother Nature's table. When in Africa with the San Bushmen, my main source of protein was porcupine. In Brazil, it was monkey, alligator and fish. In Siberia, it was reindeer brain.

The list goes on, and so should your shopping list.

Protein: How much do I need?

This is still debated by nutritionists today.

The answer? We don't know. The field of nutrigenomics – how our individual genes uniquely interact with our food – teaches us this varies from person to person. At best we can make an educated guess and start with research from the often-quoted sports nutrition bible *The Complete Guide to Sports Nutrition*.

It states that the International Olympic Committee Consensus on Sports Nutrition recommends strength and speed athletes consume 1.7g of protein per kg of bodyweight per day. This is considered the optimal amount to help the muscles repair and regrow.

But what if you're not a strength, speed or power athlete?

Maybe you're training for a marathon. Maybe you want to lose fat. Or maybe you just want to be generally healthy. Studies show this idea of 1.7g of protein per kg of bodyweight per day is still a good base to start and here's why.

Protein and endurance

Endurance athletes need just as much protein.

In research published in *The Journal of Applied Physiology* it was suggested: 'We conclude that bodybuilders during habitual training require a daily protein intake only slightly greater than that for sedentary individuals in the maintenance of lean body mass and that endurance athletes require daily protein intakes greater than either bodybuilders or sedentary individuals to meet the needs of protein catabolism during exercise.'[30]

Put simply, endurance athletes need protein to prevent their body breaking down.

Train too hard or too long and the body will enter a catabolic state. Your muscles break down, the immune system is badly affected and injuries are more likely to occur. However, get an adequate supply of protein and you're equipped with the 'building blocks' needed to recover.

Protein and immune health

In Chapter 4 we learnt the body's immune system is complex. It's a network of biological structures and processes that exist within our bodies to protect us against disease and foreign bacteria. These biological structures range from special cells and proteins to tissues and organs, and each works in harmony with the others to keep us fit and healthy.

It's basically a masterpiece that's designed to work like clockwork. But protein can help too.

This is based on research from the Memorial University of Newfoundland in Canada that states: 'Nutrition is a critical determinant of immune responses and malnutrition is the most common cause of immunodeficiency worldwide. Protein malnutrition is associated with a significant impairment of immunity.'[31]

Basically, protein keeps the body 'strong' in more ways than one.

Protein and appetite

'It is the protein content that is important in promoting short-term weight loss.'

The above quote is from *The Journal of the American Dietetic Association*.

The article said 'We speculate that it is the protein, and not carbohydrate, content that is important in promoting short-term weight loss and that this effect is likely due to increased satiety caused by increased dietary protein.'[32]

Note the word 'speculate' before you chow down on kilos of protein, but know that it does show promise for our expanding waistlines by stopping us overeating. An idea supported by the American Society for Clinical Nutrition, which states 'Potential beneficial outcomes associated with protein include increased satiety as protein generally increases satiety to a greater extent than carbohydrate or fat.'[33]

Basically, protein can be a valuable tool for those who know how to wield its power.

'Adults retained more lean mass and lost more fat mass when consuming higher-protein diets.'

NUTRITION REVIEWS [34]

THE SCIENCE OF THE STEAK
by Simon Partridge

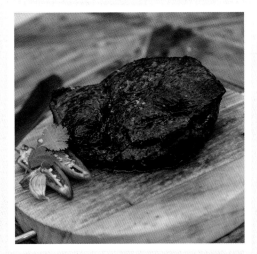

I want to give you a foolproof way of cooking your favourite steak to perfection.

So below I've given you step-by-step instructions for each delicious cut of steak to make sure you get the most from them. I always recommend cooking steak either rare or medium-rare to let the true flavours and textures of the steak naturally come out. The cooking instructions are based on a steak weighing 8oz and being approximately 1-inch thick for all cuts apart from the minute steak and fillet steak.

Also, please adjust cooking times for larger or smaller steaks as required.

FILLET STEAK

Allow the beef to breathe by taking it out of the vacuum pack and placing it on a plate. Let the steak come up to room temperature, then rub with oil and season to taste. Get your pan or BBQ as hot as it will go, then cook the steak for 1 minute on each side (including the 'edges') to seal the whole outer surface. Now place your steak in a preheated oven at around 150˚C for 5 mins (for super-rare), 7 mins (for medium) or more if you want (although we don't recommend it!). Remove the steak from the oven, place it on a plate and cover with foil for 5 minutes to allow the meat to relax and the juices to return.

If you are feeling adventurous you can try a beef wellington or even very thinly slice it raw as a carpaccio!

SIRLOIN/RIBEYE/RUMP STEAK

Allow the beef to breathe by taking it out of the vacuum pack and placing it on a plate. Let the steak come up to room temperature, then rub with oil and season to taste. Get your pan or BBQ as hot as it will go, then carefully place the steak on the cooking surface. Turn the steak every minute to achieve that caramelised outer surface and repeat so that both sides have been cooked twice (if you would like a rare steak) or three times for medium-rare. Remove the steak from the pan, place it on a warm plate and cover with foil for 5 minutes to allow the meat to relax and the juices to return.

MINUTE STEAK

Allow the beef to breathe by taking it out of the vacuum pack and placing it on a plate. Let the steak come up to room temperature, then rub with oil and season to taste. Get your pan or BBQ as hot as it will go, then cook the steak for 1 minute on each side (hence the name Minute Steak!). Remove the steak from the pan, place it on a warm plate and cover with foil for 5 minutes to allow the meat to relax and the juices to return.

>

STEAK TOP TIPS

A few more top tips to make sure your steaks are perfect:

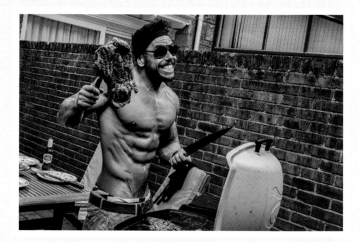

- Use a very sharp knife to cut into your steak after cooking. A blunt knife will 'shred' the meat rather than cut it.

- The resting part of cooking before and after is very important, so make sure you follow the instructions. It makes a big difference!

- Some people prefer to season the meat after cooking, but we feel that the seasoning before makes for tastier steak!

- Get yourself a good-quality heavy-based pan/ griddle.

- Get your pan as hot as you possibly can and don't add any oil to it (you are oiling the steaks instead).

- Always err on the side of caution when cooking a steak. We always suggest that you cook your steak until you feel it is underdone, then take it off the heat. The residual heat in the steak will continue to cook it after you have taken it off the pan. You can always cook it some more if it really is underdone. Once you have overcooked a steak there is no going back!

- If you are cooking your steak on a BBQ, then always allow your coals to turn that dusty white colour and the flames to die down before you place the meat on the coals. Otherwise, you will end up with a charcoaled steak!

- When cooking with a quality product, treat it with the utmost care and attention and it will repay you with the tastiest and most succulent meat ever!

FINDING YOUR FUEL | CARBOHYDRATES AND FATS

Your body gets energy from both fat and carbohydrates. Knowing this is so important because if energy levels are high, then losing fat, running marathons and lifting weights all become possible. But fail to understand it and fat loss becomes hard, impossible or often temporary and you're unable to train with any real intensity as the 'gas tank' is running on empty. So which one is better?

The honest answer is: carbohydrates, fats or both. It completely varies from person to person and kitchen to kitchen. This is the Law of Biological Individuality and it can never be ignored. That's why this section is called Finding Your Fuel.

Because after reading it you'll be able to find an energy source that works with your body and you will no longer be doomed to eat through rules, restrictions, checklists and pie charts.

Carbohydrates: The basics

Carbohydrates mainly come in the form of sugar and starch. As nutrients, we often refer to them as our body's primary fuel source. This is because we're designed to store carbohydrates in the liver, brain and muscles, where we can break down the sugar and starch into glucose, which we then use as energy to fuel our bodies and feed our cells.

Now carbohydrates, like protein, have many other roles within the body, but for now understand that we can, will and often do run well on carbohydrates.

Carbohydrates: The best sources

Carbohydrates can – and should – come from fruits and vegetables. Unfortunately, quite often they don't. Instead, people will gorge on heavily processed foods and drinks – like sweets and soft drinks – that are high in calories and low in nutrients. The result is we're often overfed but undernourished. The solution is to seek variety and stock your cupboard with fruits and vegetables in preparation for some recipes and culinary genius to follow.

Carbohydrates: How much do I need?

This depends on many factors. Technically, you can live without carbohydrates, but most conventional sports nutritionists would advise against it. This is because we've long known that a wholesome bowl of carbohydrate-rich granola in the morning is stored in the muscles as glycogen, ready for us to use later during some form of physical activity.

Research published in *The European Journal of Applied Physiology and Occupational Physiology* is equally full of praise for a hearty and simple bowl of porridge. That's because researchers from Loughborough University set out to quantify the difference carbohydrate intake made to a runner's performance. They believed that reducing the carbohydrate content in the diet would have a direct impact on performance.

Carbohydrates: Endurance

To test this, they took 18 runners and had them complete a 30-km time trial.

In the first trial, the diet of the runners was not modified at all. Then, seven days later, the runners were randomly assigned into two separate groups. Both groups consumed the same amount of calories; however, the diet of one group was predominantly made up of carbohydrates. The other group was lower in carbohydrates and supplemented with fat and a protein powder supplement to compensate for the lower carbohydrate content.

Following the experiment scientists stated 'The carbohydrate group ran faster during the last 5 km,' adding, 'Furthermore, the men in the carbohydrate group ran the 30 km faster after carbohydrate loading.'

This led to the conclusion – and widely held belief – that 'Dietary carbohydrate loading improves endurance performance during prolonged running.'[35]

An idea supported by the Scandinavian Physiological Society: 'These results suggest that muscle glycogen (carbohydrate) availability can affect performance during both short-term and more prolonged high-intensity intermittent exercise.'[36]

And the Australian Institute of Sport: 'The recommendations of sports nutritionists are based on plentiful evidence that increased carbohydrate availability enhances endurance and performance during single exercise sessions.'[37]

Carbohydrates: Carb loading

Carb loading is a tried-and-tested approach to improve performance.

As far back as the 1960s, athletes were increasing their carbohydrate intake to run faster, cycle further and lift heavier. With many weird and wonderful ways being trialled, it wasn't until recently that the art had been perfected to ensure muscles are fully fuelled to reduce the onset of fatigue.

How does it work? It's believed the average athlete can only store enough muscle glycogen – the muscle's form of stored carbohydrates – to sustain 90 minutes of exercise. After 90 minutes, our muscle glycogen levels deplete, our 'gas tank' runs low and fatigue sets in.

Sports drinks, gels and even a banana may help. But studies show that increasing your carbohydrate intake three days before could be the most effective way of ensuring you're fully fuelled. How much? To put some exact figures on all of this, research published in *The Journal of Sports Medicine* states: 'Carbohydrate intake ranges from 5 grams to 7 grams per kilogram of bodyweight per day for general training needs and 7 grams to 10 grams per kilogram of bodyweight per day for the increased needs of endurance athletes.'[38]

But let's put sports science to one side for the moment.

I feel compelled to acknowledge a culinary masterpiece that's fuelled many a marathon and obstacle race of mine. Annie's Acai Bowl is unlike anything you've tried before. It tastes unbelievable and the smell when it leaves the oven is enough to convince anyone to carb load.

THE ACAI BOWL
by Annie Mayne

Packed with as much flavour as nutrient-dense carbohydrates, this is the best way to flood the body with all the vitamins and minerals it needs. This is my all-time favourite carb-rich breakfast, lunch, dinner and/or snack.

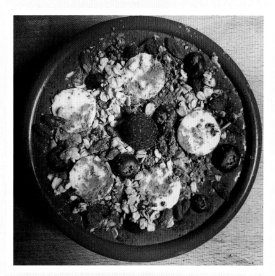

Ingredients

Serves 1

125g frozen mixed berries

1 banana

250ml coconut milk

1 tbsp chia seeds

30g Vanilla Crème whey protein 80
   from THE PROTEIN WORKS™)

90g gluten-free oats

30g acai berry powder or frozen acai

Method

1. Add all the ingredients into a blender and go nuts.
2. Make sure the mixture isn't too wet; you want it to be almost smoothie-like.
3. Transfer to a bowl and add any berry, fruit, seed or nut you can find.

	Calories	Carbs	Fat	Protein
Total	857	160g	25g	55g
Per serving	857	160g	25g	55g

Fat: The basics

'No disease that can be treated by diet should be treated with any other means.'
MAIMONIDES

We need fats in our diet to live. Hopefully, this is not news to anyone. Hopefully, the low-fat-diet-hype train has well and truly left the station. This is because it's long been shown that our bodies need fat to assist in vitamin absorption, to aid hormone regulation and even aid optimal brain function. Without it our diets and health look bleak.

Fat: The best sources

Like protein and carbohydrates, the term 'fat' is too general. There are thousands of different fats, and each arrives equipped with a number of different health benefits. From those found in meat, fatty fish, nuts and nut butters to oils and basically countless other sources. Again – worth restating – we humans are biologically wired to seek variety, and finding fats is one of my favourite kitchen-based pastimes.

Fat: How much do I need?

Here's some food for thought (bad pun intended).

The American Journal of Medicine published a brilliant piece of research looking at 'Dietary fats, eating guides, and public policy: history, critique, and recommendations.' It stated: 'Controversies over the nutrition science of dietary fat, and equally over the advice furnished to consumers about dietary fat, have confounded US nutrition policies and eating guidance for the last 90 years. This is so despite the remarkable congruence between the first US food guides (1916) and the most recent (2000 Dietary Guidelines for Americans), both of which state that dietary fats should be consumed "moderately". 39

OK, so fat's good. But what does 'moderately' look like?

'The 2002 Report of the US Food and Nutrition Board (issued jointly by the United States and Canada) quantifies this by stating that healthy dietary fat should constitute "25–35% of calories"'[40]

But 'moderately' and '25–35% of calories' don't explain the success of fat-fuelled athletes. Take elite cyclists for example.

On what grounds did research from *The European Journal of Applied Physiology and Occupational Physiology* claim that an elite cyclist's performance could be improved by a high-fat diet of 70% fat, 7% carbohydrates and 23% protein compared to a high-carbohydrate diet of 12% fat, 74% carbohydrates and 24% protein?

'These results would suggest that two weeks of adaptation to a high-fat diet would result in an enhanced resistance to fatigue and a significant sparing of carbohydrate during low-to-moderate intensity exercise.'[41]

The answer is a ketogenic (keto) diet.

Fat: Ketogenic diet

Low in carbohydrates but high in fat: the goal of the keto diet is to achieve a state of ketosis.

This is where the body produces small fuel-efficient molecules called 'ketones' as an alternative fuel for the body when blood sugar (glucose) is in short supply. Basically, they're produced in the liver from fat if you don't have any/many carbohydrates and sugars in the diet and only a moderate amount of protein – since excess protein can also be converted to blood sugar. The body and brain then use them to fuel the day ahead.

Does it work? According to the Law of Biological Individuality you may only know if you try it.

But the theory is that fat can become a more efficient fuel source for some people. This is why research published in *The Current Sports Medicine Reports* states: 'The number of gruelling events that challenge the limits of human endurance is increasing. Such events are also challenging the limits of current dietary recommendations.'[42]

The authors then add that traditionally high-carbohydrate diets have been favoured, but there are 'some situations for which alternative dietary options are beneficial'.

'Situations' like a fat-fuelled expedition to the Arctic…

Fat: Lessons from the Arctic

Long before the word 'keto' was invented we humans were undertaking fat-fuelled physical activity.

One of the earliest documented demonstrations of this was the Arctic Schwatka expedition of 1878–80, when explorers went in search of the lost Royal Navy Franklin Expedition. Sponsored by the *New York Herald* and the American Geographical Society, the team left the west coast of Hudson's Bay in April 1879, but found something they weren't expecting.

A state of ketosis…

Lead by Lieutenant Frederick Schwatka, the team stayed in the far north for two years, living with the Inuit. During this time, Schwatka lived on 'white man's' food as long as supplies lasted. But once that ran out, he and his team were forced to embrace the Inuit way of life and dine on reindeer, seal and bear.

What's incredible is that during the expedition Schwatka kept a diary that was later published by the Mystic Seaport True Maritime Adventure Series in a book titled *The Long Arctic Search*. Throughout the pages, he perfectly describes how the body survives and thrives on a high-fat Inuit diet, once adapted:

'When first thrown wholly upon a diet of reindeer meat, it seems inadequate to properly nourish the system and there is an apparent weakness and inability to perform severe exertive, fatiguing journeys. But this soon passes away in the course of two or three weeks. At first the white man takes to the new diet in too homeopathic a manner, especially if it be raw. However, seal meat which is far more disagreeable with its fishy odour, and bear meat with its strong flavour, seems to have no such temporary debilitating effect upon the economy.' [43]

Again, this was all before our current understanding of nutritional science.

But through self-experimentation, Schwatka found that by increasing the fat content of the low-carb diet – seal and bear meat is notably high in fats – you can speed up the time it takes you to achieve ketosis. How? Because your increased fat intake forces the production of ketones, which replace the carbohydrates as a source of energy.

More fat means a quicker state of ketosis.[44]

Something the Inuit have known and practised for years.

MANAGE YOUR MICRONUTRIENTS

Too often micronutrients are overlooked in a nutrition plan. Granted, we need macronutrients (carbohydrates, fats and proteins) in larger quantities within the diet and it's only these that can be used as energy. But vitamins, minerals and enzymes play a key role in energy production since enzymes require nutrient co-factors (like vitamins B1, B2, B3 and B5, and the minerals magnesium, iron and sulphur) or they simply do not function.

In short, little to no micronutrients in the diet means little to no energy in the gym and life.

KETO TACO BOWL
by Annie Mayne

100% keto friendly, each taco bowl is best served warm so it melts in your mouth. Packing over 30g of protein in every serving, it's incredibly low-carb.

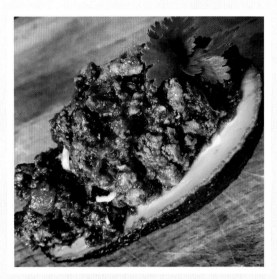

Ingredients

Serves 4

2 slices bacon

180g raw Brussels sprouts, shredded

1 tbsp olive oil

1 tbsp minced garlic

500g ground beef *

1 tsp cumin

2 tsp smoked paprika

Fresh coriander

Juice of 1 lime or lemon

2 large avocados

* For keto, select meats that have a higher percentage of fat.

Method

1. Cook the bacon until crispy. Remove from the pan, add the Brussels sprouts and cook for 4–5 minutes. Break up the bacon and return it to the pan.
2. Add the oil and garlic and cook for 3 minutes before adding the ground meat.
3. Cook until browned and add the cumin and paprika. Cook until the meat is no longer pink, then season to taste with salt and black pepper, coriander and lime or lemon juice.
4. Slice the avocados in half and remove the stones. Using a fork, mash up the flesh of the avocado, then form a large dip inside the avocado for the filling.
5. Add the sautéed sprouts and meat. Top with a garnish of your choice.
6. Get some cheese on there!

	Calories	Carbs	Fat	Protein
Total	2096	64g	160g	124g
Per serving	524	16g	40g	31g

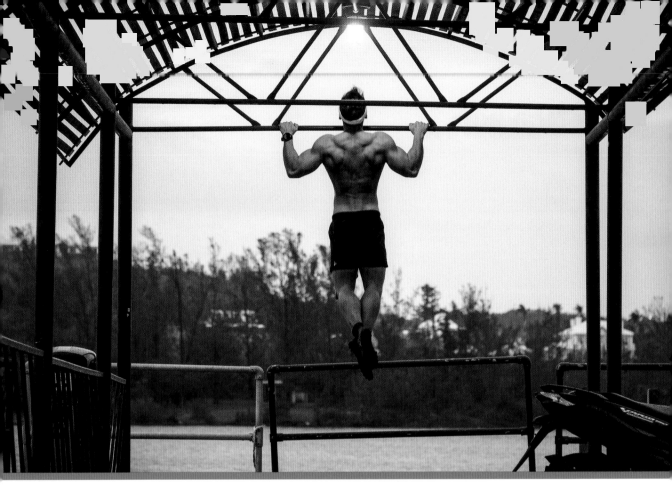

FAT LOSS | FITNESS
FOOD AND TRAINING

What's the best form of training to lose fat?

The honest answer is all of them. This is because when losing fat, your training (to keep things simple) should play one key role: to help you create a calorie deficit. Therefore, the exact type of training becomes less important.

Yes, studies show that High-intensity Interval Training 'may be more effective at reducing abdominal body fat than other types of exercise'.[45] But to quote research from *The Journal of Sports Medicine*, 'Developing programmes to aid in long-term adherence to physical activity regimes remains the most critical challenge.'[46] Basically, the training method doesn't matter; consistently training does.

Which is why we should learn to use every method described here, chopping, changing and modifying our weekly routine however we want and whenever we want.

HIGH-INTENSITY CARDIO | FAT LOSS

Sprint, rest and repeat.

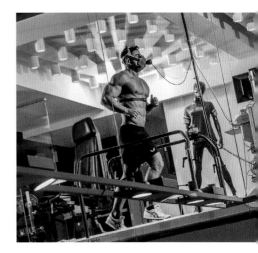

It may be one of the simplest training routines in the world, but science shows it could also be the most effective. High-intensity Interval Training (HIIT) typically involves exercising at a frenetic pace for 20 to 90 seconds followed by a period of low-intensity training or complete rest that lasts 20 to 120 seconds.

You then repeat this for a total of 10 to 20 minutes, using your weapon of choice – whether that's a bike, a treadmill or just on your lonesome up and down a hill.

Why? It burns more body fat.

That's according to scientists from Laval University in Québec, Canada,[47] who compared a 15-week HIIT programme to a 20-week endurance-training programme. After taking muscle biopsies and body fat measurements they found the HIIT programme was more effective at stoking up the body's metabolism, which resulted in greater fat loss.

Put simply, HIIT can burn more body fat in less time.

STRENGTH TRAINING | FAT LOSS

Lifting lots of heavy weight can help you burn lots of fat.

No, seriously: research published in *The Journal of Applied Physiology* showed the positive effects strength training could have on body fat.[48] Scientists took 13 untrained, healthy men and had them complete a 16-week strength-training programme. All the men improved their strength in the upper and lower body, increased muscle mass and lowered their body fat both in total and regionally around the arms, legs and stomach.

This is perhaps explained by research conducted at the Department of Food Science and Human Nutrition at Colorado State University, where they monitored the post-exercise energy expenditure in me after heavy resistance training.

What they found was that following a strenuous 90-minute weightlifting protocol, 'the subject's post-exercise metabolic rate – the rate at which their metabolism remains elevated and they keep burning calories – remained high for a prolonged period and may enhance post-exercise lipid oxidation.'[49]

Basically, weight training increases the rate at which you burn calories even after you've left the gym.

Finally, strength training improves body composition, helping you not only to lose weight, but to lose body fat and increase lean muscle.[50] To quote *The Journal of Strength and Conditioning Research*, 'It appears that the volume and intensity of this type of training is sufficient to elicit beneficial alterations in body composition,' citing the large, heavy compound movements as being responsible for these positive changes.[51]

LOW-INTENSITY CARDIO | FAT LOSS

Low-intensity training is a valuable tool (with lower 'stress') when losing fat.[52]

This is because – as we discovered in Chapter 4 – it's widely agreed among strength and conditioning experts that low-to-moderate training can have a positive effect on your immune system, while high-intensity training can have a negative effect.

What this means is while high-intensity training and strength training come with benefits like burning fat after you've left the gym, low-intensity training is a tool that shouldn't ever be overlooked in your quest to lose fat. It's low impact, low stress, just as valuable and won't leave you and your immune system waving the white flag from overtraining.

FOOD | FUN

BREAK THE RULES OF FOOD

The wait is over. Now it's time to see the dessert menu.

This is because chocolate-flavoured fat loss isn't hard. It's just forgotten. Contrary to popular belief, it's completely possible to eat 200 g of the purest, richest, dark chocolate. Every day. Every week. Every month. While your body fat never ventures further north than 9%.

Written from the kitchen, this will be your taste buds' favourite chapter.

THE POWER OF COCOA

When we talk about losing fat, the word 'chocolate' is practically dieting blasphemy.

Dubbed a nutritional sin by many dieticians, consumption of the aforementioned evil is punishable by a guilt-fuelled visit to the gym. So, by what possible dietary logic do I consume 200 g every day?

No this isn't a 'cheat meal' and nor am I gifted with a crazy metabolism. Every single day, immediately after the gym, I will religiously make my way to the kitchen, take a bar of cocoa-rich Peruvian chocolate out of the cupboard and chow down. Yes, my muscles are depleted and therefore my ability to eat and assimilate food is vastly improved, but the dessert-based wizardry doesn't stop there.

To figure out why, let's first take a look at the origins of chocolate. Trace it back far enough and you'll find it's actually a plant-based food that originates from the seed of a fruit, called the cocoa bean. Research shows cocoa, in its raw form, is naturally very high in flavanols (a natural plant nutrient). Understand this and you begin to understand the power of chocolate.

Just like the ancient Mayans.

The Mayan warrior secret

The Maya civilisation was known for its art, architecture and badass warriors who loved cocoa. Legend has it Mayan warriors would march for miles throughout the day and then charge into battle fuelled only by cocoa beans that they'd keep in a leather pouch slung around their waist. Chocolate was basically a symbol of power. A privilege of warriors and the elite that was consumed to offer the sustenance needed to tackle virile challenges.

This runs contrary to its junk-food-themed reputation, but chocolate – as the Mayans understood it – is an incredibly complex substance that contains 400–500 different compounds, each loaded with health properties that the Mayans intuitively understood.

Many years later and modern science would confirm cocoa is a phenomenally healthy superfood that's worthy of our respect and – in the case of the Mayan warriors – worship.

The sweet science

Take research from the University of L'Aquila in Italy[53] for example. They found that the flavanol content of dark chocolate 'improves insulin sensitivity in healthy persons'. In essence, what this means is your training session, coupled with flavanol-dense chocolate, has turned your muscles into giant sponges that will absorb and use anything and everything you give them.

So what's the reason for the vilification of chocolate in the first place? Why the bad press? The answer lies in the way most modern chocolate is made.

Not all chocolate arrives equipped with a magical cocoa supply. Dark chocolate, for example, is usually quite high in cocoa and may contain 70–85% cocoa. This will of course vary depending on which brand you buy. But it should come as no surprise that its caramel-layered, sugar-ridden cousins don't arrive with the same health properties.

This is because the added sugar causes insulin – the hormone related to fat storage – to shoot through the roof, cravings to occur and the wheels on our dieting wagon to fall off.

Now I just want to say I'm not some food Nazi. I won't say you should run for the hills every time a packet of caramel biscuits is opened. But just know that not all chocolate is created equal. There are some kinds of chocolate that should be included in the diet in moderation. Then there are others that could – nay should – be eaten on a daily basis.

'My doctor told me I had to stop throwing intimate dinners for four unless there are three other people.'
ORSON WELLES

ALCOHOL

'Wine is the most healthful and most hygienic of beverages.'
LOUIS PASTEUR

For years, alcohol has been portrayed as your waistline's archenemy. Considering it's a close second to dietary fat in terms of its calorie density – roughly seven calories per gram – it's easy to see why. But alcoholic drinks come in many different forms and each has a different physiological impact on the body that's far more complex than simply counting the calories on the bottle.

Which is why – contrary to mainstream calorie-themed dogma – this section of the book serves to bring to light some less well-publicised studies in the area of fat loss and moderate alcohol consumption. Now, moderate consumption must be stressed since in all studies, excessive intake has not surprisingly been linked to many health issues. In no way am I making light of any of them, but that's a separate issue altogether.

This section merely serves to give a brief insight into the vast field of alcohol research to offer a different perspective on man's favourite tipples. Not to prescribe or dictate anyone's dietary habits, just to show that the bottle of gin in your cupboard maybe shouldn't be as feared as you first thought.

So why does alcohol get such bad press?

Well, as far back as 1980 research was published in the *American Journal of Clinical Nutrition*[54] that dubbed alcohol a non-essential nutrient that contains 'empty calories'. What this means is – unlike carbohydrates, fats and proteins – the body has no nutritional need for those shots you had on Friday night. Instead, it quickly identifies the alcohol as a 'toxin', goes into biological overdrive and frantically tries to deal with it. All the time you're blissfully unaware and on your third round of drinking games with the lads.

Next, scientists from the University of Lausanne in Switzerland[55] proposed the idea that alcohol – and its toxic-like property – is actually guilty of slowing the entire fat-burning

DARK CHOCOLATE PROTEIN BROWNIES
by Hester Sabery

Presenting my ultimate Chocolate Protein Brownie recipe. A healthy, protein-packed dessert you can have completely guilt-free after the gym and a nice alternative to protein powders.

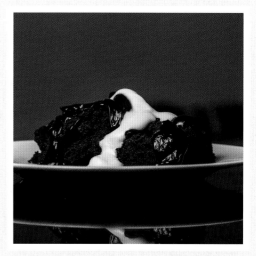

Ingredients

Makes 12

45g dark chocolate (80%), plus extra for decoration

95g organic virgin coconut oil from THE PROTEIN WORKS™

10g smooth peanut butter from THE PROTEIN WORKS™

10g cocoa powder

65g coconut flour

2g baking powder

70g Chocolate Silk whey protein 80 from THE PROTEIN WORKS™

215g honey

1½ tsp vanilla extract

3 eggs

45g chopped almonds

40g chopped cashews

Method

1. Preheat the oven to 180˚C. Grease a 20cm/8in square tin and line with baking parchment, making sure there is enough parchment either side of the tin to lift out easily.

2. Melt the chocolate, coconut oil and peanut butter over a bain-marie or heat a in microwave, stirring every few seconds until melted. Leave for 5 minutes to cool a little.

3. Place the cocoa powder, coconut flour, baking powder and chocolate whey protein in a large bowl and gently whisk to get rid of any lumps. Whisk in the honey, vanilla extract and melted chocolate, coconut oil and peanut butter mixture until blended.

4. Add the eggs one at a time and whisk well after each addition. Finally, fold in the nuts. The mixture will be very thick and fudgy.

5. Scrape the brownie batter into the prepared tin and even the mixture out. Bake for 25–30 mins until a knife inserted into the centre comes out with moist crumbs on it, but no wet batter, and the brownie is quite firm.

6. Leave to cool in the tin, then lift out the brownie. Peel away the baking parchment and use a sharp knife to cut the brownie into 12 squares. Dust with a little cocoa powder and drizzle with melted chocolate to decorate. Maybe add a few pistachios, fresh raspberries and yogurt for extra toppings!

	Calories	Carbs	Fat	Protein
Total	2726	300g	197g	104g
Per brownie	227	25g	16g	9g

process. Yet more bad news for 'calorie counters' who now live in fear that their bodies are taking a double hit of fat-burning suppression and fat accumulation from these 'empty calories'.

Now it was early research like this that led to the vilification of most – if not all – alcoholic drinks. Countless articles have since been published that compare one glass of wine to several large cookies or liken a pint of Guinness to an entire roast dinner. But this is where the problem lies, since tarring all alcoholic drinks with the same brush is wrong. Also, measuring alcohol – and all food for that matter – by its caloric content is equally as flawed.

This is because this approach presupposes that the human body needs food solely for energy and calories. This simply isn't the case. The human body is in fact a complex 'chemical factory' that processes different food substances in many different ways. Basically, calories and energy are not the only things we extract from food and they're also not the only things we extract from certain alcoholic drinks.

Let's take that refreshing glass of gin and tonic you've just politely turned down at dinner. Firstly, gin is a distilled spirit, which means – compared to other drinks – it's very low in sugar. Excellent news for the waistline since – alcohol content aside – sugar is readily stored as fat by the body. To quote research from the *Journal of the American Medical Association*, 'Several studies have found an association between sugar-sweetened beverages and incidence of obesity'.[56] Therefore, based on the evidence, it would be wise to choose a distilled spirit over those colourful, sweetened cocktails that come decorated with fruit to make them look healthy and fresh.

Next, one important hormonal factor that determines how prone we are to storing fat is our insulin sensitivity. Put very simply, when a person has poor insulin sensitivity they are more prone to storing fat as their bodies are less efficiently able to process carbohydrates. Yet scientists from the Department of Medicine and Clinical Science at Kyushu University,[57] Japan, believe that 'alcohol improves insulin sensitivity'. Again, another possible reason why you should politely accept that glass of gin between courses – you're simply giving your waistline a hormonal advantage.

Finally, let's take red wine as an example. It's been found to contain a natural, health-boosting compound known as resveratrol that's produced when the grapes used to make the wine are 'under attack' from fungus and disease. It's believed that you ingest these same disease-fighting properties when you drink a glass of red which – to quote scientists from the University of Illinois in Chicago – could have 'anti-inflammatory, neuroprotective and antiviral properties'.[58]

All these ailments are associated with the ageing process, so essentially it could – in theory – be proposed that you're keeping Father Time at bay by drinking a glass of the red stuff.

In summary, if you take an alcoholic vow of abstinence for personal, religious or health reasons – as advised by a qualified medical professional – then ignore the musings contained within this part. But if you're fit and healthy and simply deny yourself that one glass of wine with your friends on a Saturday evening because of the calorie scaremongering that's broadcast by often well-meaning organisations, perhaps reconsider.

Once again: assessing food, alcohol and calories in this way is over-simplistic and flawed.

Ultimately, this section was never meant to declare more rules and regulations to live by. There are too many cocktails, concoctions and variations for one article to address and I humbly accept my work here only scratches the surface. Instead, I hope it encourages you to become an epistemocrat of food – that is someone who holds his or her own knowledge in great suspicion.

So going forward, question all nutritional literature and don't rely on others to dictate your dietary habits. Read every label thoroughly and not just the calorie content. Lastly, above all else, don't deny yourself a fine glass of wine and good company just because of the calories.

'Compromises are made for relationships... not wine.'
SIR ROBERT SCOTT CAYWOOD

SLEEP

'Sleep is the best meditation.'
DALAI LAMA

Do you want to lose weight? Then stay in bed.

I imagine you didn't expect to hear that in this chapter. But scientists from the University of Chicago[59] have discovered that not getting enough sleep could 'hormonally handicap' you in your quest to lower your body fat. What this means is that disturbing your natural sleep pattern also disturbs your fat-burning hormones.

For this reason, if you want to learn to lose fat you must first learn the art of 'strategic sleep'.

Strategic sleep

First you must understand that sleep is the most effective rejuvenating tool we have readily available to us. Don't believe me? Take a peek at the research published in the *Journal of Psychiatry and Neuroscience*, which teaches us that our recovery-boosting growth hormone spikes during sleep.[60] Or the studies published in the *Journal of Immunology*, which found that it's during sleep that your immune system – the body's defence against disease – is re-fortified.[61]

In 1994, scientists made an amazing discovery. They found a powerful new fat-regulating hormone called leptin. Now, while modern science openly admits we've only just scratched the surface with our understanding of this hormone, we do know it has a significant impact on everything from our appetite to how much fat we store. To quote the *Journal of Neurochemistry*, 'leptin is well known as a hormone important in the central control of appetitive behaviours'.[62]

Put simply, master leptin and you master your appetite, cravings and body fat. So how exactly do we do this? Yes, you guessed it: sleep.

This is because researchers from the aforementioned study at the University of Chicago took 12 healthy men aged 22 to 30, and then closely monitored their calorie intake, appetite and hunger during two days of 'extended sleep' and two days of 'restricted sleep.'

Results revealed that during the two days when the subjects were restricted to only four hours of sleep, their leptin levels dropped by 18%. This, in turn, increased appetite by a staggering 23%. Researchers all concluded that this increase in appetite was specifically for 'calorie-dense foods' with a high carbohydrate content like chocolate, sweets and generally junk food.

Hormonal 'tug-of-war'

What's interesting is they also reported a 28% increase in a hormone called ghrelin.

Later dubbed the body's 'hunger hormone', ghrelin is produced by the stomach, and signals to the brain whether we're hungry or not. To use a sporting example, it's almost like your stomach is in a tug-of-war competition, on the one side is leptin telling your brain you're full and happy. On the other side is grehlin, which is telling your brain you're hungry and need to attack the cookie jar.

Depending on how much sleep you get may determine which team wins the 'digestive tug-of-war'. This, then, has important implications for your nutrition. Your cravings – and your ability to stick to a diet – don't actually have much to do with psychology and willpower.

'Sleep curtailment in healthy young men is associated with decreased leptin levels, elevated ghrelin levels and increased hunger and appetite.'[63]

Instead, it's much more to do with your sleep patterns and corresponding hormones.

Will this really have an impact on your body fat?

Body fat and bedtime | The study

Research published in *Annals of Internal Medicine* believes so. The title of the study says it all: 'Insufficient sleep undermines dietary efforts to reduce adiposity.'[64]

Sleep scientists wanted to see just how much hormonal disturbances from lack of sleep increased appetite, and find out whether these hormonal disturbances would manifest themselves in meaningful changes in body fat when on a calorie-controlled diet.

They took 10 overweight, middle-aged, moderately healthy test subjects…

- Participants had to stay in bed for either 5.5 or 8.5 hours per night for 14 days.
- At least three months later subjects swapped conditions.
- Food intake was restricted to 90% of resting metabolic rate.
- Meals were standardised and weighed to ensure calorie intake was controlled as tightly as possible.

Basically, our sleep scientists did everything they could to control the conditions of the study.

Body fat and bedtime | The results

- The amount of time subjects slept increased or decreased as scheduled.
- Energy consumption was near identical (about 1450 calories per day).
- Daily caloric expenditure was also nearly identical (about 2140 calories per day). That's an estimated daily calorie deficit of 700.
- Macronutrient breakdown was 48% carbohydrate, 34% fat and 18% protein.
- Both groups lost about 3 kg (6.6 lb) during the study, but…

… subjects in the group sleeping for 8.5 hours lost 50/50 fat and lean mass, while subjects in the group sleeping for 5.5 hours lost 20/80 fat and lean muscle mass. No, that's not a typing error.

Only one-fifth of the weight lost was actually fat. That's 0.6 kg of the 3 kg total.

And it gets worse for the subjects in the 5.5 sleep group. Why? Yes, you guessed it: hunger was higher. All as ghrelin levels shot through the roof and plagued their sleep-deprived bodies, which made keeping away from the cookie jar that much harder.

Body fat and bedtime | The conclusion

The above study did come with a few drawbacks.

Firstly, the subjects were sedentary and never ventured into the gym. This would of course have helped to retain muscle mass while dieting. Also, the 65 g of protein per day was much lower than the 1.7 g of protein per kg of bodyweight per day recommended by the International Olympic Committee Consensus on Sports Nutrition.

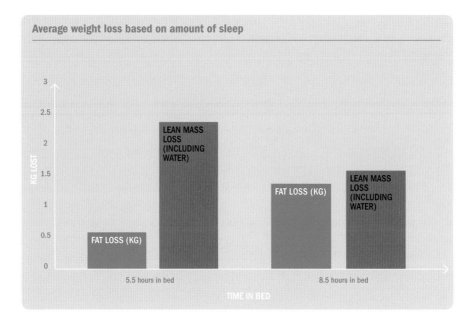

But even with the best diet and training plan, it's hard to imagine it would make that much difference and offset the hormonal changes caused by lack of sleep. At best you'd have to diet longer, struggle more and you'd just feel hungry all the time. No thank you!

Body fat and bedtime | The lesson

Sleep, snooze and grab a siesta.

It really is that simple. In view of the evidence, sleep is essential for fat loss and getting less of it means your nutrition plan may be destined to end in a biscuit-based disaster. In summary, a good night's sleep will magnify the effectiveness of your training and nutrition; a bad night's sleep will serve as a 'hormonal handbrake' to your fat loss.

If you're tired and hungry, release the handbrake and head to bed.

HOW TO WRITE YOUR OWN DIET

IN FIVE STEPS

The best diet in the world is useless unless you can stick to it, so be sure to get stuck into the meal plans and recipe section to make sure your taste buds love your diet plan as much as your waistline does.

1. Work out your basal metabolic rate (BMR)

This is the amount of calories your burn per day at rest.

To do this, use the Harrison Benedict Formula.[65]

- **For men:** 66.5 + (13.75 x weight in kg) + (5.003 x height in cm) – (6.755 x age in years)
- **For women:** 655.1 + (9.563 x weight in kg) + (1.850 x height in cm) – (4.676 x age in years)

2. Multiply by your level of activity

- Little to no exercise means multiply your BMR by 1.2.
- Light exercise a few times a week by 1.375.
- Moderate exercise 3–5 times a week by 1.55.
- Heavy exercise 6–7 times a week by 1.725.

Congratulations! You now know your daily calorie requirements.

3. Set your calorie deficit/surplus

Determine whether you want to…

- Eat more calories than you burn to store fat and set the size of your calorie surplus.
- Burn more calories than you eat to lose fat and set the size of your calorie deficit.
- Eat the same as you burn to stay the same (calorie balance).

4. Find your food ratio

This part is important. To re-quote the *International Journal of Obesity* 'Regardless of assigned diet, 12-month weight change was greater in the most adherent.' [66] Therefore the ratio of protein, fats and carbohydrates doesn't matter as long as you can stick to it. To help you find your food ratio, here are three to choose from:

- High Carb[67]: 20% protein, 10% fats, 70% carbohydrates
- Balanced Macros[68]: 25% protein, 25% fats, 50% carbohydrates
- High Fat[69]: 23% protein, 70% fats, 7% carbohydrates

5. Make your meals in grams

Now it's time to move your food from the calculator and into the actual kitchen. Protein and carbohydrates contain 4 calories per gram, while fat provides 9 calories per gram. Based on this, here's how a 2000-calorie diet looks for each food ratio:

HIGH CARB	BALANCED MACROS	HIGH FAT
Protein = (2000 x 0.2) ÷ 4 = 100g	Protein = (2000 x 0.25) ÷ 4 = 125g	Protein = (2000 x 0.23) ÷ 4 = 115g
Fats = (2000 x 0.1) ÷ 9 = 22g	Fats = (2000 x 0.25) ÷ 9 = 56g	Fats = (2000 x 0.70) ÷ 9 = 156g
Carbs = (2000 x 0.7) ÷ 4 = 350g	Carbs = (2000 x 0.50) ÷ 4 = 250g	Carbs = (2000 x 0.07) ÷ 4 = 35g

1 MAN | 3 DIETS | 1 RESULT

'Don't become emotionally attached to a nutrition or training principle; as sciences progress, so must we.'
ROSS EDGLEY

Which one do I use? Any and all of them (to prove a point).

This is because in 2013 I decided to trial each diet. Playing any and every sport I could, my body remained the same at 8% body fat. The only thing that changed was the quantities of the macronutrients I ate. Allow me to show you in a Table of Theoretical Nutritional Awesomeness based on my height, age and weight in 2013 so you can see a working example of the theory.

Worth stressing is that this is just the theory. There are thousands of other variables that influence your body's energy system. Some we know, others we don't.

These range from the cooking method[70] to the weather and corresponding temperature[71] at which the food is eaten. 'Weight' within the formula doesn't take into account muscle mass and body composition. Daily activity is so subjective. Calories expended will fluctuate day by day. Plus hundreds of other biological factors a mathematical equation can't take into account.

But should you understand the theory, **you** are ready to choose a meal plan that works for **you**, no longer blindly following one that is given or prescribed to you. Any of these might be the right diet for your body:

- 7-Day High Carb Meal Plan.
- 7-Day Balanced Macro Meal Plan.
- 7-Day High Fat Meal Plan.

Age: 27 | Height: 178cm (5ft 10) | Weight: 90kg | Total calories per day: 3823

HIGH CARB			BALANCED MACROS			HIGH FAT		
20% Protein	10% Fats	70% Carbs	20% Protein	25% Fats	55% Carbs	20% Protein	70% Fats	10% Carbs
765 calories of protein	382 calories of fats	2676 calories of carbs	765 calories of protein	956 calories of fats	2103 calories of carbs	765 calories of protein	2676 calories of fats	382 calories of carbs
191g of protein a day	42g of fats a day	669g of carbs a day	191g of protein a day	106g of fats a day	526g of carbs a day	191g of protein a day	297g of fats a day	96g of carbs a day

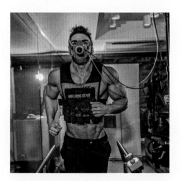

Inspired by the *Journal of Sports Medicine*[72]

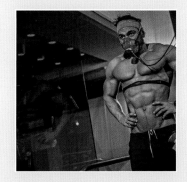

Inspired by research from the *Journal of the American Dietetic Association*[73]

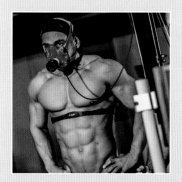

Inspired by the *European Journal of Applied Physiology & Occupational Physiology*[74]

Serving as a human guinea pig for three different diets

7-DAY HIGH CARB MEAL PLAN

HIGH CARB		
20% Protein	10% Fats	70% Carbs

	DAY 1	DAY 2	DAY 3	DAY 4	DAY 5	DAY 6	DAY 7
Breakfast	Quinoa cooked in coconut milk topped with fruit and almonds	Strawberry and pineapple protein pancakes	Oats/Porridge, with cinnamon, blueberries with a scoop of whey protein	Nourishing nut and seed bread (see below)	Protein waffles and honey	Granola, yogurt and mixed berries with a scoop of whey protein	Chia breakfast bowl (see opposite)
Lunch	Harissa-crusted chicken	Loaded potato skins (with chilli) and salad	Baked egg, chickpeas, spinach, aubergines and peppers with tortilla wraps	Salmon, cream cheese and toasted bagel	Spaghetti and meatballs	Wholewheat tortilla with shredded chicken and avocado slices	Lamb tagine and rice (see below)
Snack	Healthy biscotti and green tea	2 rice cakes and cottage cheese	Wholegrain protein muffins (see below)	Tortilla chips with chill and salsa dip	Greek yogurt with blueberries, honey and a scoop of whey protein	Sliced banana bread	Protein granola bar
Dinner	Steak burger	Grilled salmon noodle stir-fry (see below)	Baked sweet potato with cottage cheese, salsa and bacon croutons	Seafood linguine	Chicken curry and rice	Chicken, noodles and stir-fry mixed vegetables	Chilli, brown rice and mixed vegetables
Snack	Healthy protein flapjack	Natural yogurt with apple slices and granola	Oatmeal protein cookie with milk	Quinoa cooked in coconut milk covered in fruit and almonds	Lemon and quark granola and oat cheesecake	Warm bowl of porridge oats, cinnamon, raisins and a scoop of apple and cinnamon protein	Healthy protein flapjack

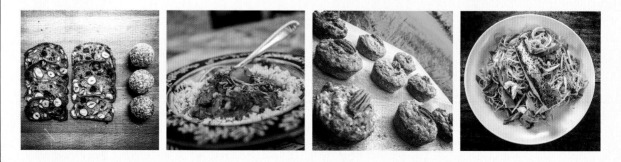

CHIA BREAKFAST BOWL
by Annie Mayne
7-day High Carb Best Meal

Made from one of the oldest superfoods in the world, chia seeds are an incredibly versatile ingredient and can be blended with any fruit to make a breakfast bowl packed with nutrient-dense carbohydrates to start your day.

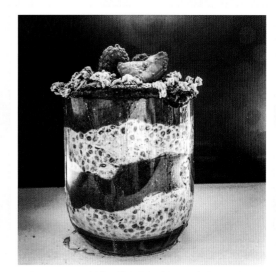

Ingredients

Serves 1

250ml coconut milk

30g strawberries, blueberries
   or other fresh fruit

2 tbsp agave syrup

½ tsp vanilla extract

32g chia seeds

Method

1. Add the coconut milk, berries, agave syrup and vanilla to a blender. Blend on high for 1–2 minutes to purée the fruit.

2. Pour the mixture into a mason jar or a small bowl/cup and mix in the chia seeds.

3. Cover and refrigerate for at least 3 hours or preferably overnight.

	Calories	Carbs	Fat	Protein
Total	492	66g	22g	10g
Per serving	492	66g	22g	10g

7-DAY BALANCED MACRO MEAL PLAN

BALANCED MACROS		
20% Protein	25% Fats	55% Carbs

	DAY 1	DAY 2	DAY 3	DAY 4	DAY 5	DAY 6	DAY 7
Breakfast	Scrambled eggs on toast	Blueberry and orange protein pancakes (see below)	Cinnamon and raisin oatmeal with a scoop of whey protein	Raspberry and blueberry protein waffles	Spinach and onion omelette	Banana and honey protein granola	Banana and coconut protein waffles
Lunch	Beef chilli stir-fry	Kidney bean chilli	Parma ham and cheese toasties (see below)	Harissa-crusted chicken with coconut rice and stir-fried greens (see opposite)	Beef kofta with bulgur and kale salad	Quinoa toast with peanut butter, avocado and strawberry jam spreads	Chicken burrito with avocado and spinach
Snack	Raw protein balls (see page 61)	Protein granola bar	Pumpkin muffins	Super green protein smoothie (see below)	Club sandwich	Protein smoothie with pineapple and Raspberry	Raw vegan brownies with a protein shake
Dinner	Roasted chicken thighs, potatoes and spring onions with a herb vinaigrette	Steak and mixed vegetables (see below)	Chicken and vegetable flat-crust pizza	Cauliflower and aubergine pizza	Steak and sweet potato fries	Beef and cheese burger	Pork, beef, pancetta meatballs
Snack	Mixed berry smoothie	Turmeric chicken salad	Chocolate acai protein bowl	Fruit and nut mix and a protein shake	Protein pumpkin pie muffins	Low-fat Greek yogurt and sliced apple	Blueberry, strawberry and pear smoothie

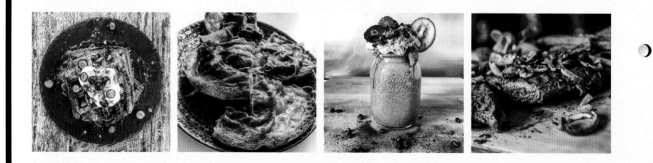

HARISSA-CRUSTED CHICKEN WITH COCONUT RICE AND STIR-FRIED GREENS

by Simon Partridge

7-day Balanced Macro Best Meal

The beauty of this recipe is it's so easy to make, tastes amazing and because of the fresh ingredients used, it has the perfect combination of protein, fats and carbohydrates on every plate.

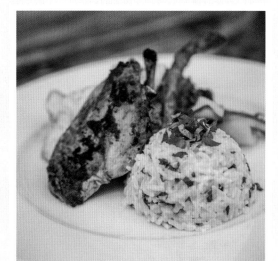

Ingredients

Serves 1

2 skin-on chicken breasts

2 tsp harissa

Salt and freshly ground pepper

1 tbsp coconut oil

100g long grain rice

1 tin coconut milk

6 spears asparagus, cut lengthways

1 pak choi, leaves separated

50g mangetout

1 courgette, thinly sliced

1 handful baby spinach

50g fresh coriander, chopped

Juice of 1 lime

Method

1. Preheat the oven to 200°C.
2. Smear the harissa on to the skin side of the chicken.
3. Season with salt and black pepper and drizzle a little coconut oil over the top.
4. Roast for 20–25 minutes. In the meantime, cook the rice. Measure your rice out in cups: if your 100g dried rice is equal to 1 cup, then add 1 cup of boiling water to it and then 1 cup of coconut milk. Add a pinch of salt and simmer for 12–15 minutes until almost cooked, then remove from the heat. Cover with a lid. Adding the coconut milk and then leaving it to rest will produce the perfect sticky rice.
5. While the chicken is cooling and the rice is resting, heat the remaining coconut oil in a wok, then add the vegetables and stir-fry for 2 minutes.
6. Add the coriander and lime juice.
7. Serve immediately. It's very simple, very quick and very tasty!

	Calories	Carbs	Fat	Protein
Total	935	53g	60g	48g
Per serving	935	53g	60g	48g

7-DAY HIGH FAT MEAL PLAN

HIGH FAT		
20% Protein	70% Fats	10% Carbs

	DAY 1	DAY 2	DAY 3	DAY 4	DAY 5	DAY 6	DAY 7
Breakfast	Avocado and scrambled eggs with crusty roll cooked with coconut oil	Full-fat Greek yogurt mixed with peanut butter	Smoked salmon, cream cheese and poached eggs	Full-fat English breakfast with avocadoes	Baked eggs with bacon and creamy kale	Simple omelette with spinach	Smoked salmon, avocado and poached egg
Lunch	Roasted veg and feta cheese salad (see below)	Chorizo, peppers and baked egg	Chicken skewers, peanut satay sauce and feta cheese salad	Loaded hasselback zucchini (with cheese, bacon and spring onions)	Chicken burger and veg	Chicken, cashew and spring onion stir-fry	Hummus, falafel and feta cheese salad
Snack	Dark chocolate peanut butter cups (see opposite)	Celery sticks dipped in almond butter	Vegan protein balls	Protein smoothie blended with almond butter	Hummus and carrot/celery sticks	Chicken pho soup (see below)	Green tea/ Coffee/Lady Grey tea mixed with a teaspoon of coconut oil
Dinner	Grilled seabass	Boiled egg, avocado and chickpea salad (see below)	Chicken meatballs with courgette and spinach	Grilled steak burger, veg and cashews	Fillet steak with sweet potato fries and greens	Venison burger with bacon, melted cheese and greens (see below)	Roasted butternut squash, goat's cheese, spinach and olive quiche
Snack	Chocolate and almond milk protein smoothie	Dark chocolate peanut butter cups	Almond and avocado smoothie	Smoked salmon, and poached egg	Coconut milk protein smoothie	Keto-friendly vegan chocolate tart	Simple omelette with spinach and avocado

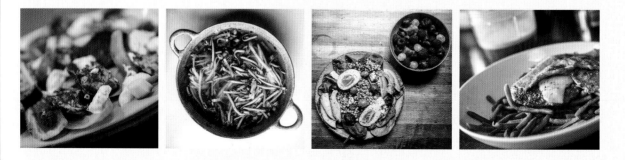

DARK CHOCOLATE PEANUT BUTTER CUPS
by Annie Mayne
7-day High Fat Best Meal

Simply the greatest snack you can have on a high-fat diet. Packed with healthy fats, these are practically a dessert and have so much energy crammed into every cup.

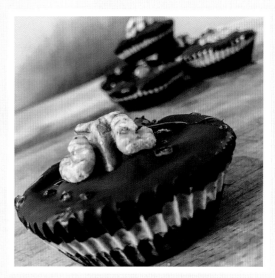

Ingredients

Makes 6

125g dark chocolate

2 tbsp (natural) peanut butter

2 tsp organic virgin coconut oil from THE PROTEIN WORKS™ (if this isn't your jam, substitute it with grass-fed butter instead. It has the same healthy fat which solidifies the peanut butter middles)

A small pinch of sea salt

6 walnut halves

Method

1. Melt the chocolate, either in the microwave or in a heatproof bowl over a pan of gently steaming water.

2. Stir until smooth, then use a spoon to drop a small amount of the chocolate into the bottom of 6 cupcake cases. (To ensure you don't have spillage, I recommend double layering the cases).

3. With the same spoon, push the chocolate up the sides of the case to create a cup. This will hold the mixture.

4. Place in the freezer for about 30 minutes.

5. In the meantime combine the peanut butter, coconut oil and salt. Stir until you get a smooth and creamy consistency.

6. Remove the chocolate cups from the freezer and add a dollop of peanut butter in the middle of each. If you can, try to leave some room around the sides so that the chocolate can cover the sides when filling. I have yet to master that, as demonstrated by my photo!

7. Cover each cup with a layer of melted chocolate, decorate with a walnut half and return to the freezer for about 2 hours, or longer if needed.

8. Remove the paper cups once set. Store in the freezer or fridge for best consistency.

	Calories	Carbs	Fat	Protein
Total	928	52g	91g	18g
Per serving	155	9g	15g	3g

CHAPTER 7
HOW TO GET BIG AND STRONG

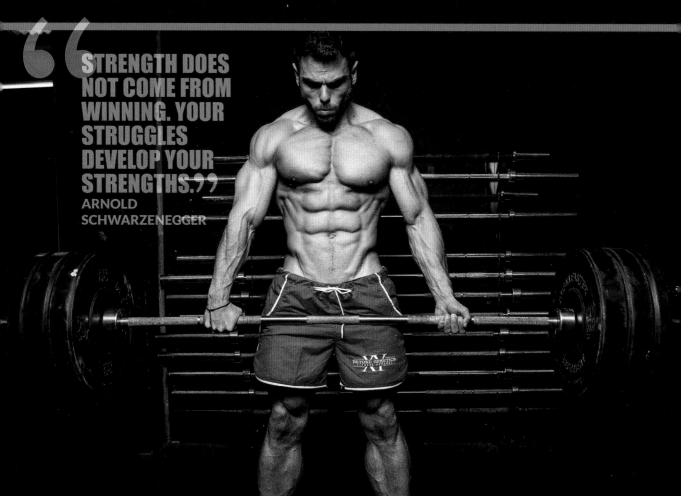

"STRENGTH DOES NOT COME FROM WINNING. YOUR STRUGGLES DEVELOP YOUR STRENGTHS."
ARNOLD SCHWARZENEGGER

HISTORY IN THE MAKING

'No citizen has a right to be an amateur in the matter of physical training… what a disgrace it is for a man to grow old without ever seeing the beauty and strength of which his body is capable.'

SOCRATES

There are many ways to build strength.

Olympic lifting, training with kettlebells, lifting dumbbells, and even using nothing but your own bodyweight will all produce improvements in strength. But when it comes to building pure maximal strength, most athletes know their squat, bench and deadlift. They're the three 'big lifts' that have long formed the backbone of many strength and conditioning routines.

Factor in the time-efficiency of barbell training – many lifters have built brutal strength with only a handful of heavy sets per week on each of the three lifts – and you realise that the powerlift rules when it comes to building maximal strength. So even if you don't compete at it, you have a deep-rooted respect for those who do. Those herculean men who bend bars, defy gravity and lift ridiculous amounts of iron off the floor. But among the long list of decorated champions and world record breakers there's one name that repeatedly pops up. That name is Andy Bolton.

Born on 22 January 1970 in Dewsbury, England, Andy himself is built like most things in Yorkshire – large, robust and insanely strong. Yes, this is partly down to genetics – you can't solely train and eat your way to a 182-cm, 160-kg (6-ft, 352-lb), muscle-bound frame. But what's amazing about Andy is that he's an absolute scholar of strength. Ever modest, he says 'I won't bore you with all the details, other than I started strength training at 18 years old and have been doing so for over 20 years. In fact, I've been competing in powerlifting for over 20 years. Over the course of my career, I have always spent a lot of time learning. I've read hundreds of books and articles on strength training. I've been to dozens of seminars and worked with some of the world's best strength coaches.'

Basically, Andy was gifted with raw strength, but is equally the sum and substance of over 20 years of research and methodology that formed this endless pursuit to be the strongest man ever to lift a barbell.

Was he the strongest?

I'm slightly biased. Andy's been a good friend of mine for years. He was there for my first 290-kg deadlift, 280-kg squat and 180-kg bench. So anything I write I acknowledge is slightly influenced by the 'time under the iron' we've shared.

But personal loyalties aside, seven WPC World Champion titles, two WPO Champion titles and a place cemented in history as the first human to ever deadlift 1000 lb (455 kg) strongly suggests so. So for all these reasons let me detail what I've been lucky enough to learn from training with one of the strongest humans in history.

Which all begins by reliving the most famous day in powerlifting history.

Andy Bolton | The World's First 1000-lb Deadlift

The date is 4 November 2006. The location is the WPO Semi-finals in Lake George, New York.

Heavy metal music is thunderously broadcast from some heavy-duty speakers. It merges with the noise of the frenzied crowd and the commentator can barely be heard. He doesn't need to be. Everyone in that building knows what's about to be attempted is historic. Words aren't needed.

1003 lb – 71½ stone – 455 kg is placed on the bar.

Without a moment's hesitation Andy steps onto the lifting platform. The crowd cheers. He lifts. Then, for one epoch-making moment, the bar seems to defy the laws of physics and physiology. It leaves the ground and the crowd erupts in a state of lifting elation. Catharsis is complete. Large men run on stage hugging other incredibly large men.

Andy stands there. His back blue from all the blood vessels that have nearly exploded through his skin as the commentator shouts over the cheers of spectators, 'You can always tell your grandchildren… where you were… when Andy Bolton lifted A THOUSAND FREAKIN' THREE!'

Was Andy emotional? Yes. Very. Was he surprised? No, not in the slightest.

Some time after that day he told me, 'For 19 years, all my life had been geared to that moment. Even when I wasn't training for it I was living it. Eating for it. Studying for it. I even thought about it in my sleep.'

He would always add, 'If I didn't make that lift it would have almost not made sense to me. I was so sure I was going to do it. Not one doubt ever entered my head. So when I stood there in front of everyone with 1003 pounds in my hand it just felt normal.'

After the lift social media erupted. Everyone sensed they'd just seen something special.

This is because raising a weight from the ground is one of humanity's oldest trials of strength. It's arguably the most primitive display of human power and now Andy can lay claim to being the greatest in history.

With a deep respect for Strongman pioneers like Geoff Capes, Andy says, 'The "strongest man" guys are amazing. I can't pick something up and run with it like they can. But they're strength athletes. When it comes to picking it up to start with, no one's stronger. Deadlifting is a test of true strength, without involving other things like stamina and balance.'

I of course wouldn't argue with either. Fortunately I didn't have to, as this chapter fuses the teachings of both.

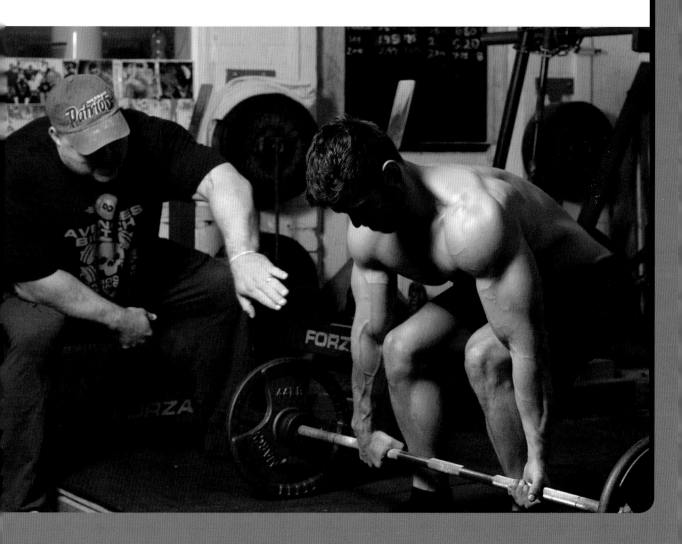

The Strength, Speed and Power Pyramid of Priority

Strength, speed and power are closely related. You must understand this if you are to become a bigger, stronger and more powerful version of yourself. This is because:

- Strength is the body's ability to generate force.
- Speed is the rate at which someone moves.
- Power is the product of strength and speed.

Now you can't be powerful if you're not fast, which is why…

- Those who are naturally strong need to work on getting faster.
- Those who are naturally fast need to work on getting stronger.

How do we become more powerful? By following The Strength, Speed and Power Pyramid of Priority, and dedicating time to maximal strength training, plyometric training and ballistic training – something we do over this chapter and the next with some of the strongest and fastest humans in history.

HOW TO USE IT

This is a hierarchical (progressive) way that illustrates how to focus your efforts.

- The lower parts make the biggest difference to your strength.
- The higher parts make a meaningful contribution to your speed, and therefore, power.

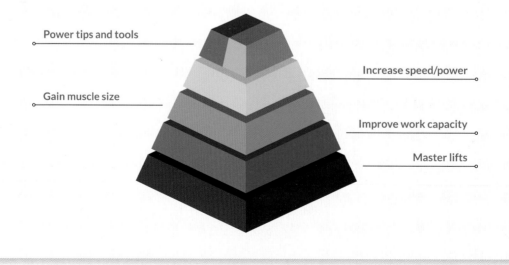

To keep things simple and focused on the training aspects, I have excluded food from the pyramid. But read back over 'Finding Your Fuel' (page 152) and 'Protein' (page 148) and the recipes for the World's Strongest Marathon and Tree-athlon (pages 61, 221 and 223) if you're unclear about the key role nutrition plays in becoming stronger.

The top part of this (and every pyramid) is infinite and forever evolving. This is why they are all open-ended and may never have a peak, because our understanding and exploration of the human body should never be 'capped' or concluded.

This is of course theoretical. It varies from person to person. There are also other things to consider, like joint health and age-related factors. But if you master lifts, improve work capacity, increase muscle size and increase speed and power you will become a stronger bigger, faster and more powerful version of yourself.

It's that simple…

MASTERING LIFTS

TRAINING FOR STRENGTH

It's 6 December 2010, four years after Andy's historic lift.

At this moment in my life I am obsessed with strength. All my training in the gym and everything I ate in the kitchen was designed to make me a more powerful version of my current self. I was bench pressing 170 kg, squatting 230 kg and deadlifting 260 kg, but was far from content, which is why Andy had invited me to train at Rall's gym in Leeds, England.

A sacred place of strength, it is where this chapter was written and is also where Andy had trained for over 20 years. Hidden away down the backstreets, it's nestled between a boxing gym and a car mechanic's and would be hard to find if it wasn't for the huge men outside flipping giant tyres and lifting inhumane amounts of iron.

Walking through the doors the entire gym exudes what I call 'Yorkshire hospitality'. It's hard to explain, but what I mean by this is your first visit will feel like a firm handshake. You're basically very welcome to train, but don't expect any bells, whistles or designer brands. This is a place completely void of pomp and pretence. Everything and everyone is real, raw and honest.

You will find no ornaments, only instruments.

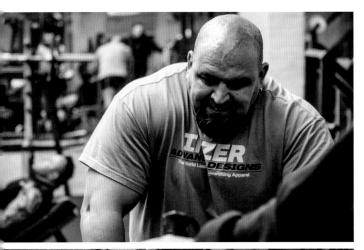

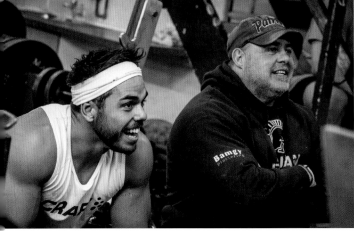

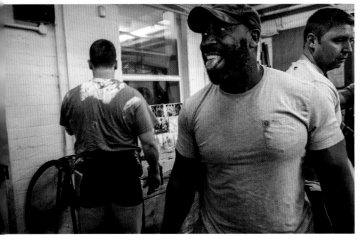

Me, Andy and the team throwing some iron plates around

This explains why the grey paint peels off the walls, also why there are holes in the roof that leak when it rains. Basically, if there is any spare budget it will be spent on new equipment or just more weight. Everything has a purpose. Nothing is unnecessary and peeling paint and leaking roofs won't stop you getting stronger.

But the tour was over and it was now time for Andy to introduce me to my new training partners.

THE WORLD'S STRONGEST TRAINING PARTNERS

The strongest squad I've lifted with…

There was no hierarchy and no ego. But when Andy spoke everyone listened. Forgoing any formalities, it took him exactly five seconds to initiate me into the group:

'This is Ross. He's lifting with us today,' he said as he unpacked his knee wraps from his bag.

Ten very large men nodded affirmatively in my direction.

Among them were Mark Steele and Romanian-born Lighean Marian Aurel. Both standing 193 cm and easily weighing over 130 kg, they were instantly recognisable. Bursting onto the scene of Strongman, they had both stormed through the British Championships and now every strength-based gym all over country knew their names.

They were also the two gentlemen previously seen outside throwing giant tractor tyres around.

Also there was the 125-kg World Powerlifting champion Dave Carter. For every year between 1988 and 2007 – except for 1996 and 1998 – he held the deadlift world record. He was also the only man I've ever seen pause midway through lifting 330 kg and smile to everyone in attendance. In short, squads don't come much stronger than this, which is why I'm so nervous.

Stepping into the old, rusty squat rack my first lift would determine if I was granted a second invite back to Rall's gym. 200 kg was loaded onto the bar and onto my shoulders… along with the weight of expectation.

Taking a deep breath, I unracked the bar. Adopting a solid stance, my shins were vertical and heels planted to the floor. As I lowered the weight the 'crease of my hip' finally hit just below the top of my knee. Ladies and gentlemen, I was now 'in the hole'. A lonely place at the bottom of the squat where the only person you can rely upon is yourself. It's also a place you don't want to dwell too long.

If you do, you may never get out.

Still holding my breath, I keep my abs tight. Back is straight, shoulders are back and head is forward. Beginning my ascent, my technique was far from pretty, but at least the bar was moving. Success. I was out of 'the hole'. Finishing the lift wasn't pretty. It was slow and I grinded out the lift before locking out. It's what we call a 'bar fight'. Basically, my maiden lift at Rall's was done purely on nerves, adrenaline and pride, and was void of any good technique. I look to Andy for approval, but I already know the verdict.

'What was that?' he said, laughing.

'Last time I checked it was called a squat,' I replied.

'It looked like a squat, but that definitely wasn't a squat,' he said with his giant arm around my shoulder. 'You're quite strong, but you'll only ever lift so much with raw strength. We've lots of work to do on your technique if you're to ever lift to a serious standard, but it's not a bad start.'

There aren't many places where a 200-kg squat is deemed 'a good start', but I didn't mind. I was the runt of a very strong litter and I was OK with that. I received a second nod of approval from the team and an open invite back to Leeds.

The dilapidated gym was my new home.

The secret to strength

It's not **what** you lift, but **how** you lift.

See, strength – at its most basic level – can be defined as a muscle's ability to produce force. Well, this force can vary greatly throughout a particular lift and range of movement. To keep things simple, let's continue with the squat example.

The force generated by the muscles to 'lock out' the final part of the squat will be very different to the force needed to get out of 'the hole' at the bottom of the lift. Basically, muscle force and tension vary throughout all movements. So for you to become strong during a particular lift, it's:

Your muscles' ability to generate force combined with coordinated neuromuscular activation.

Or, put simply, how effective you are at generating force at the right times during the lift.

From 'lock out' to 'the hole', technique is everything, and there's a huge skill to the squat, bench and deadlift, which is why incredibly specific, highly frequent and utterly purposeful practice will mean the faster your nervous system will master and store the movement pattern.

Even Andy had to refine and perfect this over years.

On this note, a story cemented in strength folklore surrounds a 19-year-old Andy Bolton. A trainee roofer at the time, he walked into the gym having never seen a barbell and ripped a 260-kg (573-lb) deadlift off the floor. It was insane, natural, pure strength.

But even when gifted with this genetic strength advantage he knew he needed specific, purposeful practice to add another 195 kg (430 lb) onto his lift to become the first man in history to raise 1003 lb above his knees.

'Training can be defined as the process by which genetic potential is realised. In conclusion, elite-sporting performance is the result of the interaction between genetic and training factors.'
BRITISH JOURNAL OF SPORTS MEDICINE[1]

So that's what he did. After 20 years his nervous system had mastered lifting patterns better than anyone else in history. He had successfully practised himself strong.

FIVE WAYS TO PRACTISE YOURSELF STRONG

1. Visualise every lift

Visualise how the movement is supposed to look and feel. Imagine as many details as possible. How the bar feels in your hands, the weight on your feet and load on your back. Andy would often tell me he'd dreamed of that 1000 lb over a million times. It was so well ingrained in his central nervous system that when he did it the entire lift just felt normal. He'd perfected this visualisation over years.

After the set, analyse it. How did it feel? How did it look? What could be improved upon? Repeat that process for each set.

Simply doing the movements helps, but to gain proficiency with the lifts as quickly as possible, practice needs to be deep and purposeful to cement the skills and keep bad habits from developing.

2. Lift without ego

When starting out, remove your ego.

Again, it's not **what** you lift, but **how** you lift. The weights you use need to be light enough that you're in control of the load, yet heavy enough to force the body to perform the correct movement pattern. A loaded barbell squat is very different to an unloaded bodyweight squat. So although there's no set, concrete law, generally speaking, coaches recommend using a weight between 60–80% of your 1-repetition maximum.

If you're a complete beginner and don't know what your 1-repetition maximum is, just identify the heaviest weight that you feel very comfortable with and then work with 15% less than that.

3. Always lift, never fail

If you're just learning to lift you need to avoid failure on your sets.

The more you struggle and strain to grind out a repetition, the more your technique breaks down. For example, let's say you're doing sets of five. The first three might be beautiful. Your form might be immaculate and the repetitions flawless. On the fourth set you might feel the form breaking down. You're wobbly and shaky. But by the fifth set your technique looks barely recognisable from the first three.

You're ingraining the proper motor pattern you want to learn with 60% of your work. But you're ingraining something completely different with the other 40%. That means it will take longer to master the proper technique. By staying at least three repetitions away from failure you continue to make this form of incredibly specific, highly frequent and utterly purposeful practice useful.

Worth noting is that to get in enough work while avoiding failure – work capacity – performing multiple sets of low repetitions is best. The fewer reps you do each set, the less fatigue you'll develop from your first rep to your last rep, and the shorter the time you need to be locked in and focused on your technique will be.

4. Don't dilute your strength

If you dilute your training, you dilute your strength.

This links back to Chapter 2 and the SAID principle (Specific Adaptation to Imposed Demands). Your body will adapt specifically to the demands you place on it, which is why it makes perfect sense that if you want to get stronger you should probably practise strong stuff.

This is also related to the work of Robert Hickson and his idea of 'concurrent training'.

For those not familiar with concurrent training, this is where an athlete trains more than one fitness component (strength, speed or stamina) at equal amounts of focus, all within the same workout. In Hickson's view – supported by research from the field of molecular biology and his own experiences – this approach will produce less than optimal results.

To understand this, here's a brief backstory.

Robert Hickson was a keen powerlifter who had followed a traditional strength-training protocol for most of his athletic career. This was until he went to study in the laboratory of Professor John Holloszy. Holloszy is considered the 'father of endurance exercise research' and every lunchtime he would leave the Washington University Medical Campus and run through the nearby Forest Park.

Keen to make a good impression, Hickson decided to break from his usual training protocol and accompany Holloszy. But weeks into his new routine he discovered the strength and size of his muscles were decreasing. This was despite the fact that he was still doing his strength training at the same frequency and intensity. When Hickson approached Holloszy with his strength and conditioning dilemma, Holloszy suggested this should be his first study.

So, in his new laboratory at the University of Illinois in Chicago, that's exactly what he did.[2]

In an article published in 1980 in the *European Journal of Applied Physiology and Occupational Physiology*,[3] Hickson concluded that concurrent training dilutes your effectiveness to improve a specific component of fitness (e.g. strength or stamina). Your body doesn't know whether to become stronger or more enduring, since the 'potency' of your training a specific component is lost.

It's not important to understand the intricacies of each for now. Just know that, according to research from the Division of Molecular Physiology at the University of Dundee, strength training and endurance training bring about very different adaptations within the body. Combining both forms of training 'blocks each other's signalling' to adapt.

5. Get 'tight' to get strong

Andy often says 'The secret to becoming instantly stronger is tightness'.

This sounds odd, I know. But for all the lectures I've attended on the topic of sport biomechanics, Andy has a unique way of keeping things so simple. When he says 'tightness' he's referring to your body's ability to get tight, rigid and strong when you squat, bench and deadlift.

Here's why this is important. The tighter you get, the more force you generate, and the more force you generate, the more weight you can lift. Why? It's all because of Sherrington's Law of Irradiation. This law states that when you contract one muscle hard, the muscles around it and connected to it contract hard as well. Now you can see why anyone who thinks the bench press is a 'chest exercise' or that the squat is a 'quad' exercise is sadly mistaken and throwing strength away for free.

The idea of isolating certain body parts is not the way to go if you want to build maximal strength.

'A muscle working hard recruits the neighbouring muscles and if they are already part of the action it amplifies their strength. The neural impulses emitted by the contracting muscle reach other muscles and "turn them on" as an electric current starts a motor.'
SHERRINGTON'S LAW OF IRRADIATION

Which is why the squat, bench and deadlift are total body exercises. From this point forwards treat them as such and embrace 'tightness'. Commit to tensing your body as hard as possible on every set and every rep you perform. If you do this, you will be rewarded with instant strength gains and the quickest possible strength gains from week to week.

THE SQUAT

'The squat is a great lower-body developer, but – as you just found out – it's really a total body exercise, working every muscle you have, albeit with an emphasis on the legs.'
ANDY BOLTON

People are squatting wrong. According to Andy 'Too many complain about back pain, knee pain and even shoulder and elbow pain when squatting. I'd say 95% are doing it wrong.

But if people spent more time learning the right technique, as opposed to just mindlessly pumping out the reps, they could squat pain free. Improving strength and reducing injury at the same time.'

Enter Andy's Three-point Squat Plan:

- How to set up.
- How to lower the weight.
- How to lift the weight.

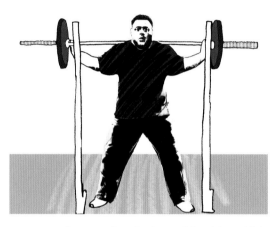

How to set up

When the bar is in the rack position, it should be in line with your mid-chest.

Too high and you have to calf-raise it off the rack, too low and you have to do a quarter squat to unrack the bar. Neither option works safely, especially as you get stronger and the weights get heavier.

Grip the bar with the narrowest grip you can that doesn't cause elbow pain (you'll have to experiment with this).

Step under the bar with a hip-width stance, placing your feet directly under the bar. Your shoulders should be pulled back and down, your chest should be out, your upper back tight and your lower back in a neutral position.

Take a deep breath of air, get as tight as you can and unrack the bar.

To unrack it, simply stand straight up with it. Now step back 20–25 cm (4–6 inches) with your left foot and then do the same with your right foot.

Your stance should be shoulder width or slightly wider, your toes turned out somewhere between 5 and 35 degrees depending on your flexibility.

You are now ready to squat.

How to lower the weight

Pause. Take some air in. Get as tight as possible.

Push your knees out slightly and 'sit back' as you descend.

Aim to keep your shins as vertical as possible. They will shift forwards somewhat, but should feel like they stay pretty vertical.

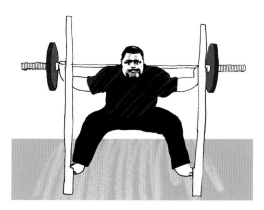

Under no circumstances should your heels leave the floor.

When the crease of your hip is just below the top of your knee (when viewed from the side) you have hit the bottom of the squat… you are 'in the hole'.

How to lift the weight

Do not breathe out when you're in the hole. This will cause you to lose tightness and therefore you'll lose strength and greatly increase your injury risk. Keep the abs as tight as possible and squeeze the bar hard.

As you come up, avoid letting your knees cave in and carry on looking straight ahead or slightly up.

Keep your upper back tight with your shoulders back and down throughout.

When you reach lockout, stay tight.

Take in more air and either step forwards and rack the bar or descend into another rep.

On the descent, move as quickly as you can while maintaining complete control of the bar (Note: This may not actually be very quick at all.)

On the ascent, drive the bar upwards as hard and as fast as you possibly can. Think speed, speed, speed. That said, never compromise technique for speed. Nail your technique first and then add speed in once you become a competent and efficient squatter.

THE BENCH PRESS

'Every man (and some women) wants a bigger bench. Who hasn't been asked the famous question: How much do you bench?'
ANDY BOLTON

The first step towards building a massive bench press is (again) technique.

Andy says 'The way most bodybuilders (even the pros) and most gym rats bench is a disaster. The typical 'flat back, flared elbows, touching the upper chest' style of benching is a nightmare for the shoulders. It beats them up and will lead to injury sooner or later. I've seen it happen too many times. Not only that, it's weak, too.'

He adds, 'There's only one way a self-respecting human being should bench and that's powerlifting style. Don't worry, it'll build just as much muscle as the style that destroys your shoulders, but it'll also let you lift way more weight and massively reduce the risk of injury.'

Enter Andy's Three-point Bench Press Plan...

- How to set up.
- How to lower the weight.
- How to lift the weight.

How to set up

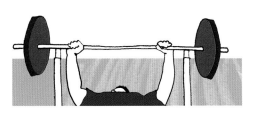

Lie on the bench so your eyes are directly under the bar.

Grip the bar with your hands slightly wider than shoulder-width apart. If you have a history of shoulder pain or injuries, take a narrower grip – index fingers 2.5 cm (1 in) from the smooth part of the bar.

Spread your feet as wide as you can, drive your knees out and tense your glutes as hard as possible. This creates a stable base. (Think in terms of a pyramid – they didn't build them with a narrow base so you shouldn't bench with a narrow stance either.)

Pinch your shoulder blades together and force your chest out to create a slight arch in your back. (The more you arch the shorter the range of motion, but the greater the risk of back injury.) However high you decide to arch, your shoulder blades must be pulled back and down and your chest must be forced out.

(No 'flat back' benching allowed here – it's rough on the shoulders.)

Take a deep breath into your belly, and with the help of a spotter if necessary, contract your lats hard and pull the bar out of the rack. Pull it out until it's directly over your nipple line.

You're now in the start position and ready to take the bar for a ride.

How to lower the weight

While you push your feet into the floor, drive your knees out and keep your glutes as tight as possible.

Bring the bar down in a straight line so that it touches your nipple line.

As you descend, grip the bar, keep your lats tight and ensure your shoulders stay back and down. Do not bounce the bar off your chest.

Maintain control at all times.

How to lift the weight

As the bar touches your chest, ensure everything is tight.

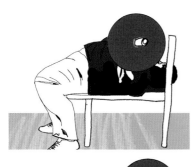

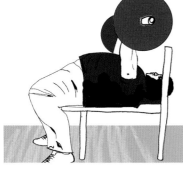

Holding your breath, immediately drive the bar off your chest and towards lockout.

Push the bar in a straight line or slightly towards your face. Do not push it way back towards your face, as this can be rough on the shoulders.

If you want, breathe out at the sticking point – while keeping tight. Otherwise, breathe out a little at the top.

Take in some more air and descend into another rep.

THE DEADLIFT

'The deadlift is a brutal test of strength. There's a bar on the floor; your mission is simply to grab it with straight arms and then stand up straight with it in your hands.'
ANDY BOLTON

In theory the deadlift sounds pretty simple, but the first thing I learnt from Andy was that when pulling big weights, the reality is very different. 'There's very little margin for error. When shifting a lot of poundage you can injure your back and pop a bicep faster than you can imagine,' he says. 'But learn the correct technique and those dangers can be more or less eliminated.'

Enter Andy's Three-point Deadlift Plan:

- • How to set up.
- • How to lift the weight.
- • How to lower the weight.

How to set up

Approach the bar with a hip-width stance.

Point your toes straight ahead or turn them out very slightly.

Be sure to deadlift wearing lifting slippers or go barefoot.

Relax your upper back. Keep your lower back neutral and hinge at the hips. Then (with little knee bend) lower yourself to the bar.

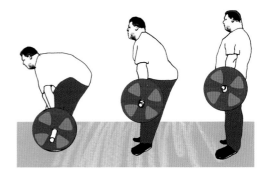

Take a deep breath of air into your belly and pull yourself down to the bar until it's touching your shins and your hamstrings feel tight and loaded. Your upper back can be rounded, but your lower back must still be in a safe, neutral position.

At this point you have two choices:

Grip Option 1: Use the Olympic lifting hook grip. The hook grip is double overhand, but the index and middle fingers cover the thumb. This is pretty uncomfortable at first, but you'll get used to it.

Or… **Grip Option 2:** Use the powerlifting style mixed grip where one hand is in the same overhand position as the double overhand grip, but the other hand is under the bar, palm facing backwards. If you use this mixed grip, be sure to switch hand placement on every set to avoid uneven upper back development.

How to lift the weight

Now, with a firm grip, drive the bar off the floor as hard as you can, keeping the bar as close to your body as possible.

When the bar gets just past your knees, drive your glutes forwards to lock the bar out. Stand perfectly erect at lockout – do not lean back.

How to lower the weight

Take a sip of air and descend quickly.

Alternatively, drop the bar, reset your stance and grip, and pull another rep.

GETTING STARTED WITH STRENGTH TRAINING
FREQUENTLY ASKED QUESTIONS

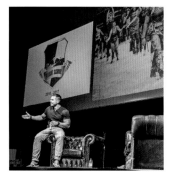

'I've built my 1214-lb squat, 775-lb bench and 1008-lb deadlift by writing my own strength-training programmes. Believe me, it took about 10 years of trial and error to get really good at writing strength-training programmes that produce results for me and those I coach.'

ANDY BOLTON

Throughout 2017 I was asked to talk… a lot.

The format was typically the same. I'd be put on stage. Handed a microphone and a can of Red Bull. Then I'd speak for hours fuelled on copious amounts of caffeine and questions from the crowd. But interestingly, at every event I would always get asked the same question from someone new to training:

'How do I start strength training?'

Which is why, when sat in the armchair during a talk to sports science students, I decided to write the four simple objectives your first strength training should serve to achieve.

- To make strength training a habit.
- To increase work capacity so you're able to train and positively recover from workouts.
- To build kinaesthetic and muscular awareness and to 'know your body'.
- To become proficient with the movements.

It's that simple, which is why your first workout shouldn't be too rigid. Instead, as long as it achieves the above and follows the principles of the Beginner's Strength Plan below, you'll get stronger.

THE BEGINNER'S STRENGTH PLAN

1. How many sessions per week?

Generally speaking, training each lift 2–4 times per week is best. Note the word 'generally' since (again and as always) this doesn't account for biological individuality. But the reason for this is because firstly, you need enough time to practise those movements. Secondly, the repair and regrowth of the muscles – a process known as muscle protein synthesis – stays elevated for new lifters for 36–48 hours.

So 2–4 sessions per lift, per week, means you're spending a lot of time actually building muscle. Once you've mastered the above there's no point continuing with your 'training wheels' and 'L plates'.

You'll just plateau and end up bored since most of the strength gains you make on a beginner's programme come from neurological improvements – your nervous system learning the lifts you're doing.

2. How fast will I improve?

When you first start training it's possible you have enough muscle to squat 100 kg (220 lb).

But in reality, you can only squat 75 kg (165 lb) since your nervous system doesn't 'understand' the lift yet. You haven't learnt those motor patterns. But as the weeks progress you should be able to add lots more to the bar – weekly – until you're warming up on 100 kg.

Your muscle mass may only have increased by 10–20%, but your squat went up to a much greater degree because your nervous system adapts to stressors much faster than your muscles do. When you hit a wall and your lifts stop going up as quickly, it's because you're finally bumping up against the limits of how much you can lift with your current muscle mass.

To continue getting stronger you must move up a class and graduate to intermediate.

3. How soon can I add serious weight?

It, of course, varies from person to person.

But as mentioned before, your primary goal when first training should be to practise the skills of strength with 60–80% of your 1 repetition maximum. Stick with this weight until you no longer see improvements week on week and begin to struggle and 'grind out' the lift. This means the easy strength progress you get from gaining proficiency with the lifts is about to run out, so it's time for a change.

This could be anywhere between two and four months.

Also, it can happen for different lifts at different times. Is your bench progress slowing, while your squat and deadlift are still shooting up? Then change your bench training, but keep training your squat and deadlift the same way until they too are maxed out. But once it does, you need to learn how to use the basic Repetition/Weight Scheme.

4. Calculate your One-Rep Max (1RM)

You don't have to actually test your 1RM to know it.

This is good news since testing it every week would leave you exhausted. Instead, the basic table on the left can help you estimate the percentage of your 1RM you should be using to achieve a certain amount of repetitions in your workout. To keep things simple, if you bench press 100 kg for 1 repetition then (based on the table) you should be able to perform 4 repetitions with 90 kg, 8 repetitions with 80 kg and so on.

Some workouts are set up differently.

They might detail the number of repetitions you should be performing. That's fine; instead, you look at the number of repetitions and then use the corresponding percentage of your 1RM. You're simply using the table below to do the conversion in a slightly different way.

Remember that each exercise has its own one-rep max.

These are only estimates. The lower your rep count, the more accurate your one-rep max estimate will be.

Calculate your one-rep max (1RM)

Repetitions	% one-rep max (1RM)
1	100
2	95
3	93
4	90
5	87
6	85
7	83
8	80
9	77
10	75
11	73
12	70

THE WORLD'S FITTEST BOOK | 199

Do you need more muscle?

'To feel strong, to walk amongst humans with a tremendous feeling of confidence and superiority is not at all wrong. The sense of superiority in bodily strength is borne out by the long history of mankind paying homage in folklore, song and poetry to strong men.'

FRED HATFIELD, Powerlifting: A Scientific Approach

To answer this question you need to understand two forms of strength.[4]

Absolute strength: This is the greatest force that can be produced by a given muscle under involuntary stimulation. Note the word 'involuntary' as this is commonly measured through electrical stimulation of the nerves supplying the muscles to make them contract as hard and as powerfully as humanly possible. Yes, I've done this in the lab. Yes, I can confirm it's not pleasant.

Competitive strength: The ability of the muscles to produce the greatest force possible through a voluntary contraction. This time note the word 'voluntary' since this is performed during competition and it's not surprising this isn't as powerful as being electrocuted. Instead it's the maximum force you can produce simply by getting psyched up.

The difference between these two is known as your **strength deficit**.

If there's a small difference between them it shows you're using the muscle mass you have to its full neurological potential. Basically, all your muscle fibres are being used and firing.

You're 80 kg (176 lb) but squatting 200 kg (440 lb). You've a good power-to-weight ratio. You're maxing out your muscles' neurological potential. You're like a scooter that's managing to reach 70 mph with the small 'engine' (muscle) working overtime and you need to add more muscle to get stronger. You need more Structural Strength Training.

But, if there's a big difference between them it shows you're not using your muscle mass to its full, neurological potential and all the muscle fibres aren't being recruited.

You're 100 kg (220 lb) and squatting 150 kg (330 lb). You've a bad power-to-weight ratio. You're like a supercar car with a giant engine that's being driven at 50 mph. You are not using your muscle mass to its full, neurological potential and need to drill technique to do this. You need more Functional Strength Training.

So, are you a scooter or a supercar?

When you know the answer you will be better able to design your training programme and decide whether you need to get big, strong or both. Worth noting is that strength training is always a combination of Structural and Functional Strength Training, but if you know your Strength Deficit you will know which one to focus on.

USE YOUR 'TRAINING STRENGTH'

Finally, scientists identified a third kind of strength.

Training strength: Typically measured by your single-repetition maximum. This is the weight that – in the training room – you can lift for one repetition on the squat, bench or deadlift, but without 'substantial emotional excitement' like your 'competitive strength'.

The difference between competitive strength and training strength is therefore **intensity**.

Intensity is defined as a certain percentage of someone's maximum lift. Working off your competitive strength might not be a great idea since the high levels of nervous and emotional stress incurred require days or even weeks to recover from. For this reason – and remembering the Law of Progressive Overload – it's far better to work with your training strength maximum.

To quote Andy, 'Always lift but never fail. Leave a rep in the tank.'

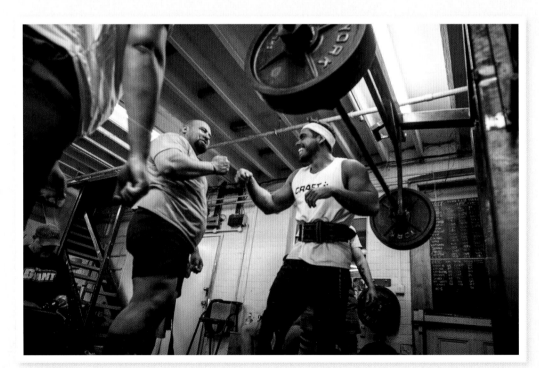

MORE MUSCLE OR MORE STRENGTH?

FIND OUT WHAT YOU NEED

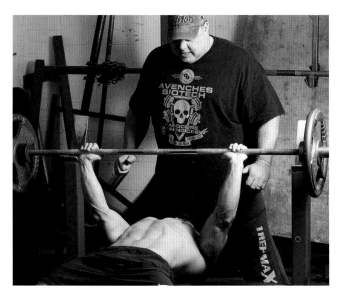

'Discipline is doing what you hate to do, but nonetheless doing it like you love it.'
MIKE TYSON

It's 15 December 2011 and one year since my first visit to Leeds.

For 12 months I had religiously spent, 'time under the iron' practising my lifts. Eating and sleeping powerlifting, I was now (semi) competent and would perform quite well on the international stage for my weight. All because, as Andy had promised, I had practised myself stronger, adding 10 kg to my bench (180 kg), 50 kg to my squat (280 kg) and 30 kg to my deadlift (290 kg).

Which meant there was good news and bad news.

The bad news is all the 'low-hanging fruit' had been picked. I was now relatively well drilled in lifts, and motor patterns had all been learnt. As a result I was now fresh out of those gains in strength that come from neurological improvements, technique and practice that saw me improve week on week.

So what's the good news?

Basically, I had graduated. I was now capable of walking into any strength-based gym in the world and putting up impressive numbers. But now it was time to get bigger and stronger. My focus under the bar should be to:

- Continue making small and gradual improvements in strength that come from refining technique.
- Increase work capacity.
- Avoid injury.
- Increase muscle mass.

Putting pen to paper we began writing programmes, each governed by these goals.

1. Increase strength | More practice

You can always perfect your technique.

So now would be a good time to change the training intensity of your main lifts. To do this make sure you do very little work below 70% of your one-rep max and very little above 90% one-rep max. Do this to continue improving your technique and skill lifting heavy weights.

Next, try keeping the volume for your main lifts low to moderate and (again) don't fail.

Leave a repetition or two 'in the tank'. This is because your main lifts will put a lot of strain on the body (leaving you 'beat up'), which can then limit how much total training volume you can handle per session and per week. But in reality, you don't need lots of high-quality, heavy work to improve neurological factors. That's why this type of training is known as Functional Strength Training. It's powerlifting-centric training, used to improve the muscles' strength.

2. Increase strength | Work capacity

This was well covered in Chapter 5 so I won't repeat myself.

Instead, just note how much of a recurring theme it is and aim to include more variety in your workouts. Not only will this allow you to focus and work harder on your main lifts, it's also less boring and increases work capacity. So learn to front squat, overhead press, close-grip bench, pause squat, sumo deadlift and don't be afraid of 'bodybuilding-centric' movements.

Yes, that means bicep curls aren't just for the beach.

3. Increase strength | Avoid injury

Closely related to bodybuilding-centric movements and work capacity is injury prevention.

There is always the risk of injury as you push the body to become bigger, stronger and more powerful, but a major reason to make your training more 'bodybuilding-centric' is that bodybuilding-style training has a very low injury rate compared to other strength-based sports.

If you look at the table opposite you'll see a list of studies that detail the different injury rates in strength-based sports. Studies were only included where an injury rate per 1000 hours of training was calculated and presented.[5 6 7 8 9 10 11 12]

Study	Sport	Injury rate per 1000 hours	Most common regions
Winwood	Strongman	5.50	Low back
Keogh (2006)	Powerlifting	4.40	Shoulder
Quinney (1997)	Powerlifting	3.70	Low back
Calhoun (1999)	Olympic weightlifting	3.30	Low back
Hak (2013)	CrossFit	3.10	Shoulder
Raske and Norlin (2000)	Olympic weightlifting	2.60	Low back
Raske and Norlin (2000)	Powerlifting	2.60	Shoulder
Haykowsky (1999)	Powerlifting	1.10	Low back and shoulder
Siewe (2011)	Powerlifting	1.00	Shoulder
Eberhardt (2007)	Bodybuilding	1.00	Not specified
Brown (1986)	Powerlifting	0.84	Shoulder
Siewe (2014)	Bodybuilding	0.24	Shoulder

4. Increase strength with muscle mass

The strongest athletes are often the biggest too.

Generally speaking, they have large muscles and they know how to use them. This is supported in thousands of studies, including one published in *The European Journal of Applied Physiology*[13] that found muscle thickness was strongly correlated to elite powerlifters' performance in all three lifts.

The Journal of Sports Medicine and Physical Fitness[14] agrees, and found one of the strongest predictors of strength in national-level lifters was muscle mass per unit height. Bigger is (often) stronger.

Basically, think of muscle mass as potential strength.

If you gain mass, you may not get stronger right away, but you have the potential to be. If you stay the same size, you have a cap on how strong you can get. Which is why bodybuilding-centric training can (again) be so valuable and why this type of training is called Structural Strength Training. It's bodybuilding-centric training, used to improve muscle size.

This is why it's wise to get most of your training volume from 'accessory', bodybuilding-centric lifts for major muscle groups by performing sets of 10–20 repetitions for 3–5 sets and training each muscle/movement two to three times per week.

Many coaches recommend accessory lifts over lighter sets of bench, squat and deadlift to keep training specificity high for the main lifts. This is because lifting lighter weights for higher repetitions develops a different motor pattern than lifting heavier weights for lower repetitions.

You (again) don't want to 'dilute' your main lifts.

How do we make muscle?

There are three ways to build muscle. These can be identified as **Mechanical Tension**, **Metabolic Stress** and **Muscle Damage**. Each comes with their own set of advantages, but worth noting is that muscular humans throughout history had learnt to use all three, either in a single workout or 'cycling' through them over the course of a week/month.

	Mechanical Tension	Metabolic Stress	Muscle Damage
Description	Mechanical Tension is created when the muscle generates force to lift heavy things.	Metabolic Stress ('the pump') is created by maintaining constant tension on the muscles by reversing directions just short of 'lockout'.	Muscle Damage is created by slow negatives, extended range of motion and high tension in the stretched position of the muscle.
(Most) used by	Powerlift	Bodybuilding	CrossFit
Maxim	'Just lift heavy things'	'Get a good pump'	'Mix it up and shock the body'
How to train it (Training variables)	Weight used: 80–90% 1RM	Weight used: 60–70% 1RM	Weight used: 70–80% 1RM
	Sets: 3–8	Sets: 3–4	Sets: 2–5 (depending on frequency)
	Repetitions: 3–8	Repetitions: 12–20+ (to failure)	Repetitions: 8–12
	Rest: 2–3 minutes	Rest: Less than 60 seconds	Rest: 1–2 minutes

Build muscle | Mechanical tension and metabolic stress

Mechanical Tension and Metabolic Stress compete in a tug-of-war.

More of one typically means less of the other. This is because when you add weight to the bar you generate more forces and therefore create more Mechanical Tension in the muscles. But this also means you can't do as many repetitions. Therefore Metabolic Stress in the muscles is lower.

Lower the weight on the bar and the opposite happens. You're now able to perform more repetitions and produce more Metabolic Stress. But with less weight you can't generate as much force, therefore Mechanical Tension in the muscles is lower.

Which is why so many bodybuilders use a variety of lifts to target both. Or will use the previously mentioned 12–20 repetition range in the table above, since the weight is:

- Manageable enough that you can maintain good technique and care for your joints.
- Heavy enough to create tension, but also produce a good range of motion with no 'cheat' in form.
- Light enough that you can work close to failure and not 'burn out'.

But (again) let's think beyond the 'average' muscle with Muscle Damage.

Build muscle | Muscle damage

Have you ever triumphantly lifted a weight only to drop it thinking your work here is done?

Of course you have. There's something satisfying about grinding out a rep and then proudly dropping the weight to signal to the weights room you've won that particular bar fight. But a study conducted at the University of Florida, USA, has found that dropping the weight could in fact halve your efforts in the gym.[15]

That's because you're only performing a concentric muscle contraction. If you imagine a bicep curl this is where the biceps are contracting but the muscle itself is shortening. By dropping the weight you completely neglect the eccentric muscle contraction. During a dumbbell curl this is the lowering phase of the exercise where the bicep is lengthening.

To quote the University of Florida study, 'More important is the dramatic effect of eccentric strength training on overall muscle strength.'

An idea supported by research published in *The Journal of Applied Physiology*, which stated 'Eccentric training can further enhance maximal muscle strength and power. In skeletal muscles, these functional adaptations are based on increases in muscle mass and number of sarcomeres (muscle fibres).'[16]

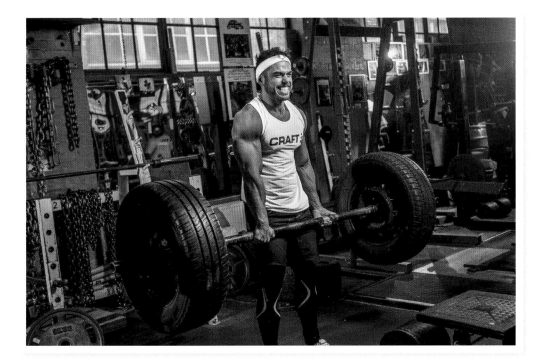

THE WORLD'S MOST MUSCULAR HUMAN

HOW TO BUILD SIZE

No man understood the above better than Dorian Yates, one of the greatest bodybuilders ever to grace the stage. I've had the honour of interviewing the six-time Mr Olympia Champion on a number of occasions as he explained to me in great detail how a boy from Birmingham, England, was able to build more muscle and lose more body fat than any other human on earth between 1992–97.

'Each workout is like a brick in a building, and every time you go in there and do a half-ass workout, you're not laying a brick down. Somebody else is.'
DORIAN YATES

In his prime, the 178-cm (5-ft 10-in) Yates weighed around 130 kg (286 lb) off-season.

Closer to a competition, though, he would step onto the scales at 118 kg (260 lb) with a body-fat level that was so low he looked as if he was carved out of granite.

He basically loved, lived and breathed Mechanical Tension, Metabolic Stress and Muscle Damage. In a sport of extroverts who relished the opportunity to show off the results of their hard work, Yates was one of few who loved the hard work. He would simply turn up, unzip his tracksuit, walk on stage and unassumingly leave the competition with the trophy in his gym bag.

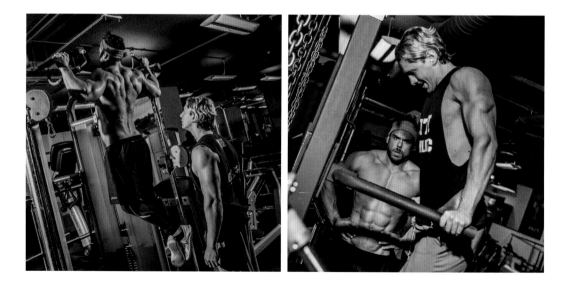

'I didn't mind posing on stage, but it wasn't my favourite part,' he says. 'I enjoyed working out the best way to train, studying nutrition and doing my own diet and learning all about every aspect of this. To me that was the best part of the challenge.'

As a scholar of bodybuilding, Yates pioneered a new method of exercise called 'high-intensity training'. Expanding on the work of former Mr Olympia Mike Mentzer and Mentzer's coach Arthur Jones, he created his own system that focused on reaching maximum muscle stimulation through short, high-intensity workout sessions rather than long workouts.

His goal was never to build strength, but always to build size.

FIVE LESSONS FROM THE WORLD'S MOST MUSCULAR MAN

1. High-intensity training | Metabolic stress

Yates was a big fan of using drop-sets.

This is where you perform any exercise to failure – or just short of failure – and then drop the weight/resistance and continue for more repetitions with the reduced poundage. For each exercise, his workouts would typically involve one or two warm-up sets and one working set.

Just one working set might seem surprising, but Yates says, 'I'd perform a set with 100% energy to 100% failure, then beyond to 100% fatigue – and I won't do another set until I feel that the muscles have recuperated 100%, however long that takes. One set at that extreme intensity does the muscle-building job. For anyone trying this system, if you feel you can attempt a second set, you couldn't have been pulling out all the stops during the first set.'

Because the focus is on working the muscles to complete failure, another set becomes impossible to do with the same intensity. Which is why your 5-Day Strength Routine (pages 210–13) contains fewer work capacity-specific movements, but more drop-sets and super-sets – to complete failure – to increase intensity but lower the volume and time of the entire session.

2. Go big to grow big | Mechanical tension

Inspired by his powerlifting days, Dorian always recommended big movements.

'The most effective exercises for stimulating muscle growth are multi-joint movements like the squat, bench press, deadlift, chin-up and dip. The musculature of the human body was never meant to work in isolation. All the compound movements put a great deal of stress on the muscle in the mid-range of motion, which is usually their sticking point as well.'

But he also stresses the importance of using smaller, isolation movements.

'If you lock out your knees at the very top of a squat, you'll note that there's no longer any stress on the quads, hams and glutes. In the middle of the rep, there is tremendous stress on that whole area. Isolation exercises are more effective at providing stress at either the full stretch or the peak contraction of the movement.'

Using shoulder training as an example he says, 'To fully tax the length of any given muscle, you should perform both a basic compound movement and an isolation exercise. An overhead press would provide plenty of stress to the anterior or front head of the deltoids, but very little for the lateral heads. That's why I always did some type of lateral raise in addition to presses.'

He concludes, 'Isolation movements do have their place, as they allow you to work the muscle from various angles. Therefore the key point is that you do need both types of exercises for best growth results.'

3. Repetition/weight scheme | Muscle damage

Yates believed there was a more effective way to build muscle than only lifting the most weight.

This was an idea supported by researchers from the Lundberg Laboratory for Human Muscle Function and Movement Analysis at Göteborg University. Their aim was, 'to identify dose-response relationships for the development of muscle hypertrophy by calculating the magnitudes and rates of increases in muscle cross-sectional area induced by varying levels of frequency, intensity and volume, as well as by different modes of strength training.'[17]

Put more simply: what type of repetition range, volume and intensity builds the most muscle?

What the scientists concluded was that using a moderately heavy weight – approximately 60–75% of your one-rep maximum – and performing this lift until failure elicited the best results for muscle hypertrophy. This is not to say lifting maximal loads is not without its merits, but generally speaking lifting with sub-maximal weight to failure builds most muscle.

It's true that in Yates's famous training DVD he's seen throwing around inhumane amounts of metal. But when asked if he's among the strongest bodybuilders in the world, he replies, 'I don't think so. I've seen some of the poundages that [eight-time Mr Olympia] Ronnie Coleman uses and I don't think I could ever duplicate that. Ronnie's probably stronger than me. He comes from a powerlifting background.' He also adds, 'But this wasn't my goal. My goal was to put the optimal amount of weight and stress on the muscle to elicit the most muscle hypertrophy.'

4. Time to grow | Metabolic stress

This idea was supported by 2012 research published in the *Journal of Physiology* that wanted to, 'determine if the time that muscle is under loaded tension during low-intensity resistance exercise affects the synthesis of specific muscle protein fractions'.

In plain English: will more time lifting the weight during a set produce more, better-quality muscle?

To find out, the researchers got eight men to perform three sets of unilateral knee extension exercise at 30% of one-rep max. Some participants completed the exercise slowly, lifting for a total of six seconds. Others performed the same exercise, with the same weight, but completed the action in one second.

The results?

After the participants ingested 20 g of protein and the researchers monitored how the body absorbed and used it, they found 'myofibrillar protein synthetic rate was higher in the slow condition group compared to the fast one'.[18]

In simple terms, the muscles in the group that experienced more time under tension experienced a greater degree of protein synthesis – the repair and re-growth of the muscles.

In summary, that is how one man rewrote the blueprint for building muscle.

5. Rest and recovery

Train hard, but recover harder!

This is what I learnt from Dorian. He tells me, 'Training at maximum intensity is a good thing, but too much can be detrimental. Eventually your nervous and adrenal system would burn out and you would become grossly overtrained. The remedy that I found for this was to cycle my training. I determined that I could train all-out, to failure and beyond, for periods of five or six weeks before starting to feel run-down.'

He adds, 'At that point, I would take two weeks and stop my sets just short of failure. This was enough to allow full recuperation and "recharge the batteries" so I could launch into another intense training phase. Still, it is important to note that without maximum intensity, maximum results in terms of growth can never be achieved.'

Which is why you will notice that I only recommend you follow this 5-Day Strength Routine for a maximum of four weeks – based on Dorian's recommendation – to avoid the Exhaustion Phase.

YOUR 12-WEEK STRENGTH WORKOUT

Training notes

'To get stronger you must get smarter.'
ROSS EDGLEY

- The sessions of this workout are based around your primary powerlifting movements.
- The number of workouts, sets, repetitions and volume increases from weeks 1 to 12 to increase work capacity.
- Your 3-Day Routine is built around your squat, bench and deadlift.
- Your 4-Day Routine is built around your squat, bench and deadlift, but includes a shoulder press session.
- Your 5-Day Routine is built around your squat, bench and deadlift, but includes a shoulder press and arm session

Regarding the routine itself:

- The 3-Day Routine is heavily orientated to Functional Strength Training where we:
  - Unlock the neurological potential of the muscle mass we already have by practising ourselves stronger.
  - Increase the strength of our muscles through powerlifting-centric movements.

This is all based on the type of specific training Andy Bolton has done for over 20 years.

- The 4-Day Routine fuses Functional and Structural Training:
  - We're trying to increase work capacity by introducing more repetitions, sets and variety into our training.
  - We use both powerlifting-centric and bodybuilding-centric movements.
  - Our goal is to improve our body's ability to positively tolerate more strength-based training.
- The 5-Day Routine emphasises Structural Training:
  - We're trying to increase the size of the muscles by emphasizing bodybuilding-centric movements.
  - This will in turn increase the 'potential strength' of the muscles.
  - It was a routine I wrote following thousands of workouts with thousands of bodybuilders.
- This workout is ideal for any athlete wanting a solid strength-conditioning routine.

	3-DAY ROUTINE	4-DAY ROUTINE	5-DAY ROUTINE
	WEEKS 1–4	WEEKS 5–8	WEEKS 9–12
KEY FOCUS	Practise technique Increase muscle strength Functional Strength Training Powerlifting-centric	Practise technique Increase work capacity Functional & Structural Improve muscle size & strength	Practise technique Increase muscle size Structural Strength Training Bodybuilding-centric
WORKOUT	Monday: Bench Press Tuesday: REST Wednesday: Squat Thursday: REST Friday: Deadlift Saturday: REST Sunday: REST	Monday: Bench Press Tuesday: Deadlift Wednesday: REST Thursday: Squat Friday: Shoulder Press Saturday: REST Sunday: REST	Monday: Bench Press Tuesday: Deadlift Wednesday: Arms Thursday: Squat Friday: Shoulder Press Saturday: REST Sunday: REST
MAIN GOAL	Refine and improve technique to unlock the neurological potential of the muscle mass you have and increase strength.	Improve work capacity by introducing more repetitions and sets, therefore improving your body's ability to tolerate more strength training.	Emphasise 'bodybuilding-centric' movements to improve the size of your muscles and therefore their 'potential strength'.

3-DAY ROUTINE | WEEKS 1–4 | MONDAY: BENCH PRESS

Exercise	Reps	Sets	Rest	% One-Rep Max	Focus
Bench Press	5	3	120 secs	87%	Functional Strength
Close Grip Bench	8	3	90 secs	80%	Functional Strength
Dumbbell Fly	12	3	60 secs	70%	Structural Strength
Tricep Pushdown	20	3	60 secs	60%	Structural Strength
Tyre Flip	10	4	60 secs	Load with hard but achievable weight	Work Capacity

3-DAY ROUTINE | WEEKS 1–4 | WEDNESDAY: SQUAT

Exercise	Reps	Sets	Rest	% One-Rep Max	Focus
Squat	5	3	120 secs	87%	Functional Strength
Leg Press	8	3	90 secs	80%	Functional Strength
Leg Extension	12	3	60 secs	70%	Structural Strength
Calf Raise	20	3	60 secs	60%	Structural Strength
Backwards Sled Drag	20 metres	4	60 secs	Load with hard but achievable weight	Work Capacity

3-DAY ROUTINE | WEEKS 1–4 | FRIDAY: DEADLIFT

Exercise	Reps	Sets	Rest	% One-Rep Max	Focus
Deadlift	5	3	120 secs	87%	Functional Strength
Pull-up	8	3	90 secs	80%	Functional Strength
Bent-over Row	12	3	60 secs	70%	Structural Strength
Barbell Curl	20	3	60 secs	60%	Structural Strength
Battle Ropes	60	4	60 secs	-	Work Capacity

4-DAY ROUTINE | WEEKS 5–8 | MONDAY: BENCH PRESS

Exercise	Reps	Sets	Rest	% One-Rep Max.	Focus
Bench Press	5	5	120 secs	87%	Functional Strength
Floor Press	8	3	90 secs	80%	Functional Strength
Incline Bench Press	12	3	60 secs	70%	Structural Strength
Ring Dip	12	3	60 secs	70%	Structural Strength
Prowler Push	20 metres	3	60 secs	Load with hard but achievable weight	Work Capacity

4-DAY ROUTINE | WEEKS 5–8 | TUESDAY: DEADLIFT

Exercise	Reps	Sets	Rest	% One-Rep Max	Focus
Deadlift	5	3	120 secs	87%	Functional Strength
Pull-up	8	3	90 secs	80%	Functional Strength
Bent-over Row (Underhand Grip)	12	3	60 secs	70%	Structural Strength
Barbell Drag Curl	20	3	60 secs	60%	Structural Strength
Kettlebell Swing	20	5	60 secs	60%	Work Capacity

4-DAY ROUTINE | WEEKS 5–8 | THURSDAY: SQUAT

Exercise	Reps	Sets	Rest	% One-Rep Max	Focus
Squat	5	3	120 secs	87%	Functional Strength
Front Squat	8	3	90 secs	80%	Functional Strength
Calf Raise	20	3	60 secs	60%	Structural Strength
Forward Lunge	20 metres	4	60 secs	Load with hard but achievable weight	Work Capacity
Backward Lunge	20 metres	4	60 secs	Load with hard but achievable weight	Work Capacity

4-DAY ROUTINE | WEEKS 5–8 | FRIDAY: SHOULDER PRESS

Exercise	Reps	Sets	Rest	% One-Rep Max.	Focus
Standing Barbell Press	5	3	120 secs	87%	Functional Strength
Front Dumbbell Shoulder Raise	12	3	90 secs	70%	Structural Strength
Side Dumbbell Shoulder Raise	12	3	90 secs	70%	Structural Strength
Battle Ropes	20	3	60 secs	-	Work Capacity

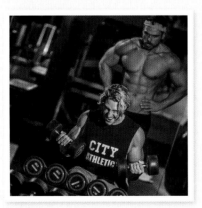
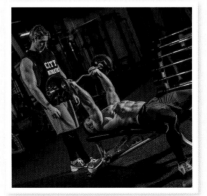

Building strength with Shaun Stafford, good friend and fitness legend

5-DAY ROUTINE | WEEKS 9–12 | MONDAY: BENCH PRESS

Exercise	Reps	Sets	Rest	% One-Rep Max	Focus
Bench Press	5	5	120 secs	87%	Functional Strength
Incline Bench Press	12	3	60 secs	70%	Structural Strength
Ring Dip	12	3	60 sccs	70%	Structural Strength
Dumbbell Fly	20 – Final set to failure	5	60 secs	60%	Structural Strength
Wide-grip Push-up	20 – Final set to failure	5	60 secs	60%	Structural Strength

5-DAY ROUTINE | WEEKS 9–12 | TUESDAY: DEADLIFT

Exercise	Reps	Sets	Rest	% One-Rep Max	Focus
Deadlift	5	3	120 secs	87%	Functional Strength
Bent-over Row	8	3	90 secs	80%	Functional Strength
Wide Pull-up (Overhand Grip)	12	3	60 secs	70%	Structural Strength
Farmers Walk	20 metres	5	60 secs	Load with hard but achievable weight	Work Capacity
Shrug	20 – Final set to failure	5	60 secs	60%	Structural Strength

5-DAY ROUTINE | WEEKS 9–12 | WEDNESDAY: ARMS

Exercise	Reps	Sets	Rest	% One-Rep Max	Focus
Pull-up (Neutral Grip)	5	3	120 secs	87%	Functional Strength
Incline Dumbbell Curl	12	3	60 secs	70%	Structural Strength
Seated Dumbbell Drag Curl	12	3	60 secs	70%	Structural Strength
Weighted Dip	5	3	120 secs	87%	Functional Strength
Tricep Pushdown	20 – Final set to failure	4	60 secs	60%	Structural Strength
Z-bar Triceps Extension	20 – Final set to failure	4	60 secs	60%	Structural Strength

5-DAY ROUTINE | WEEKS 9–12 | THURSDAY: SQUAT

Exercise	Repetitions	Sets	Rest	% One-Rep Max	Focus
Squat	5	3	120 secs	87%	Functional Strength
Leg Press	8	3	90 secs	80%	Functional Strength
Calf Raise	20 – Final set to failure	3	60 secs	60%	Structural Strength
Bulgarian Split Squat	20 – Final set to failure	3	60 secs	60%	Structural Strength
Forward & Backward Lunge	20 metres	4	60 secs	Load with hard but achievable weight	Work Capacity

5-DAY ROUTINE | WEEKS 9–12 | FRIDAY: SHOULDER PRESS

Exercise	Repetitions	Sets	Rest	% One-Rep Max	Focus
Standing Barbell Press	5	3	120 secs	87%	Functional Strength
Front Dumbbell Shoulder Raise	12	3	90 secs	70%	Structural Strength
Side Dumbbell Shoulder Raise	12	3	90 secs	70%	Structural Strength
Face-pull	20 – Final set to failure	3	60 secs	60%	Structural Strength
Hang Power Clean & Press	20 – Final set to failure	3	60 secs	60%	Structural Strength

THE WORLD'S STRONGEST MARATHON |
Silverstone Race Track, England

RUNNING A MARATHON PULLING A CAR

The World's Strongest Marathon was officially invented on 22 October 2015.

I remember the date well. That's because, weighing a solid 92 kg, I entered my home gym in Stamford, England, to tell Geoff Capes about my plan to run a marathon (26.2 miles) pulling a 1.4 tonne car around Silverstone's iconic race circuit to raise money for the Teenage Cancer Trust.

Sitting among his team of junior shot putters – each throwing around ridiculous amounts of iron on the weightlifting mats beside us – he turned to me. Looked me up and down. Paused to consider his response. Then delivered a reply that was as brutally honest as it was invaluable.

'You're too small,' he said.

Standing 178 cm (5 ft 10) tall I'm certainly no Hercules, but at 92 kg I wouldn't call myself 'too small'.

But then again Geoff was 198 cm (6 ft 5 in) and weighed 146kg (23 stone) in his prime. He could also run the 200 metres in 23.7 seconds, was a national-level cross-country athlete in his youth and to this day still holds the record for the truck pull. For all these reasons and more I decided to sit cross-legged and humbly listen.

He then critiqued my (small) boy-sized body and taught me the physics of Strongman.

Opposite is what I wrote in my training journal.

THE TRAINING

Remember the training principles behind The World's Longest Rope Climb (page 97)?

I was able to manipulate my training and forms of muscle contraction – solely performing concentric contractions – so I was never sore, injured or in need of a rest day. Well the exact same principle was applied to The World's Strongest Marathon training routine.

Again, this was based on research conducted by the Department of Health and Human Performance at Oklahoma State University[19], which found constant concentric contractions (when the muscle is under tension but shortening) could be a valuable tool in building strength, while also reducing muscle soreness.

The physics of Strongman

Isaac Newton was a very clever man. An English mathematician and physicist, he is widely recognised as one of the most influential scientists of all time. He was also a former pupil at my school – King's School Grantham, England – which is why I was very familiar with his Laws of Physics. Laws that I found would have a profound impact on my marathon.

See, Newton's First Law of Motion states, 'An object at rest stays at rest unless acted upon by an external force.'

What this means is to get an object to move you need force. In my case the 'object' is a 1.4-tonne car and to get it to move I need my body to generate a lot of 'external force'. Now force is calculated using this equation:

Force = Mass × Acceleration

It's clear that I need either:

1. More Acceleration: I need my legs to work harder and faster; or
2. More Mass: I need to bulk up.

I now understood what Geoff meant. My 92 kg frame was no longer good enough and according to Isaac Newton I might be destined to fail.

Leaving the gym, I thanked Geoff for all his help, said goodbye to his child shot-putting prodigies, then headed back to Cheshire in search of calories, a gym and something very heavy to pull a very long distance.

'At mile 20, I thought I was dead.
At mile 22, I wished I was dead.
At mile 24, I knew I was dead.
At mile 26.2, I realized I had become too tough to kill.'
MARATHON RUNNERS (TRADITIONAL)

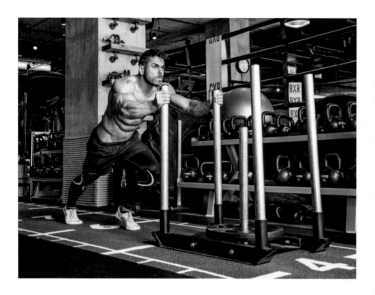

'There is a significant amount of mechanical stress accrued during this part of the lift. Since mechanical stress is thought to be the chief factor stimulating muscular adaptation, researchers have concluded that the eccentric portion of a lift is that which induces many of the adaptations from resistance training. However, the damage produced by eccentric muscle action has the potential to cause a significant amount of soreness, fatigue, and inflammation.'

But luckily for me – and my legs – one of the best examples of an exercise that requires constant concentric contractions is pulling a car for a marathon (or, on a smaller scale, sled pulls). If you think about the action, the resistance is constant during the concentric phase – the muscles tense and shorten during each stride – with a much less intense and demanding eccentric contraction where the leg is in tension but lengthening in stride.

Could I still build muscle this way?

Yes, it seems so. A study printed in the *Journal of Strength and Conditioning* found eight weeks of concentric-only exercise significantly increased quadriceps' cross-sectional size (3.3%) and strength (39.7%).[20] A few years later, research published in the same journal showed that 12 weeks of concentric training increased quadriceps' strength by 15.5%.[21]

Therefore, sled drags were my new best friend. Adding more miles and more weight each week and combining them with The 3-Day, 4-Day and 5-Day Strength Training Routines contained in this chapter, I became a bigger and stronger version of myself. I'd created a workout that allowed me to:

- Build as much muscle as possible.
- Improve strength as much as possible.
- Enhance work capacity as much as possible through the Law of More.

After a month of embracing the Law of Progressive Overload I had graduated from sled, but wasn't ready for a 1.4-tonne car yet. The solution? Visit Everton Football Club's School of Science, find a tractor and ask an old friend from Loughborough University for help.

THE TRACTOR

It's 1pm on 4 November 2015 at Everton Football Club's training facility.

Known as the 'School of Science', it's widely regarded as being one of the greatest football training facilities in the Premier League. Many of football's finest have passed through these academy doors and the immaculately green fields remain steeped in rich heritage and history.

But today was a little different.

Today some of the country's best coaches and players watched in both amazement and amusement as their Head of Strength and Conditioning sat on a tractor and was pulled around the grounds by yours truly. Answering to the name of Matt Taberner, he was a renowned coach, but an even better friend.

While many thought the marathon was 'sporting suicide', he had faith, which is why he convinced the groundskeeper to lend us his tractor, found a harness and attached it to the front, and was now sitting on the back with a stopwatch, cup of tea and notepad.

'Right, let's just put the harness on and take the tractor for a little jog,' he said.

'Nice and steady. That way we'll know where we're at and how much work we have to do.'

He made it sound so easy and for the first mile I thought so too. But deep into mile 2 the problems began.

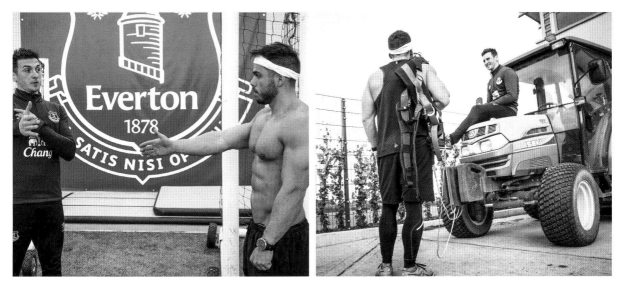

Matt Taberner introducing me to 'Tractor Training'

My legs filled with lactic acid and no longer worked. The harness chafed and removed the skin from my shoulders. Even the feeling in my hands was a forgotten memory as blood was either cut off by the rope or stuck somewhere between my feet and knees.

At 2.8 miles in, the tractor came to an abrupt halt.

It didn't matter how much I pulled: it appeared the Laws of Physics had spoken. Unhooking the rope I collapsed on the floor and lay face-down on the grass. I was in trouble. Exactly 12 weeks away from pulling a 1.4-tonne car 26.2 miles for charity and many of the donations already agreed.

I eventually rolled over to see Matt sipping his tea. He then said something I wasn't expecting, 'Do you want a cup of tea? The club kitchen does the best home-made protein flapjack.' Remembering Geoff's advice, I nodded. I needed to get bigger... a lot bigger!

We then went through my training programme with a fine-tooth comb and The World's Strongest 7-Day Diet Plan was created. Designed to increase size and strength while producing the work capacity of a thoroughbred horse. And all wrapped in calories and Strongman principles.

THE DIET

When, what and how much more should I eat to increase lean muscle?

In theory, it's simple. Cast your mind back to Chapter 6 and how we calculated your Maintenance Calorie Number. Now take that number and eat more of it. Do this, achieve a calorie surplus, make sure you strength train and you will gain muscle.

This is because if you remember it takes roughly **3500 calories to burn or store one pound of fat.**

Well, to gain muscle it takes roughly **2500 calories to synthesise one pound of muscle.**

Now, gaining muscle also requires you to gain weight (a little fat) too. This is just how a calorie surplus works, since it can't be all roses and ripped biceps.

So if we want to gain 1 lb (450 g) of pure muscle per month, we might also need to gain 1 lb of fat (creating a combined total of 2 lb extra bodyweight). To do this we will need to increase our calories by 6000 per month (based on the 2500 calories needed to synthesise one pound of muscle and 3500 calories needed to store one pound of fat).

Over 30 days this equates to an extra 200 calories per day. For a 1 lb increase in muscle mass per month, target 2 lb of weight gain and increase your daily calorie intake by 200.

So why aren't we all gifted with the right-sized arms, legs and chest we all want? Because we are not using the idea of a calorie surplus correctly, that's why.

Calorie surplus: Word of warning

The idea of a calorie surplus is too often misused.

People, in a quest to build muscle, may enthusiastically visit their gym with a doughnut in one hand and an ice cream in the other in the vain hope they'll nutritionally induce 20-inch biceps. Sadly, it doesn't quite work like that.

It would be nice if it did. But like or not, we must adhere to the research published in *The Journal of Obesity Surgery*:

'It is a common belief that clinical vitamin or mineral deficiencies are rare in Western countries because of the unlimited diversity of food supply. However, many people consume food that is either unhealthy or of poor nutritional value that lacks proteins, vitamins, minerals and fibre. The prevalence of vitamin deficiencies in the morbidly obese population is higher and more significant than previously believed.'[22]

People's diets are basically high in calories, but low in nutrients, which is why the quantity and quality of the food I ate before and after training was so important. Allow me to explain with an explanation of my two favourite recipes from The World's Strongest Marathon.

The diet | Before training

Remember 'Finding Your Fuel' (page 152)?

During The World's Strongest Marathon I fuelled my training on mountainous amounts of vegan-friendly, nutrient-dense carbohydrates. Why? Because, it's not about the quantity you eat, but also the quality.

Quality of food

Research published by the American College of Sports Medicine states that plant-based diets 'high in unrefined plant foods are associated with beneficial effects on overall health, lifespan, immune function and cardiovascular health.'

It also points out: 'Whether a vegetarian or vegan diet is beneficial for athletic performance has not yet been defined.'[23] But research from the *International Journal of Sports Nutrition and Exercise Metabolism* might support this idea.

'Ultra-endurance exercise training places large energy demands on athletes and causes a high turnover of vitamins through sweat losses, metabolism and the musculoskeletal repair process. Ultra-endurance athletes may not consume sufficient quantities or quality of food in their diet to meet these needs. Consequently, they may use oral vitamin and mineral supplements to maintain their health and performance.'[24]

And it is echoed by *the International Journal of Sports Nutrition*: 'Additionally, micronutrient needs may be altered for these athletes while dietary intake is generally over the Recommended Daily Allowance because of high caloric intake.' [25]

Basically, there should be a massive emphasis on 'quality of food', vitamins and minerals. Something vegan athletes – like my ice-bathing friend Tim Shieff – have known for years. Generally speaking, vegan diets are higher in dietary fibre, vitamin C, iron, magnesium, folic acid, vitamin E and phytochemicals, and lower in calories, saturated fat and cholesterol.

Quantity of food

Before training I would always have additional carbohydrates to hand.

This is based on research from the University of Queensland where strength athletes were subjected to a carbohydrate-restricted diet to analyse its effects on performance. After a 2-day carbohydrate restriction programme athletes performed three sets of squats with a load of 80% of one-rep max.

They found the carbohydrate restriction programme caused a 'significant reduction in the number of squat repetitions performed'.[26]

This led sports scientists to conclude carbohydrate restriction could reduce your strength potential in the weights room, which is something I didn't want when running a marathon with a car on my back. Which is why I would never start training unless I had a backpack full of home-made granola bars.

The diet | After training

What you eat after training will determine whether you recover efficiently.

This is because all the sweat and toil in the gym won't make you bigger and stronger without proper nutrition. Training merely provides the necessary stimulus to get bigger; it's what you eat afterwards that will determine if your muscles grow. Just ask scientists from the School of Biomedical Sciences at Victoria University, Melbourne, Australia, who discovered athletes increased more muscle mass when using proper 'nutrient timing'.[27]

What's this? 'The strategic consumption of protein and carbohydrate after each workout', which they found 'represents an effective strategy that enhances the adaptations desired from training.'

How much protein and carbohydrate?

This, of course, depends on the rest of your day's food intake, but the often-quoted nutritional bible, *Nutrient Timing: The Future of Sports Nutrition* recommends a 2:1 or 3:1 or 4:1 ratio of carbohydrates to protein. This simply means after training (and depending on your size, type of training and therefore nutritional requirements), eat:

GRANOLA ENERGY BARS
by Annie Mayne

Easy to make and easier to eat, these are packed energy-rich snacks that help you meet your elevated needs for carbohydrates, vitamins, minerals and micronutrients.

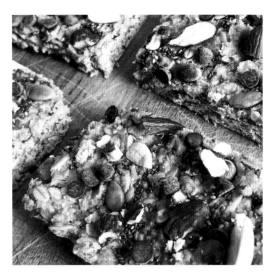

Ingredients

Makes 12

180g porridge oats

45g pumpkin seeds

30g golden linseeds

60g puffed brown rice cereal

45g raw almonds

30g chia seeds from
THE PROTEIN WORKS™

45g dried cranberries

30g goji berries

100g organic virgin coconut oil
or butter (whichever is on hand)

100g light brown sugar

150g honey

1 tsp ground cinnamon

75g dark chocolate, chopped

Method

1. Preheat the oven to 180°C.
2. Spread the oats, pumpkin seeds and linseeds out on a roasting tray. Toast them in the oven for 8–10 minutes.
3. Line a 20 cm (8 in) square tin with baking parchment.
4. Tip the cooled oats and seeds into a large bowl with the puffed rice cereal, almonds, chia seeds, dried cranberries and goji berries. Mix it all together.
5. Place the coconut oil, sugar and honey in a pan and heat gently until the sugar has dissolved. Bring to a boil and let it bubble for 1 minute. Remove from the heat, then add the cinnamon. Pour this all over the oat mixture. Allow to cool for 10 minutes.
6. Stir through the chocolate.
7. Turn the mixture into the tin and spread it out in an even layer. Pack it down well: you can use your hands, a glass or anything to get stuck in.
8. Refrigerate for at least 1 hour until completely cold.
9. Cut into 12 slices. If you clingfilm each individual bar you can store them at room temperature for up to two weeks. They keep for up to one month in the fridge.

	Calories	Carbs	Fat	Protein
Total	4067	547g	208g	166g
Per serving	339	46g	17g	14g

- 60 g carbohydrates and 30 g protein for a 2:1 ratio of carbohydrates to protein.
- 90 g carbohydrates and 30 g protein for a 3:1 ratio of carbohydrates to protein.
- 120 g carbohydrates and 30 g protein for a 4:1 ratio of carbohydrates to protein.

All to kick-start the repair and re-growth of the muscles.

An idea echoed by research published in the *Journal of Physiology*[28] *and Journal of Sports Medicine.*[29]

THE WORLD'S STRONGEST MARATHON: THE START

1am on 22 January 2016 on Silverstone's iconic racetrack.

For months I had been training and eating myself bigger. Today we would find out if it had worked. It was pitch black and so cold the rain threatened to turn to snow as thin layers of ice formed on the ground. None of this was ideal, but there was now no turning back. The event had been well documented in the media the week before, which meant I was leaving here either victorious or in an ambulance.

At the security gate the guards didn't even ask for ID. They just smiled from the warmth and comfort of their security booth. Waving me through the barrier, they wished me luck and said the Stowe Circuit building was open and had coffee and biscuits waiting for me.

To this day I don't know if coffee and biscuits are ideal pre-marathon food. To this day I don't care. I will forever be grateful to the staff at Silverstone for that one small gesture as the coffee served to both wake me up and warm me up while I unpacked the harness and food supplies from the car and waited for the team to arrive.

PROTEIN-PACKED PANCAKES
by Annie Mayne

The best thing about this recipe is once you make one, it's easy to make lots. Also, the ingredients and toppings can be easily tweaked to change the carbohydrate-to-protein ratio depending on what you want and what your body needs.

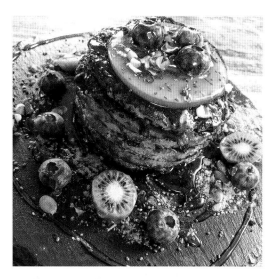

Ingredients

Makes 12

1 banana

2 eggs

90g Banana whey protein 80 from THE PROTEIN WORKS™

250ml coconut milk

45g gluten-free oats

1 tbsp chia seeds

Method

1. Mash up the banana. Add the eggs and whisk.
2. Add the protein powder and coconut milk. Whisk some more.
3. Fold in the oats.
4. Make sure your frying pan is steaming hot! Add 2 tbsp of mixture at a time and cook for 2 minutes on each side until lightly browned.
5. Feel free to add a variety of treats as toppings – I've used chia seeds, but you can take your pick from fruits, nuts, berries, honey, etc... go wild!

	Calories	Carbs	Fat	Protein
Total	802	95g	25g	54g
Per serving	67	8g	2g	5g

Thankfully – before the magnitude of the task ahead dawned on me – I didn't have to wait long.

Just 10 minutes later, James Ruckley, Christie Wright and Karina Grimes walked through the doors. Forming the greatest marathon-car-pulling team ever assembled. They were also the only marathon-car-pulling team ever assembled. All close friends of mine from the obstacle racing community, they were each brilliant athletes themselves, but today had selflessly decided to put their training to one side and help their strange friend pull a car for a marathon.

Christie was chief physiotherapist. Possibly with the hardest job, she was tasked with keeping my body from breaking and would later spend hours massaging the cramp from my left bum cheek (the right one remained oddly strong).

Karina was head of morale and food. She had more stamina than she did food and I would later be grateful for both. Covering miles throughout the day, she ran back and forth from Stowe Building to find me calories, carbohydrates and fats in any and every form.

Finally, there was my driver James. A giant hero of the World's Strongest Marathon, he should have been at home studying for his medical exams. Instead, he'd driven 300 miles to Silverstone – with a bag full of books, caffeine and cake – and was now sitting in the driving seat revising, eating and occasionally steering when we hit a corner.

1:30am and I am standing on the racetrack. Coffee was drunk. Biscuits were eaten.

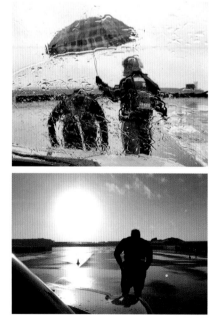

Twelve weeks had passed since I stood before Geoff Capes and had my physique critiqued. Granted, I still wouldn't be mistaken for a Strongman competitor, but I had managed to eat and lift myself bigger, stronger and heavier.

As a result my legs now tested the elasticity of the fabric in my trousers. My newly sized shoulders cushioned the car's harness that once dug into the bone on my shoulder blades. And my chest served as counterweight to use against the car's complete reluctance to move.

The handbrake was off and I was away. The first five hours were actually OK. With each lap my pacing improved and my strides became short yet powerful and efficient. We began to memorise every lump and bump in the track, so knew when to take it easy and when to pick up the pace to keep the car in constant motion and my legs from seizing up.

But 8:00am arrived, the sun came up and the problems began.

Stowe Circuit is 1.281 km in length (0.796 miles) and has five turns in total. But it's also completely open to the elements. There is no shelter from the rain and no buildings to block the wind. What this means is the rain virtually falls horizontally and is blown directly into your face.

Also the ground is purposely made to be so incredibly smooth. This is of course perfect for a Formula 1 car travelling at over 200 mph, but far from ideal when your feet feel void of any grip as they battle the wind and rain.

8:48am – only four miles in – and so begins my darkest hour.

MY DARKEST (MARATHON) HOUR

What little grip I had in my feet is now nowhere to be found.

Out of desperation I resort to crawling on my hands and feet and attempt to 'claw' my way around the circuit. Whether it was the cold, the fatigue or a mixture of both it's clear I wasn't thinking straight. I even tried removing my gloves to see if that would give me more grip in my hands.

It didn't, for those wondering. It just left me with very sore and very numb fingers.

It was at this point that the team pulled the handbrake and called an emergency meeting. Even now I'm so glad they did since I've no doubt I would still be out on that fourth corner if they hadn't.

They then convinced me to eat, rest and wait out the weather. Unfortunately, this was a waiting game we were never going to win since it's January and so we're right in the middle of a British winter. But for the moment I was glad to lie down, have my legs massaged by Christie and be hand-fed granola by Karina.

9:45am and the lactic acid (finally) begins to leave my legs.

Standing up, I walk to the window, only to see the rain still relentlessly pouring onto the track. Worse, the sky was completely grey with not a single break in the clouds. With time now ticking away – and media arriving shortly – things weren't looking good and the entire marathon was in jeopardy.

But heroes come in many forms and it was at 10:05am that mine appeared on the horizon.

He wasn't on a white horse. Nor was he wearing a cape. Instead, my knight in shining armour arrived complete with a giant woollen hat, three layers of coats and big, thick trousers that made him walk funny. Also, instead of a trusty shield for protection, he came wielding a giant umbrella and two pairs of gloves that made his hands look comically big.

This was my hero. This was my older brother. 'What are you doing in here? That car's not going to pull itself is it?'

At this point I should mention Scott is often brutally honest, but at this point he was also brutally right. I smiled. He nodded. The team agreed.

The harness was attached and we went back out into the rain. Only this time Scott walked every metre in front of me carrying his giant umbrella to shield me from the wind and rain. It was the strangest slipstream Silverstone had ever witnessed, but we were moving and it was working.

3pm and the rain stopped. The clouds lifted and so did the spirits of the entire team. We had taken the worst Silverstone – and the British winter – could throw at us and we were still moving.

I unhooked the harness. Continued to eat anything and everything Karina gave to me. Then looked at Scott who was carrying a GPS tracking watch to clock the miles.

'How far was that?' I asked, exhausted. 'That's exactly 18,' he said, looking at the watch.

'18 miles isn't bad,' I said with a huge sigh of relief and feeling semi-proud of myself. I was over the worst of it.

'No, 18 miles isn't bad mate...' He paused. 'But you did 18 km.' He then burst out laughing. I couldn't help but laugh too.

I'd been working to 26.2 miles and the entire time Scott was working towards the equivalent in kilometres (42.2km to be exact). Every time he said, 'Another 1 down!' I was thinking, 'Wow another mile! I am motoring on this marathon.'

Turns out, not so much! But I didn't mind. Morale was now high and the sun was (semi) shining.

Also members of the Silverstone Racing Club had come down to see the spectacle and take pictures. I should mention that Silverstone has a rich history of motor sport dating back to the 1940s. Now, 18 km in – and half-way approaching – I was glad I wouldn't now join that history as the guy who collapsed on Stowe Circuit, tangled in a harness, after saying he could pull a car for a marathon.

No one wants to be that guy.

THE END

Hours and miles passed.

Members of the media and racing club arrived, took pictures and then quickly left after realising that, with a top speed of 3 mph on the slight downhill segment of the track, the sport of marathon car pulling was not a spectator event. The only people that remained were my support team.

Day turned to night and at 5:30pm Silverstone circuit became strangely tranquil: completely silent and illuminated only by the lights coming from the main building's paddock. My lactic-ridden body almost felt at peace as my brain released whatever endorphins it had left to cope with the fatigue. I entered an almost meditative state: I wasn't sleeping but I wasn't fully awake either.

At 37 km down my support team doubled. Just when I needed them my mum, girlfriend, auntie and her girlfriend arrived to walk the last 5.2 km with me.

Needless to say, it wasn't quick and it wasn't pleasant. But after 19 hours, 36 minutes, 43 seconds – and an unholy amount of 'harness chafing' – I had managed to pull a 1.4-tonne car 26.2 miles around Silverstone's racetrack. But what started out as a strange – yet well-intentioned – idea to raise money for charity, actually turned into something so much more.

All because as the event trended worldwide for 18 hours, my social media became a melting pot for ideas as inquisitive marathon runners and strongmen all exchanged fitness theories. In our own small way we had explored How To Get Big and Strong to the extreme.

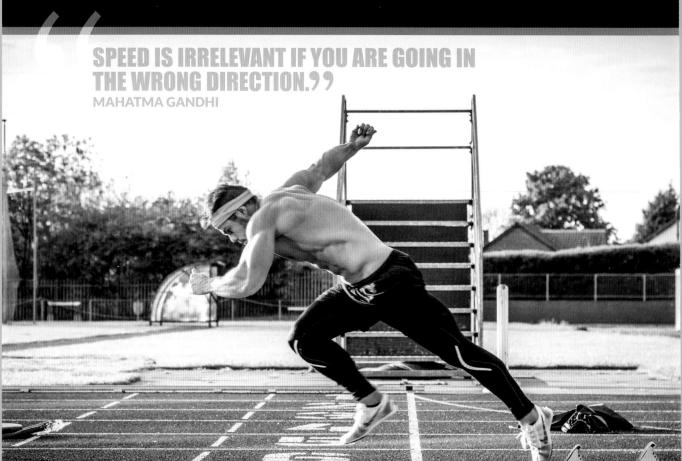

CHAPTER 8
HOW TO INCREASE SPEED AND POWER

"SPEED IS IRRELEVANT IF YOU ARE GOING IN THE WRONG DIRECTION."
MAHATMA GANDHI

THE WORLD'S FASTEST TRACK WORKOUT

The fastest workout I've ever attended took place on 14 October 2015 at Brunel University.

But I must stress it wasn't just fast. No, it was Olympic-standard fast.

To this day I have never seen so many specimens of speed assembled onto one athletics track, from 100-metre specialists like James Ellington to nationally decorated 400-metre champions Margaret Adeoye and Nigel Levine. I was basically the only one without a World Championship selection to my name and the only one not training for the Rio 2016 Olympics.

My coach? Celebrated in sprinting circles, he answered to the name of Linford Christie.

Now 56 years old he stands 185 cm (6 ft 2 in) tall with a body still virtually void of fat. His big shoulders and broad chest remain a by-product of the custom-built frame he used to win all four major competitions open to a British athlete: the Olympic Games, the World Championships, the European Championships and the Commonwealth Games.

A feat no man has achieved since.

Was I nervous? Yes. Was I the slowest there? Yes, it was very likely.

But what I lacked in speed I made up for in unbridled enthusiasm. I knew it was a privilege to train under one of the fastest men in history, so I put my spikes over one shoulder – and my fears to one side – and headed over to the track to begin stretching with the team.

I had 10 new training partners in total.

All different shapes and sizes, but each possessing outstanding pace that they perfected and refined on the University's hallowed ground. Brunel University – on the outskirts of London – has a rich sporting heritage. You can't simply arrive and train there. No, you must be invited.

Everything about it looks and feels elite.

The hall is filled with the distinct smell of a rubber synthetic track that's best described as overpowering. The sound of weighted sled drags that echoes around the walls is simply intimidating. Finally, the sight of long jumpers performing one-legged, 50-inch box jumps in the corner can only be described as humbling.

In that moment I made peace with the fact that when it came to sprinting I would be dead last. But I didn't mind. This is because the session would actually start in the gym. What this means is with a (mildly) impressive squat, bench and deadlift – from the time spent under the iron in Leeds – I knew there was a chance I could (semi) impress under the bar…

Even if my sprinting was far below Olympic standard.

The Strength, Speed and Power Pyramid of priority

The foundations of your Strength, Speed and Power Pyramid of Priority are now strong.

Now it's time to make the rest of the pyramid fast! To recap: strength, speed and power are closely related. You have to understand this if you are to become a bigger, stronger and more powerful version of yourself. This is because:

- Strength is the body's ability to generate force.
- Speed is the rate at which someone moves.
- Power is the product of strength and speed.

Now you can't be powerful if you're not fast, which is why those who are naturally strong need to work on getting faster.

Which is exactly what we do in this chapter.

Power tips and tools

Gain muscle size

Increase speed/power

Improve work capacity

Master lifts

HOW TO INCREASE SPEED AND POWER

RATE OF FORCE DEVELOPMENT

To increase power you need to understand **rate of force development** (ROFD).

This is possibly one of the most underappreciated areas of applied science when it comes to your gym routine. Defined as the body's ability to generate the greatest amount of force in the shortest time possible, the faster your ROFD the quicker and more explosive you and your movements become.

To use an example, let's consider the athletes performing a 200-kg deadlift.

Now both Athlete A and Athlete B are capable of producing 200 kg of force, but lifter A has a significantly faster rate of force development. What this means is it may take Athlete A just two seconds to produce the required force to get the bar moving and off the floor and four seconds to lock it out at the top of the lift.

However, Athlete B has a slower rate of force development, which means they take four seconds to get the bar moving and another four to lock it out. Ultimately, what this means is that Athlete B takes longer to complete the lift and might therefore fatigue before fully locking out.

How do we improve ROFD? Train under the guidance of Linford Christie, that's how...

This is because it's obvious the team at Brunel were **fast**.

But what few people know is that they each had a powerful bench press and squat too. Why? They understood how to take 'conventional' strength training and turn it into something that could build blistering speed on the track.

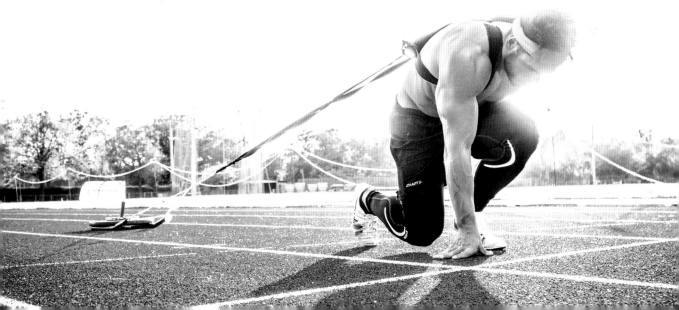

See, gyms all over the world are filled with athletes comparing strength metrics. The weight of their bench, the depth of their squat and the sheer rep volume of a savage deadlift session they just completed. Each one serves as a topic of debate among athletes in the locker room as they proudly share every detail.

But why does fast and explosive power output get such little airtime?

Why are gyms not filled with men and women comparing their lifts in metres per second? Or nostalgically reliving an amazing ROFD they produced during last week's bench press session? The answer is that sadly, not enough people understand the principles of speed training. But studies show that once you do it could add another important dimension to your routine.

A (QUICK) HISTORY OF SPEED TRAINING

Speed training has been around as long as we humans have been moving.

But huge advancements were made during the 1950s in the old Soviet Union. A time when Soviet athletic endeavours were unrivalled and considered to be at the cutting edge of sports science. During this period the American coaches noticed that just before competitions the Soviet athletes were performing jumping-based drills.

This all seemed a little odd. It was completely different to the traditional static stretching that the rest of the world's athletes were doing on the sidelines – touching their toes and bending their knees[1].

So what were the strange Soviet athletes doing?

Well, aside from winning they were using the pioneering work of the strength genius Dr Yuri Verkhoshansky and a training protocol he called the **depth jump**.

Improve speed in seconds

The depth jump can improve your speed in seconds. Put simply, Verkhoshansky would have athletes drop off a box, land on the floor – absorbing the shock – and then instantly jump as high as they possibly could. Later labelled 'shock training' in reference to the body's ability to absorb the shock/impact, it was believed that one short-term adaptation to the depth jump was a higher vertical jump compared to a static jump.

Research would later reveal this was because Verkhoshansky was able to 'play around' with the elasticity of the muscles and tendons by positively manipulating the body's stretch-shortening cycle.

The stretch-shortening cycle is essentially where the muscles contract eccentrically (the muscles lengthen), which is followed by an immediate concentric contraction (the muscles

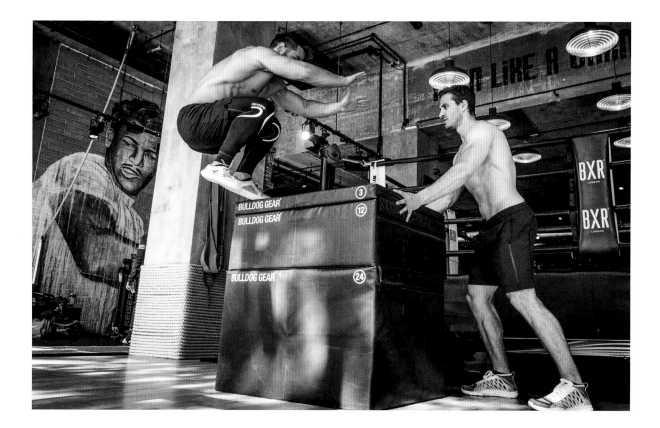

shorten). This – based on research from the School of Kinesiology at the University of Zagreb in Croatia – has been shown to improve the concentric phase, resulting in increased force production and output.

This explains why during a depth jump athletes were able to jump higher. They effectively used the 'elastic energy' built up during the eccentric phase (when landing) to help them during the concentric phase (the jump itself).[2]

Interestingly, Verkhoshansky also found that the training adaptations to this form of training weren't solely short term. In a study published in 1989 in the *National Strength and Conditioning Journal* he discovered that elite athletes undertaking a depth jump programme gained 15% in their maximal strength, which paved the way for more research in the area.[3]

This all sounds great, you must be thinking.

Well, it must be noted that while many of Verkhoshansky's teachings still hold true today, there is now a difference between earlier plyometric principles and the modern usage in sports science. This is because Verkhoshansky's 'shock training' was originally confined to improving jumping performance, while modern sports science uses plyometric principles to increase overall muscular speed and power.[4]

Basically, it goes beyond just improving the height of an athlete's jump.[5]

SECRET TO POWER | STRETCH-SHORTENING CYCLE

The stretch-shortening cycle used for shock training forms only a small part of Ballistic Resistance Training.

Ballistic training is a type of weightlifting characterised by movements in which the athlete tries to apply the maximal force to the resistance with the goal of lifting, moving or projecting it as quickly as they can. The possibilities extend far beyond improving your vertical jump (with the utmost respect to Verkhoshansky) and this is where things become really interesting. Consider that every time you perform a conventional squat or bench your body naturally decelerates at the top of the movement. In fact, it's believed in a one-repetition maximum lift, as much as 24% of the lift time is spent decelerating.[6]

For a lift at 80% of your one-repetition maximum, deceleration can increase to as much as 52%. Even if you perform repetitions quickly ('speed reps') the speed decreases at the end of the concentric motion. It's a protective mechanism put in place by our joints that stops our shoulders from becoming detached from our bodies during quick bench press.

Ballistic training virtually eliminates this deceleration.

Compare a bench press to a plyometric push-up where your aim is to throw yourself into the air, and you'll see that same protective mechanism goes out the window. Instead, it means achieving maximal acceleration, optimal power, a fully firing nervous system and optimal activation of fast twitch muscle fibres.

For these exact reasons, learn to go ballistic.

USING SPEED FOR STRENGTH

Speed can make you strong!

This might sound odd, but research published in the *Journal of Strength and Conditioning Research* investigated 'the additive effects of ballistic training to a traditional heavy resistance training program on upper body strength'. Seventeen resistance-trained men were selected and assigned into two groups.

One group followed a traditional strength-training protocol for eight weeks while the other combined traditional strength training and ballistic training. This consisted of a conventional bench press coupled with plyometric push-ups (where the athlete's hands leave the floor during the upward-concentric phase).

Following the eight weeks the athletes' one-repetition maximum was measured on the bench press and results revealed that although both groups improved, the traditional strength training group increased by 7.1% on average compared to 11.6% for the ballistic strength training group. Scientists concluded: 'The inclusion of ballistic exercises into a heavy resistance training program increased 1 repetition maximum bench press and enhanced power.'[7]

For this reason, if you want to increase your bench press numbers try hitting the gym mats in an effort to perfect your plyometric push-up. Science shows your chest will be more powerful when you do.

USING SPEED FOR INSTANT STRENGTH

Speed can be used to generate instant improvements in strength.

Don't believe me? Let me explain with one of the best – and most unlikely – examples of using speed and the stretch-shortening cycle to improve strength. All thanks to my old friend (again) Andy Bolton.

This is because if you watch a video of his first 1000-lb deadlift – WPO Semi-Finals in Lake George, New York, on 4 November 2006 – you'll see he grips the bar, performs three hamstring stretches and then on the third stretch he begins to lift. This is because he knows that performing two brief stretched, eccentric contractions can help to improve the subsequent concentric contraction.

For him that meant 1000 lb came off the floor and he became immortalised in the record books as one of the strongest men ever to live.

FASTER (BETTER?) MUSCLES

Sports science teaches us that there are two types of muscle fibres in our skeletal muscle.

These are Type I fibres and Type II fibres that can be further subdivided into Type IIa and Type IIb. Type I fibres are also more commonly known as 'slow twitch' muscle fibres and these are the muscle fibres required for forms of long endurance training. They've a much slower contractile speed and have a smaller cross-sectional area, which means they're not good for filling your T-shirt or shifting some iron in the gym.

But they are much more resistant to fatigue.

Now Type II muscle fibres are more commonly known as 'fast twitch' muscle fibres and it's these that have a faster contractile speed and a much larger cross-sectional area. You basically want lots of these when trying to lift heavy in the gym since they're responsible for generating power. And also their larger cross-sectional size looks better on the beach.

This partly explains why Olympic sprinters are seen stretching the limits of their Lycra with their giant quads on the start line while their marathon counterparts struggle to fill their chosen attire. This is why if your goal is to improve the size and appearance of your muscles you should probably listen to the findings from scientists at the Department of Kinesiology at McMaster University, Hamilton.

They measured muscle activation during periods of ballistic training using electromyographic technology (EMG). What they found was: 'A selective activation of fast twitch motor units may occur in ballistic contractions under certain movement conditions.[8]

What this means is based on this research –and that published in *The Journal of Strength and Conditioning Research* – ballistic training could make you a more powerful athlete who fills their gym kit that little bit better.

THE WORLD'S FASTEST TRACK WORKOUT |
Loughborough University, UK

HOW TO BUILD MORE SPEED

A few weeks after my maiden voyage to Brunel, I was becoming a semi-decent sprinter.

I say 'semi' because my technique on the track needed work, but my Rate of Force Development in the gym was improving by the week. Which is why Linford sent me back to the motherland of Loughborough University to meet my new training partner, so I could continue to refine my running.

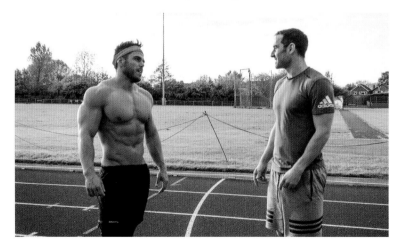

So here I am…

Back on home soil I head to the indoor athletics track housed at the High Performance Athletics Centre to meet a speed-based specimen who answers to the name of Ashley Bryant.

Called the HiPAC for short, the Centre is hard to describe since it's filled with sports science beyond my comprehension. But it's basically a £5 million state-of-the-art athletics venue that has shiny silver equipment, high jumps, long jumps, pole vaults and a track that was made from the same material they used to create the London 2012 Olympic Games stadium.

It's home to many of Britain's best athletes. Ashley was basically a few of them rolled into one. A former student of Linford's, he had learnt to become very fast and very powerful over many sports and many movements. At the age of 22 he was the best decathlete in the country, but amazingly was also ranked in the Top 10 for the long jump and several other single events.

He was an athletic weapon and although very welcoming, he couldn't help but exude this sense of physical superiority. He was basically the kid always picked first, at every sport, in every school, in every playground.

'So Ross, how much sprint training have you done?'

Lacing up my spikes, I paused before answering. I knew he'd trained at Brunel. I also knew he ran 7.12 seconds for the 60 m, 11.02 seconds for the 100 m and 48.10 seconds for the 400 m. I had to pick my words carefully since I didn't want to overpromise and disappoint. But also didn't want to undersell myself.

'A little, but not a lot…'

'I'm not slow, but not rapid…'

'You might be impressed, but not overwhelmed.'

Laughing, he said, 'Ah OK, I see. Then let's get on the track and build some "overwhelming" speed.' I nodded and we trained.

'BUILD OVERWHELMING SPEED'

Now Ashley (like the team at Brunel) was **fast**.

But few people know he was also a genius when it came to speed strength and conditioning. He had so many tools, tips and tricks in his arsenal to manipulate his body's speed of movement, which is why – thinking outside of the squat – he started the session by introducing me to a tried-and-tested Soviet Union weapon of speed…

Resistance Band Training!

Used in strength and conditioning as far back as the 1970s, resistance bands even featured in Professor Yuri Verkhoshansky's book entitled *Fundamentals of Special Strength-Training in Sport* (1997). A book that's still widely used by fitness experts today, but what are they and how will they help to unlock supreme speed?

Resistance is useful

Resistance bands are just elastic bands that can be used to add resistance to movements.

But what's important to note is that it's 'progressive' resistance. What this means is the more the band is stretched the higher the resistance. This is a key characteristic that makes it very different to free weights where the resistance remains virtually the same as dictated by gravity.

This unique property of resistance bands is perhaps the main reason they've become so widely used in strength and conditioning. Experts believe the linear variable resistance provided by bands – the way it gets harder the more it's stretched – mimics what's known as the 'strength curve' of most muscles. A 'strength curve' is a term used in kinetics.

Kinetics is the study of the body's motion, which details how a muscle's strength will change over a range of motion. Taking the commonly used bicep curl as an example, notice how you're particularly weak during the lower range of the exercise; however, as your hand (and the bar) move towards the shoulder, the strength of the biceps increases.

Now, if you performed a bicep curl with a free weight you'd find you were limited in how much weight you could lift during the lowest part of the lift, your weakest point. But if you added some progressive resistance in the form of a resistance band attached to the bar, you'd add more resistance at the strongest point in your range of motion, therefore adding more resistance to better stimulate strength adaptations[9].

To put it simply, you make the bicep work harder over the entire range of motion.

Training better and harder?

Firstly, this is an idea supported by stories exchanged over the water fountain in the gym.

Many people I've trained with talk about a stronger 'burning sensation' and greater muscle fatigue that indicates a greater number of muscle fibres have been worked throughout the entire range of motion. But putting stories of broscience to one side, this subjective feedback of greater strength adaptations is also supported by objective studies.

Take research from the College of Exercise and Sport Sciences at Ithaca College, New York, as an example. This set out to determine if weight resistance combined with resistance bands would provide different strength and power adaptations to free weights alone.

Scientists took 44 trained athletes from the basketball, wrestling and hockey teams and then randomly divided them into either a 'control group' or an 'experimental group'. Both groups completed an identical training programme, but the control group used conventional, free weights whereas the experimental group used a combination of free weights and resistance bands.

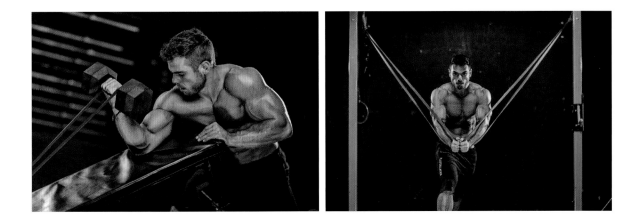

Following seven weeks of training, subjects were then put through a series of tests to see if there was any improvement in their one-repetition maximum back squat and one-repetition maximum bench press as well as their peak and average power. Results revealed that the experimental group, using resistance bands and traditional weights, showed a greater improvement in their bench press, squat, peak and average power[10].

This led the researchers to conclude: 'Training with resistance bands may be better than using free weights alone for developing lower- and upper-body strength, and lower-body power in resistance-trained individuals.' They added, 'Long-term effects are unclear, but resistance band training makes a meaningful contribution in the short-term to performance adaptations of experienced athletes.'

In summary, while this research isn't suggesting you attach bands to anything and everything, it does support the idea of using them for a short period of time to mix up your training and overcome plateaus[11].

Range of motion

Another benefit of using resistance bands is their functionality.

Unlike weights, they don't rely on gravity to provide resistance and can instead be worked over different ranges of motion. For athletes this is particularly important since it allows them to train certain movements, under resistance, over more functional ranges of motion that better mimic those experienced during sport-specific activities.

Illustrating the importance of sport-specific ranges of motion is a study published in a 1998 issue of the *American Journal of Sports Medicine*. It reported a significant improvement in the shoulder strength and speed of serve in collegiate tennis players who trained using elastic bands.[12]

As you can imagine, trying to replicate that same action and resistance with a dumbbell alone would be quite hard, if not impossible, and certainly wouldn't yield the same results.

Furthermore, researchers from Louisiana State University found a resistance band training programme strengthened the rotator cuff muscles of baseball pitchers better than a free-weight-based regime. Again, as you can imagine a resistance band would be far better at mimicking that range of motion compared to throwing dumbbells around the weights room.[13]

Put simply, this is all because free weights can only really apply resistance in a vertical plane, thanks to gravity. But resistance bands help you operate over a horizontal plane that could better replicate swinging a racquet or throwing a ball.

Rate of force development

But the most important training adaption when using bands is they improve rate of force development (ROFD).

A study conducted at the Department of Mechanical Engineering at the University of Minnesota, Minneapolis, USA, set out to examine how the use of elastic bands in resistance training can increase performance-related parameters such as ROFD.

Researchers took 20 trained male volunteers and had them perform a free-weight back squat exercise with and without elastic bands. They found that ROFD was significantly greater with the use of bands and concluded, 'Results indicate that there may be benefits to performing squats with elastic bands in terms of rate of force development. Practitioners concerned with improving rate of force development may want to consider incorporating this easily implemented training variation.'[14]

Compensatory (squat) speed

As well as Andy Bolton, another man who used the science of speed for strength was Dr Fred Hatfield.

One of the first humans to squat 1000 lb, he was a big advocate of accelerating through the lift – something he called 'compensatory acceleration training'. This is a training method that involves trying to move the weight as quickly as possible throughout the entire lift. If we take the simple equation **Force = Mass x Acceleration**, the more we accelerate, then the more force we can put into a movement.

What this means is we need to move a lighter weight faster in order to equal the force we put into moving a heavy weight. Here is Dr Hatfield's description:

'If you're applying a thousand pounds of force at the bottom of the lift and then as leverage improves you continue to apply a thousand pounds or less, you're not accomplishing as much as you can. Instead, you'll see that as leverage improves you're able to apply twelve hundred pounds of force, fourteen hundred pounds of force up near the top. The secret though is that you're applying as much force as you possibly can exert all the way through the lift. That means you're spending more time under maximum tension. That means you're going to make progress much faster than you could otherwise.'[15]

But there's a problem. Take the squat as an example. Most people will start slow at the bottom of the movement – where the leverage is not as good – and then speed up as they hit the top of the movement. If the weight is light enough, their speed will actually throw the bar up in the air at the top, but having the bar fly off the shoulders is an injury waiting to happen.

This is why the work of legendary strength coach Louie Simmons at Westside Barbell, who pioneered the use of bands on the bar, is so valuable.

A band will exert the most force at the end of the lift so the athlete must accelerate throughout the entire movement. There's no room for 'coasting' through the movement and maximal force must be used throughout to keep the bar moving. Basically there's nowhere to rest, coast or hide when lifting heavy with bands.

THE WORLD'S FASTEST WORKOUT CONTINUED
HOW TO LIFT 1.3 METRES PER SECOND

Months passed and I was now fast.

Not yet achieving blisteringly Olympic pace, but fast enough to raise an eyebrow down at the High Performance Athletics Centre at Loughborough University. But I wanted more speed, so I was told by Ashley to visit Powerbase Gym on campus and ask for Tommy Yule.

Now Tommy is hard to explain, but try to imagine a genius, academic, athletic coaching hybrid.

When he was competing in Olympic Weightlifting he won five Commonwealth Games medals, was the British record holder, was British Champion six times and represented Great Britain at the 2000 Olympic Games.

Then, as a strength and conditioning coach for British Athletics, he coached Olympic, World and Commonwealth Games medallists across three Olympic cycles and has a Masters' degree in Engineering Science from the University of Oxford on his mantelpiece.

But how would Olympic Weightlifting make me faster?

Traditionally seen as a sport reserved for the iron-monsters that dwelled in specialist gyms throughout the old Soviet Union, China and Bulgaria, it's perceived as highly specialised

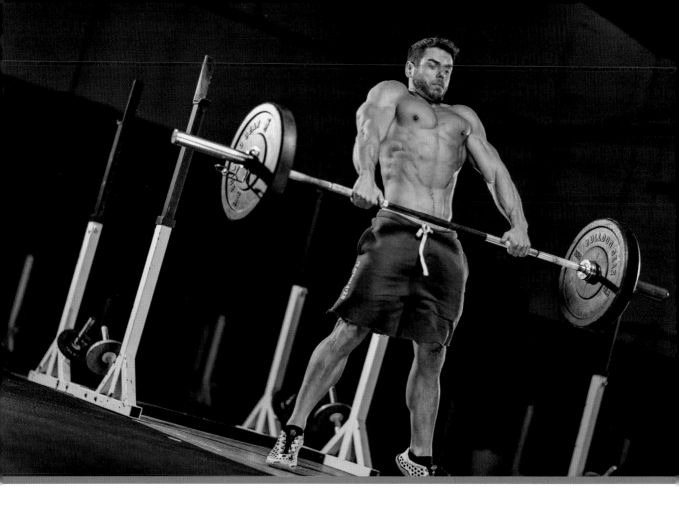

and only practised by a few. But for those prepared to embrace it, a whole host of benefits awaits. This is what I learnt listening to Tommy talk as he threw superhuman amounts of weight above his head.

OVERVIEW: OLYMPIC LIFTING

Olympic-style lifting is easy to explain, hard to do.

It's a weight training discipline in which you attempt to lift the biggest weight possible – in the form of a barbell and weight plates – above your head. It's argued that the modern version can trace its origins back to Europe in the 19th century and the first male champion, by the name of Edward Lawrence Levy, was crowned in 1891 at the World Weightlifting Competition.

It then featured during the early Olympics in various forms, including the often-forgotten one-handed lift, but eventually the International Olympic Committee decided on the current format. This includes two competition lifts: the snatch and the clean and jerk.

Each athlete gets three attempts at each lift and then judges add the total from both the snatch and the clean and jerk to get an overall result. All of which takes place within a specific bodyweight category. A far cry from the one-handed lifting format of the early Olympics.

So, that's the origins of this age-old discipline, but what about the technique?

At this point I should mention that I am a keen practitioner of Olympic-style lifting, but not an expert. I use it solely as a training tool to develop power, which is why, to analyse the movements themselves, I have recruited Tommy's Olympic Lifting protégé who answers to the name of Sonny Webster.

Born in 1994, he's basically a younger, stronger and more mobile version of me who has quads the size of anti-tank missiles and an Olympic Games to his name. His lifts can only be described as 'powerfully poetic' to watch; hence I've recruited him to demonstrate the perfect clean and jerk and snatch.

Clean and jerk

The clean and jerk begins with the barbell on the floor. The athlete must then put that weight overhead in two separate motions: clean it to the shoulders (pause) and then jerk (thrust) it overhead so the arms are fully locked out. Believed to be the single best lift for developing strength, speed and power, the entire movement requires a big pull for the clean. A powerful front squat to come out of the squat position. Finally, a herculean jerk to finish with the barbell above your head.

The set-up

- Set your feet hip-width apart and place them directly under the bar.
- Bend over (back straight) and grip the bar with a shoulder-width grip.
- Drop your hips into the squat position.
- Keep the back flat, hips higher than your knees and arms straight.
- Look straight ahead.

The pull

- Start the movement by powerfully pulling the bar with your legs, hips and back.
- Keep the bar close to your shins, but don't make contact with your shins or knees as it rises.
- As it passes your thighs it may brush them making light contact.
- Finish the pull by triple-extending your ankles, knees and hips as you rise onto your toes.

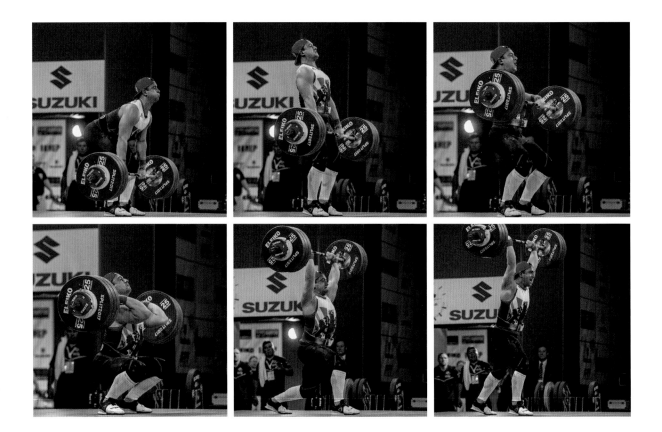

Receiving the bar

- Your body will now be fully extended.
- Immediately shrug your shoulders and 'pull' yourself under the bar.
- The goal here is for you to travel as fast as possible below the barbell.
- Move into a full squat as the bar passes your chest as fast as possible.
- Thrust your elbows out in front of you and turn your wrists over.
- Ensure you receive the bar on top of your clavicles and deltoids.

The stand

- Only once you have the bar under control can you begin to stand.
- Do this by driving your heels into the floor.
- Many people complicate this part of the lift, but it's simply a front squat.
- Note that your torso might lean forward slightly and your hips may shift backward.
- But it's important that the bar must always stay over your ankles as you stand up.

The jerk

- Now finish the movement by bending your knees and hips about 5–10 cm.
- Next, generate as much force as possible by powerfully extending your knees, hips and elbows.
- Thrust the bar overhead, remembering to lean your head back as the barbell travels above your shoulders.
- As the barbell passes your head, 'split' your legs (one forward and the other back).
- Lock the arms (and bar) overhead as both feet land at the same time.
- Return your head to the neutral position so the bar is directly over your ears (or slightly behind them).
- Finally, bring your feet back together about hip- to shoulder-width apart.
- Stand upright, controlled and motionless.
- That is one repetition.

Snatch

The snatch is unlike the clean and jerk in that it's performed in a single motion. It's considered to be one of the most explosive and powerful movements you can perform in a gym, but don't let Sonny's giant quads fool you. The snatch is not just raw power, but requires finesse, and when it's executed perfectly the heavy barbell should look light as a feather.

Worth pointing out is the perceived ease with which an athlete snatches the bar is a good indicator of their proficiency in Olympic lifts. Remember: strength is a skill and like powerlifting, it's not what you lift but how you lift it.

The set-up

- Start with your feet hip-width apart and position them under the bar.
- Bend over (back straight) and grab the bar with a wide grip.
- This should be approximately 75+ cm but will depend on your height and shoulder flexibility since some athletes will use the entire length of the bar. Get into a squat position. Back flat, arms straight and hips higher than your knees, looking ahead.

The pull

- Begin the movement by lifting with your legs, glutes and back.
- Keep the bar as close to your shins as possible without making contact.
- Avoid the knees, but don't worry if your thighs brush the bar on the way up.
- Finish the pull by triple-extending your ankles, knees and hips as you rise onto your toes.

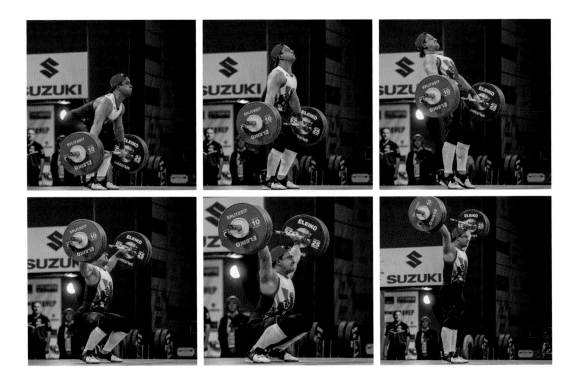

Receiving the bar

- With your back now extended, shrug your shoulders and 'pull' yourself under the bar.
- Move into a full squat position.
- Once the bar passes your head, turn your wrists over and push the bar to a full lockout.
- Do this by driving with your shoulders and triceps and don't worry if your feet position moves to a shoulder-width jump.
- You're now in a full squat with your torso extended, arms locked and bar directly over (or slightly behind) your ears.

The stand

- Only once you have complete control of the barbell can you begin the stand.
- Extend your knees and hips and ensure the bar always stays directly over your ankles and hips.
- Stand upright, controlled and motionless.
- That is one repetition.

MORE POWERFUL MUSCLES

Remember that you have two types of muscle fibres in your skeletal muscle.

To recap, these are Type I fibres (slow twitch) and Type II fibres (fast twitch) that can be further subdivided into Type IIa and Type IIb. The latter have a faster-contractile speed and a much larger cross-sectional area. You basically want lots of these when trying to lift heavy in the gym since they're responsible for generating power.

So how do you develop these? The simple answer is Olympic Lifting. This is because research conducted at the University of Memphis, Tennessee, USA, found that, 'when competitive lifters were compared, those typically utilising the heaviest loads (90% of their 1-rep max or higher), that is weightlifters and power lifters, exhibited a preferential hypertrophy of type II fibres when compared with bodybuilders. This data suggests that maximal hypertrophy occurs with loads from 80–95% 1-rep max.'[16]

Granted, bodybuilders are the foremost experts in the field of muscular hypertrophy – an increase in the size and growth of muscle cells. Also the same study did state that bodybuilders experienced hypertrophy, 'equally in both type I and type II fibres'. But this does raise an interesting point that if you want to increase the size and strength of your muscles by targeting the larger Type II muscle fibres, Olympic-style lifting could form an integral part of your programme.[17]

That's not to say you should ditch conventional forms of hypertrophy training to concentrate solely on your snatch and clean and jerk. Studies show that's a lot of stress to put the body under if you're not specifically training to compete in Olympic Lifting.[18] But in theory it makes sense to drill the technique and then incorporate them once or twice a week.

Anabolic ('muscle-building') hormones

Olympic-style lifting produces more anabolic, 'muscle-building' hormones. According to scientists from the Department of Sport and Exercise Science at the University of Auckland, New Zealand, the powerful and intense nature of Olympic Lifting produces similar spikes in testosterone and growth hormone to those experienced during large bodybuilding-type training.[19]

This is supported by researchers from the Institute of Biomedical Engineering at Imperial College, London, who reported a direct correlation between spikes in anabolic hormones and one-repetition maximum lift in Olympic lifters.[20] Again, that's not to say that if you repeatedly clean and jerk 100+ kg above your head week in and week out you're going to be walking around permanently anabolic with elevated testosterone levels. Remember the Law of Progressive Overload? This could be the Exhaustion Phase just waiting to happen.[21] But including Olympic-style lifts in your training – again just once or twice a week – has been shown to send a natural, anabolic surge of hormones through the body.

YOUR 12-WEEK SPEED AND POWER WORKOUT

REPETITION AND WEIGHT EXPLAINED

When training for speed the weight, repetitions, rest and sets all change. It's important to note this subtle difference because force and speed have an inverse relationship: as you put more weight on the bar the force goes up, but the speed at which you lift comes down (see the graph opposite).

Maximum Strength Training

Training in this 'zone' means we train heavy! Since, as we know, maximal strength is the amount of force generated through a specific movement, examples include the squat, bench and deadlift at 90–100% of your one-repetition maximum.

Strength–Speed Training

Training in this zone requires an athlete to move less weight than when training for maximum strength, but move it at a faster velocity. Examples include Olympic lifts (snatch, clean and jerk and snatch press) at 80–100% of your 1RM.

Peak Power Training

Training in this zone means we train heavy and fast! Delivering peak power output, these exercises produce the greatest amount of force in the least amount of time, and examples include the pull variations of the clean and snatch, jump squats and medicine ball throws at 30–80% of your 1RM.

Speed–Strength Training

Training in this zone means we train speed, but with weight! The goal is to move faster than we do during Strength–Speed Training, so examples include plyometric drills like high hurdle jumps and light-loaded jump squats using 30–80% of your 1RM.

Maximal Velocity Training

Now we want to move the body, muscles and joints as fast as possible. This type of training can be very sport specific, but let's take sprinting as an example. Running 100 metres as fast as you can will represent 100% of your maximum speed, but perform that same 100-metre sprint downhill and therefore assisted (known as 'supramaximal sprinting') and you're now performing above your 100% maximum speed. This training zone is classified as being at less than 30% of your 1RM.

The Force-Velocity Curve

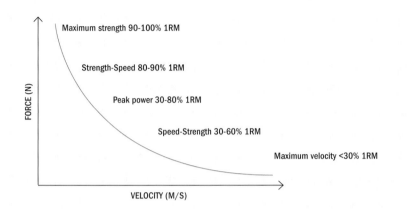

SPEED, FORCE AND WEIGHT EXPLAINED

So, what part of the graph should you train in?

The answer is all of them. These different training zones are just guidelines to various intensities and can be manipulated to fit the athlete in hand. They have been developed by coaches for educational purposes in order to show the effects different exercises and intensities have on athletic performance.

How long athletes spend at each training stage depends on three things:

- **Training age:** (As we know) if you're a newbie to training you have to spend more time improving strength before you refine your speed. This is because strength is highly correlated to power and improvements in strength for a beginner can also improve speed.

- **Specific sport:** Your choice of sport will determine what strength/speed qualities you need. This is just common sense, but a rugby player will need more strength work than a football player. But that doesn't mean a footballer shouldn't improve their strength and part of the strength and conditioning coach's job is to analyse and programme an athlete's training accordingly.

- **Time of season:** This will again change from sport to sport and athlete to athlete, but commonly during the preparatory period, a stronger emphasis should be on developing strength. Then as the season continues, a more specific approach should be taken and a greater emphasis placed on speed.

But (again) all athletes should train along the force–velocity curve.

Training notes

- The sessions of this workout are biomechanically divided. This means your 'push', 'pull' and 'lower-body' movements are performed in different sessions.
- Each workout uses the primary powerlifting movements to form the 'backbone' of the programme.
- The number of repetitions is kept low with plenty of rest between sets.
- This allows enough time to recover, so each movement is performed fast and is as powerful as possible.

Regarding the routine itself:

- The 3-Day Powerlifting/Ballistic Training Hybrid Programme:
    - Is performed weeks 1–4.
    - Combines conventional strength training with ballistic throws and jumps.
- The 3-Day Powerlifting/Resistance Band Hybrid Programme:
    - Is performed weeks 5–8.
    - Combines conventional strength training with resistance bands.
- The 3-Day Powerlifting /Olympic Lifting Hybrid Programme:
    - Is performed weeks 5–8.
    - Combines conventional strength training with Olympic Lifts.

This workout is ideal for any athlete wanting a solid strength and speed conditioning routine.

	3-DAY ROUTINE	**3-DAY ROUTINE**	**3-DAY ROUTINE**
	WEEKS 1–4	**WEEKS 5–8**	**WEEKS 9–12**
KEY FOCUS	Practise technique Combine conventional strength training with ballistic throws and jumps	Practise technique Combine conventional strength training with resistance bands	Practise technique Combine conventional strength training with Olympic Lifts
WORKOUT	Monday: Push Tuesday: REST Wednesday: Lower Body Thursday: REST Friday: Pull Saturday: REST Sunday: REST	Monday: Push Tuesday: REST Wednesday: Lower Body Thursday: REST Friday: Pull Saturday: REST Sunday: REST	Monday: Push Tuesday: REST Wednesday: Lower Body Thursday: REST Friday: Pull Saturday: REST Sunday: REST
MAIN GOAL	Refine and improve technique and increase rate of force development (ROFD) by using a powerlifting/ ballistic hybrid programme.	Refine and improve technique and increase ROFD by using a powerlifting/resistance band hybrid programme that embraces progressive resistance.	Refine and improve technique and increase ROFD by using a powerlifting/Olympic Lifting hybrid programme.

POWERLIFTING/BALLISTIC HYBRID PROGRAMME | 3-DAY ROUTINE

This workout is a fusion of strength and speed genius.

It takes inspiration from the above research and blends it with my experiences training at Brunel and Loughborough as well as the time I'd spent under the iron in Leeds with Andy Bolton. It combines traditional strength training with speed training and includes *Maximum Strength Training, Strength–Speed Training, Peak Power Training, Speed–Strength Training and Strength-Speed Training.*

All to bring about neuro-musculoskeletal adaptations that make you a quicker and more powerful athlete.

WEEKS 1–4 | MONDAY: PUSH

Exercise	Reps	Sets	Rest	% One-Rep Max	Focus
Medicine Ball Throw	5	3	120 secs	30–60%	Speed-Strength
Plyometric Push-up	8	5	120 secs	30–80%	Peak Power
Bench Press	5	5	120 secs	90%	Strength
Push Press	8	3	120 secs	80–90%	Strength-Speed

WEEKS 1–4 | WEDNESDAY: LOWER BODY

Exercise	Reps	Sets	Rest	% One-Rep Max	Focus
Depth Jump	5	3	120 secs	30–60%	Speed-Strength
Weighted Jump Squat	8	5	120 secs	30–80%	Peak Power
Squat	5	5	120 secs	90%	Strength
(Sled) Prowler Push	8	3	120 secs	80–90%	Strength-Speed

WEEKS 1–4 | FRIDAY: PULL

Exercise	Reps	Sets	Rest	% One-Rep Max	Focus
Tyre Flip	5	3	120 secs	30–60%	Speed-Strength
Backward Medicine Ball	8	5	120 secs	30–80%	Peak Power
Deadlift	5	5	120 secs	90%	Strength
Dynamic Bent-over Row	8	3	120 secs	80–90%	Strength-Speed

POWERLIFTING/RESISTANCE BAND HYBRID PROGRAMME | 3-DAY ROUTINE

We are now ready to wield the power of resistance bands.

Born from knowledge and some elasticated rubber, this workout has been created to offer a different form of progressive resistance to your training to help overcome plateaus in power, strength and speed by ultimately increasing your ROFD by loading the muscles above their habitual level in new ways.

The bands can also be used to train far more functionally than conventional weight training alone.

WEEKS 5–8 | MONDAY: PUSH

Exercise	Reps	Sets	Rest	% One-Rep Max	Focus
Resistance Band Push-up	8	3	120 secs	80–90%	Strength-Speed
Bench Press	5	5	120 secs	90%	Strength
Banded Fly	12	3	120 secs	80%	Strength*
Banded Front Delt Raise	12	3	120 secs	80%	Strength*
Resistance Band Tricep Pushdown	8	3	120 secs	80–90%	Strength-Speed*

WEEKS 5–8 | WEDNESDAY: LOWER BODY

Exercise	Reps	Sets	Rest	% One-Rep Max	Focus
Weighted Vest Box Jump	8	5	120 secs	30–80%	Peak Power
Leg Press	5	5	120 secs	90%	Strength
Weighted Lunge	10	5	120 secs	80%	Strength
Band Resisted Squat	8	3	120 secs	80–90%	Strength*

WEEKS 5–8 | FRIDAY: PULL

Exercise	Reps	Sets	Rest	% One-Rep Max	Focus
Band Assisted Pull-up	5	3	120 secs	30–60%	Strength*
Deadlift	5	5	120 secs	90%	Strength
Band Resisted Barbell Curl	12	3	120 secs	80%	Strength*
Band Resisted Single Bicep Curl	12	3	120 secs	80%	Strength*

* Progressive resistance

POWERLIFTING/OLYMPIC LIFTING HYBRID PROGRAMME | 3-DAY ROUTINE

Olympic lifts have been included in this workout for two reasons:

1. To highlight any weak links in the kinetic chain

For example, you might be able to grind out a deadlift, maybe even a squat, but the reality is you can't do this with a snatch and all the joints and muscles must be firing at their optimal level to complete one.

2. Prepare the body with neural recruitment/activation

Basically, the high level of muscle motor recruitment needed for an Olympic lift preps the body, muscle and joints to then lift big during a deadlift or squat.

You can of course design a programme that will solely focus on improving your clean and jerk and snatch, but the beauty of this particular workout is that the weight you lift is less important than the training response we're trying to achieve: to make you a faster and more powerful version of yourself.

WEEKS 9–12 | MONDAY: PUSH

Exercise	Reps	Sets	Rest	% One-Rep Max	Focus
Split Jerk	5	3	120 secs	30-60%	Speed-Strength
Bench Press	5	5	120 secs	90%	Strength
Standing Barbell Press	12	3	120 secs	80%	Strength
Resistance Band Tricep Pushdown	12	3	120 secs	80%	Strength*

WEEKS 9–12 | WEDNESDAY: LOWER BODY

Exercise	Reps	Sets	Rest	% One-Rep Max	Focus
Depth Jump	5	3	120 secs	30-60%	Speed-Strength
Front Squat	5	5	120 secs	90%	Strength
Weighted Jump Squat	8	5	120 secs	30–80%	Peak Power
Overhead Lunge	12	3	120 secs	80%	Strength

WEEKS 9–12 | FRIDAY: PULL

Exercise	Reps	Sets	Rest	% One-Rep Max	Focus
Snatch	5	3	120 secs	30-60%	Speed-Strength
Deadlift	5	5	120 secs	90%	Strength
Jump Shrug	5	3	120 secs	30-60%	Speed-Strength
Band Assisted Pull-up	5	3	120 secs	30-60%	Strength*
Band Resisted Barbell Curl	12	3	120 secs	80%	Strength*

* Progressive resistance

CHAPTER 9
HOW TO IMPROVE ENDURANCE

"ENDURANCE IS ONE OF THE MOST DIFFICULT DISCIPLINES, BUT IT IS TO THE ONE WHO ENDURES THAT THE FINAL VICTORY COMES."
BUDDHA

THE ART OF STAMINA

'Tomorrow is another day, and there will be another battle.'
SEBASTIAN COE

Standing at 178 cm (5 ft 10 in), my short limbs weren't destined for Olympic rowing gold. Also, weighing in at 95 kg my relationship with gravity meant that the Tour de France yellow jersey or a top 10 finish at the London Marathon wasn't very likely either. But what I lack in naturally gifted endurance I make up for with unbridled enthusiasm.

Why is this important? Because everything you read in this chapter is stuff I have learnt. It's completely void of any genetic advantage or physiological predisposition to be good at endurance events. That means if my portly pint-sized frame can learn the art of stamina and endurance, so can yours.

By applying these principles you can run, row, swim and cycle further than you ever thought possible. So let's start with separating endurance fact from endurance fiction.

ENDURANCE | FACT VS FICTION

There is no best way to train for endurance.

This is why – after analysing thousands of studies from years of research – scientists from the Department of Sport, Health and Exercise Science at the University of Hull stated there is no universally agreed consensus on the best way to train for endurance sports. They concluded that: 'There is insufficient direct scientific evidence to formulate training recommendations based on the limited research.' [1]

Basically, endurance is an art form, not an exact science.

The skills and stamina of the world's best athletes remain a mystery. Yes, there are common themes and shared secrets. But no, there isn't a set blueprint, which is why I embarked on an eight-year-long experiment to expand on the 'limited research', living and learning from those men and women who have perfected this craft. This chapter travels from the African plains of Namibia, to the rugged fell mountains of Keswick, in England's Lake District, then ends at the iconic Rowing Club of Cambridge University.

Was the mileage brutal? Yes! Was the quantity of food amazing? Absolutely!

But I dramatically improved my lung capacity, lactic threshold and movement efficiency, and created the Endurance Pyramid of Priority to compete in marathons, triathlons and obstacle races around the world. Sometimes carrying trees and cars, sometimes not.

The Endurance Pyramid of Priority

Building this idea of everlasting endurance is easy in theory, but hard in reality.

But for most endurance-based sports it will happen in five distinct parts: Improve Mechanics, Find Your Fuel, Build Consistency, Add Volume and Increase Intensity. These five aspects are intricately interrelated and you cannot reach your endurance potential unless you execute each one and understand how it is bound to the others.

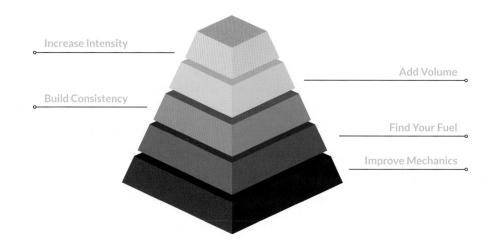

Increase Intensity

Add Volume

Build Consistency

Find Your Fuel

Improve Mechanics

HOW TO USE IT

This is a hierarchical (progressive) way that illustrates how to focus your efforts:

- The lower parts make the biggest difference to your endurance.
- The higher parts make a meaningful contribution to your endurance.

The top part of this (and every pyramid) is infinite and forever evolving. This is why they are all open-ended and may never have a peak, because our understanding and exploration of the human body should never be 'capped' or concluded. This is especially true for endurance.

IMPROVE MECHANICS

Mechanics is basically technique and your ability to move properly through core movements. Whether running, rowing, swimming or cycling, you must learn to move within these sports in the most efficient and effective way based on science and research, learning from experts and champions, but combined with your own height, weight, limb size and biological individuality.

FIND YOUR FUEL

Endurance and fuel are so closely related. You might be able to run, swim or cycle efficiently with good Movement Mechanics, but you won't run, swim or cycle far without good choices of fuel. This is why research from the Nutrition Department at the University of California stated, 'Nutrition during the 4-hour period before competition can significantly affect performance.'[2]

BUILD CONSISTENCY

Building training consistency is like 'dietary adherence' in Chapter 6. You have to be consistent in performing the mechanics of the movement. If you stop or decide to swim, cycle or row randomly a few times a month, then the efficiency you developed will all but be forgotten. So (like a meal plan) never underestimate the power of simply sticking with it.

ADD VOLUME

You Improve Mechanics by doing lots of it. It's that simple. Short and intense bursts of training are great (and we talk about them in the 80/20 Polarised Training part), but you will only develop crisp and efficient technique by increasing the distance or duration of your workouts.

INCREASE INTENSITY

The Law of Progressive Overload taught us that stress and stimuli are the keys to adaptation. Which is why, once you have built consistency and added volume to your movement mechanics and are sufficiently fuelling the sessions, next you must increase the intensity of your workouts so the stress and stimuli cause the legs, lungs, heart and body as a whole to adapt to endurance training.

THE WORLD'S OLDEST RACE | Namibia
RUNNING FOR DINNER

'Every morning in Africa, a gazelle wakes up and knows it must outrun the fastest lion or it will be killed. Every morning in Africa, a lion wakes up and knows it must run faster than the slowest gazelle or it will starve. It doesn't matter whether you're the lion or the gazelle – when the sun comes up, you'd better be running.'

CHRISTOPHER McDOUGALL, Born to Run

The Ju-Wasi tribe have forged superhuman stamina.

How? Living as hunter-gatherers for thousands of years, the most detailed analysis of African DNA to date reveals they are likely to be the oldest population of humans on earth. Therefore they've been perfecting the art of endurance longer than any other civilisation[3]. Not to win medals, not to set records, but to secure survival in one of the harshest climates on Earth. Covering a marathon a day in 39°C and on sand with barely any food or water, their ability to track and hunt animals into exhaustion has become legendary.

This is called 'persistence hunting'.

It involves chasing after your dinner until it collapses to the floor and onto your dinner plate. No weapons are needed. You just need patience, years of tracking experience in the African bush and a profound understanding of human versus animal endurance.

I had none of the above, but as my body adapted under the blistering African sun on a diet of porcupine, berries and fibrous root vegetables, I came to learn lessons that I've since applied during every marathon, triathlon and obstacle race I've ever done. One day, one mile and one stride at a time.

THE WORLD'S WORST BUSHMAN

1 August 2008 is a day my stomach and feet will never forget.

I was on my travels (again). This time tasked with documenting the life of the San Bushmen on the sun-bleached African plains of Namibia. Considered one of the world's greatest hunter-gatherer civilisations ever to have existed, they were currently sat around a campfire boiling tea and plotting the day's hunt.

They talked in an ancient form of communication that consisted of clicking sounds and maps drawn in the sand with a stick, so I had absolutely no idea what was being said. But the occasional gesture in my direction led me to believe they were planning what to do with the short, stocky, overweight trainee San Bushman they'd just adopted. Yours truly.

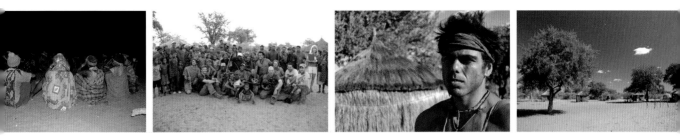

My newly adopted San Bushman family

I didn't blame them either. I must have looked so odd. I hadn't had a haircut for seven months, didn't speak a word of Afrikaans and weighed 30 kg more than their heaviest tribesmen. It's possible I was the world's worst wannabe Bushman they'd ever come across.

But what I lacked in bush skills I made up for in a complete willingness to be accepted, which is why, only moments after arriving, I found myself emerging from a mud hut wearing nothing but a pair of home-made flip-flops and a traditional 'tribal thong' that barely covered my modesty.

Eager to blend in, I found it (semi) worked.

The proverbial ice was broken. Never before had my genitals received such rapturous applause. Invited to sit among the men of the tribe, I gratefully accepted and delicately sat on the hot sand.

However, my victory was short-lived. Handicapped by the language barrier, it seemed once the novelty of my bright white scrotum had worn off there was very little else to do. Without any means of communicating, the only other way to win the respect of my hosts was to hunt.

Hunt fast. Hunt swift. Hunt far.

Moments later I had my chance. It was dinnertime and as I was handed a knife and water bottle it was clear I was joining the 'shopping trip'. Instructed to 'Gently drink as much water as was comfortable' I did as I was told and then re-filled my 800 ml bottle to the brim.

It's 7am, the temperature is rising and I have no idea when I'll see fresh water again.

But to show I'm ready – and if I'm honest to hide my nerves – I jump to my feet. Then I began to bounce around on my toes like a boxer pre-fight. But my fellow tribesman remained seated and calm, each one uninterested in partaking in any form of warm-up.

Why? Because they knew we had a long day ahead.

You know the saying, 'It's a marathon… not a sprint? Well, in Africa when living with the San Bushmen, it's more fitting to say, 'It's a hunt… not a marathon.' Little did I know it would be more than 15 hours before my lips found food and my skin felt shade again.

'THE FAT ONE'

The head of the Ju-Wasi tribe was a man called Duee.

He was 168 cm (5 ft 6 in), slim, svelte and had the largest wrinkles and laughter lines I've ever seen. Engrained into his face from years of hunting in the scorching dry seasons, they went from his eyes to his mouth. It seemed his skills as a great African hunter were matched only by his sense of humour.

This is why upon meeting me he immediately found my oddly shaped body hilarious.

Poking my chest, he found my 'moobs' particularly amusing. So did the entire tribe. I couldn't explain that my ample 'heavage' was a by-product of years of powerlifting, since covering marathons a day on root vegetables, berries and very little meat meant anyone over 60 kg (130 lb) was practically obese in the Namibian wilderness. Henceforth I was affectionately dubbed 'The Fat One'.

But I didn't mind. I felt accepted. Plus, I loved how every Ju-Wasi tribesman was truly happy living in one of the most hostile places on earth. So if my moobs added to that joy I was happy to oblige.

It's now 7:15am and the boob-based jokes stop.

An eerie sense of anticipation surrounded the village. Women and children emerged from their huts to say goodbye to their hunting pack and the serious and sombre look on their faces lead me to believe I – 'The Fat One' – should begin taking this far more seriously than I had been doing. The hunt had begun and with it my baptism of endurance…

THE ART OF ENDURANCE | TECHNIQUE

We were 10 miles into the hunt.

I didn't know where we were going or what was on the menu. The only thing I knew – as I dragged my feet at the back of the group – was that my technique was vastly different to that of the seasoned San Bushmen. Each and every one had perfected this way of moving across the sand with such speed and elegance. It verged on poetic to watch.

They glided across the African bush. I made holes in it.

Their steps made no sound. Mine were heard from miles away.

They were barely breathing. I sounded like an asthmatic antelope.

Back home in England the above mattered far less.

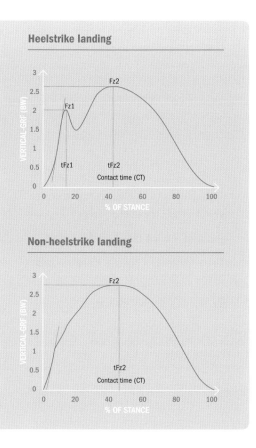

Heelstrike landing

Non-heelstrike landing

I'd even managed to win a few cross-country titles way back in my youth with the above clumsy running form. But out here it's different. My lumbering technique was announcing our arrival to the very animals we were trying to hunt, which meant returning to the village empty-handed was a real possibility.

I was one fat liability.

What's worse is, Duee had noticed. He noticed everything.

Signalling to the group to stop, he circled to the back of the pack. Looking me up and down, now my moobs weren't the only thing he was concerned about. Pointing to my footsteps, he made elephant noises to show my tracks bore an unfortunate resemblance.

He then pointed out each of the San Bushmen's footprints. They were smaller, shallower, swifter and shorter.

So what was I doing wrong? Why did I have 'elephant feet'?

THE ART OF ENDURANCE | FOOT PLACEMENT

The answer is foot placement. We humans all walk, jog, skip and run in different ways. These movements are called 'human gaits and are the different ways in which we can move, either naturally or from specialised training. One key variable in running gait analysis is how our feet strike the floor.

Typically these variations can be categorised:

- **Heel strike:** Where the heel of the foot lands first.
- **Midfoot strike:** Where the heel and ball land simultaneously.
- **Forefoot strike:** Where the ball of the foot lands first.

Now different striking patterns exert different forces – and stress – on the body. If you look at the first graph where the runner heel strikes, you'll notice an initial peak that shows the vertical ground reaction force (GRF). This is where a runner lands on the outside of the heel and 'jabs' their foot into the ground with a sudden impact.

Ouch! This is because the heel doesn't absorb any impact.

It is just bone.

But runners who land on the forefoot – shown in the second graph on page 261 – create relatively little impact force on the feet, and that first peak of this graph, where the heel was 'jabbed' into the ground, is non-existent. No ouch! This is because the ankle flexes and absorbs the impact. You're now using your ligaments, tendons, ankle and foot's architecture like Mother Nature intended.

A study conducted at Harvard University in 2012 found: 'Competitive cross-country runners incur high injury rates, but runners who habitually heel strike have significantly higher rates of repetitive stress injury than those who mostly forefoot strike.'[4]

Duee didn't need a graph or Harvard study to understand any of this.

Like his ancestors, he'd intuitively understood this for years. As a result, he was your perfect fast forefoot striker who drifted and danced his way around the bush. In comparison, I was your archetypal heavy heel striker who fumbled and stumbled his way through the African wilderness.

But why was I heel striking when it's potentially more harmful on my knees, ankles, ligaments and tendons?

To quote the same research from Harvard University, 'Humans have engaged in endurance running for millions of years, but the modern running shoe was not invented until the seventies.' Once they arrived on our shelves, they came complete with elevated and cushioned heels, which in turn encouraged heel strike running.

But before their arrival – and for most of human evolutionary history – runners were either barefoot or wore minimal footwear, which meant we would forefoot strike or midfoot strike. Without the heel-based support and padding, running with a heel strike was just outright painful and we were unable to sustain it over long distances.

LEARNING 'FASTER FEET'

This explains why the Ju-Wasi were running softer, but why were they running faster?

The answer is because running is a skill. This sounds odd, but it's a movement pattern, so more efficiency means more speed and less energy spent. This is why I was always found at the back of the group, trying my best to hide my exhaustion while my teammates glided across the sand with impeccable forefoot form and without a single drop of sweat.

Essentially, any runner looking to improve their speed first needs to improve their form.

Now it must be noted that technique will of course vary from runner to runner based on an individual's height, weight, bone structure and muscle mass (again the Law of Biological Individuality). Therefore, despite what many experts will claim, the idea of the perfect running form doesn't really exist.

But idea of the worst running form does.

I know, since I had perfected it. Here are some of the many errors in running technique crimes that I've committed over the years. Under no circumstances should you try any of them at home:

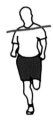
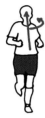
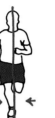
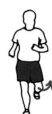
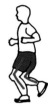

1. Dropped shoulders   2. Twisted body (showing twist to the left)   3. Narrow step width   4. Femur twists inwards   5. Swing leg facing outwards   6. Knees are deeply flexed

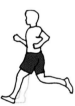
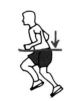
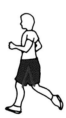

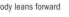

7. Leg lands too far in front   8. Low waist and lower back   9. Body leans forward   10. Restricted range of motion in hip joints   11 Lower leg tilts significantly   12. Toes point outwards after pushing off

LEARNING TO FIND YOUR FUEL

Remember the concept of 'Finding Your Fuel' (page 152)? Well, in Africa you have to find your 'fuel' from anywhere and everywhere.

It doesn't matter if it comes from the fats found in animal skin and nuts or the carbohydrates found in berries and root vegetables. Your body is so incredibly resourceful, and 20 miles into my first hunt I learnt first-hand that it can (and will) find energy and hydration from just about anything.

And by 'anything' I do mean anything!

Drinks at the 'bar'

This is because before we looked at the menu I was told we needed to visit the bar.

Easier said than done. This is because August is right in the middle of the Namibian dry season and our water bottles had been running on empty for the past 10 miles. So, while fuel was needed, hydration was necessary.

Duee motioned a drinking action with his hand. I nodded enthusiastically. In my head I had images of a green and lush oasis opening up on the African savannah where I could fill my bottle with crystal-clear water. Just like in the movies.

The reality was very different. The movies were a lie.

The elephant waterhole was 10 metres wide, around 20 cm deep and a strange blend of brown, orange and green. It was too small to be a pond, but too big to be a puddle, and the grass and foliage surrounding it were either withered, sun-bleached or chewed on by any and every animal that had passed through. Also the smell was unlike anything my nose had ever experienced before.

This is because every inhabitant within a 100-mile radius appeared to have visited, using the waterhole as both a drinks station and a toilet. It was mainly large pieces of elephant dung, but if you looked closely you could also see what the hyenas, birds and kudu had eaten for breakfast too.

What's worse is that each piece of manure was being steamed and stewed for days under the African sun. The result was a scent that was as unique as it was rancid and unforgettable. To this day it haunts my nostrils.

But before I had time to consider my options, Duee and my fellow hunters were face-down and drinking. Not even bothering to fill up their bottles just yet. I, of course, didn't possess the same Spartan-like stomach bacteria, so instead did my best to fill my bottle while avoiding as much faeces as I could. I then added a generous supply of iodine – to purify the water – and waited for it to work its magic.

Ten minutes later my delicate English stomach was ready to sample this African delicacy. The iodine had worked to kill the bacteria, but my gag reflex was far from happy. Battling the large lump of something that hit that back of my throat, I was determined not to bring it back up. I was already known for my moobs and elephant feet; I didn't want to add 'thunder chunder' to that list too.

Thankfully – and through unknown digestive physiology – I kept it down and through gritted teeth smiled and toasted Duee to thank him. He laughed and knew exactly what my head was thinking and my stomach was feeling.

FINDING OUR FUEL

Now hydrated, it was time to look at the menu. Again I (falsely) had images of zebra steak cooked over a roaring open fire, or maybe an ostrich soup that had been stewed to perfection with a collection of roasted vegetables. I was wrong. With fermented elephant faeces still rolling around in my stomach we were hot on the trail of a porcupine who'd heard us coming and buried himself deep underground.

'What now?' I asked shrugging to signify I wasn't hopeful. Looking around, all I could see was a barren wasteland. Everything was brown and torched by the sun and this was the only 'buffet' we'd seen for the past 50 miles.

But Duee wasn't giving up. Lying on the floor with his ear to the ground, he then pointed to five different places surrounding the hole the porcupine had just disappeared down. About two metres apart, my fellow hunters each knelt down and began digging with their bare hands. An ancient form of African animal chess had begun. Picking the fifth hole, I joined in the shopping trip.

Hours passed and we were now battling with the sun, our food and fatigue. Every time we dug, the porcupine moved. The only reason I ignored my ever-complaining stomach was because Duee looked ever confident the dinner bell would sound at any time.

He (as usual) was right. Checkmate!

A final hole was dug and the porcupine's tunnel exposed. With nowhere to turn it made a bid for freedom, and with its spikes flaring it shot out of the hole like a cannon. I froze, so thankfully it wasn't my hole it ran out of. Instead, it was Duee's and he delivered a spear right between its shoulder blades. We were now 30 miles from the village, but at least we would return with food.

Which is why – now safe in the knowledge that there was a 'finish line' – Duee unveiled a small bag of nuts, berries and roots, and indicated that we eat these with the skin. The fats from the animal skin and nuts combined with the carbohydrates in the berries and root vegetables would provide a dual-fuel energy source to get us back to the village.

We would then save the meat for the rest of the tribe.

How did it taste? Like slimy, furry leather, and the side helping of berries got stuck in my teeth. But it was one of the most satisfying, nutrient-dense meals I'd ever had as much-needed calories were sent coursing through my body and to my long-struggling legs and limbs.

With my senses heighted I could quite literally feel my body synthesising the energy from the food. I was experiencing something runners have known for years. That modern science had known for decades. But the San Bushmen have known this for centuries. I was experiencing the very basics of bioenergetics.

Basics of bioenergetics

Bioenergetics is the study of how the body converts food into energy.

It is why research from the Nutrition Department at the University of California stated, 'Proper nutrition during ultra-endurance races is critical for the maintenance of energy balance.'[5] Now I wasn't running an ultra-endurance race, but I knew that without food this hunt wouldn't last long.

All because (as we know from Chapter 6) the food we put in our mouths is basically chemical energy that our bodies will use when needed (like when in pursuit of a deer). It does this by converting that food into adenosine triphosphate (or ATP for short), a high-energy molecule that we use to fuel our bodies and power our muscles (along with a variety of other metabolic and life-sustaining functions in our bodies).

But how were we converting the twigs, nuts and berries we were eating en route into chemical energy (ATP) to fuel our bodies through the African wilderness?

Well, that depends on our speed and the stage of the hunt.

This is because there are three primary energy systems that produce ATP: the phosphocreatine system, the glycolytic system (anaerobic) and the oxidative system. Each of these systems can be characterised by the duration and/or intensity of the task you are performing.

ENERGY SYSTEM	DURATION
Phosphocreatine system (PC)	0–10 secs
PC and glycolytic system (slow)	10–30 secs
Glycolytic system (fast)	30 secs–2 mins
Glycolytic and oxidative system	2–3 mins
Oxidative system	3+ mins (and when at rest)

From the table above a few things should be apparent:

- Shorter duration but higher-intensity activity is powered by the phosphocreatine and glycolytic systems. This is what would happen if we spotted our dinner and were forced to sprint.

- Longer duration but lower-intensity movements are powered by the oxidative system (including rest). This is the energy system we were relying on for 98% of the hunt, covering miles and miles at a slow and steady pace.

- Throughout a hunt (like in training, sport and life) the body does a good job blending the capabilities of all of these systems to ensure you are getting the ATP you need to compete, train or survive.

Get some fat carbs

But did the fats and carbohydrates from the animal skin, nut and berry combo work so well? That is hard to say.

Sports nutritionists are still debating to this day the best food to fuel a race. What's more, throw into the mix the relatively new field of research they call 'nutrigenomics' – the study of how our genes interact with our nutrition – and consider that can of worms opened.

But one reason could be because researchers from the Centre for Human Nutrition at the University of Colorado claim, 'Glycogen (carbohydrate) storage capacity is approximately 15 g/kg body weight.'[6] To use a sporting example, this means a marathon runner who weighs 67 kg would only be able to store 1005 grams of carbs (at the most), meaning they would run out of muscle glycogen – and therefore fuel – by the 20-km mark.

Which is exactly why, as we saw in Chapter 6, research suggests the inclusion of fat in the diet (see page 152).

For good reason too, since while carbohydrates contain 4 calories per gram, fat provides a whopping 9 calories per gram. That's not to say one is better than the other, since the body processes each very differently. But when midway through a marathon, I know that having a dual-fuel supply of both can only be a good thing.

These circumstances are best described in the book *Human Muscle Fatigue: Physiological Mechanisms*. Researchers from the Department of Biochemistry at the University of Oxford stated that the energy needed to sustain exercise for a long period of time comes from the oxidisation of two fuels – carbohydrates and fats.

Interestingly, they state that the latter is a more sustainable fuel source and provides the 'largest energy reserve in the body'[7] that can provide enough energy to last about five days. In contrast, muscle glycogen reserves are limited and at most could provide energy to sustain 90 minutes of exercise.

With elephant manure in my belly and porcupine fur in my teeth, I now understood this.

MY JU-WASI GRADUATION

We arrived back to camp to a heroes' welcome.

Food was presented and clean, faeces-free water gratefully received. We then sat around the campfire as Duee entertained those in attendance with stories of my feet and gag reflex. I, of course, didn't mind and was glad to play my (small) part in the hunt. Even if it was just to provide entertainment.

Hours passed and the fire faded. I thanked Duee and my fellow Bushmen for what was an unforgettable day and then retired for the night.

Falling into my hut, my legs were throbbing, head was spinning and I still had berries and fur in my teeth. But dehydrated and with a touch of sunstroke, 'The Fat One' had survived the world's oldest endurance race. Not through technique, but through sheer determination and moob-based man pride. This was the starting point of my eight-year-long quest to master endurance, which is why, returning home, I headed to the mountains of Keswick in England's Lake District. Immersing myself in a sport that dates back to the 19th century, I hoped the history and heritage of fell running could provide me with answers to the questions I'd had since Africa.

My mentor? Friend and World Obstacle Racing Team Champion James Appleton. The human equivalent of an elite mountain goat. Attempting to keep up with him almost killed me. But I would return from the glacial ribbon lakes and rugged fell mountains of northern England a changed man, a better athlete and a mildly competent, semi-skilled fell runner.

THE GREATEST RUNNERS YOU'VE NEVER HEARD OF | Lake District, UK

FELL RUNNERS

To understand James Appleton, you must understand fell running.

A sport wrapped in mystique, it's sometimes referred to as mountain running. But to me this is too simplistic. Instead, I describe it to people as running over some of northern Britain's most remote and rugged terrain in a competition that's like 'cross-country running on speed and steroids'. Then at the end of this description I always deliver a caveat: nothing can truly prepare you for the reality.

It has a sporting culture unlike anything you've experienced. It crosses terrain unlike anything you've run on. It has a dress code unlike anything you've seen, but above all else,

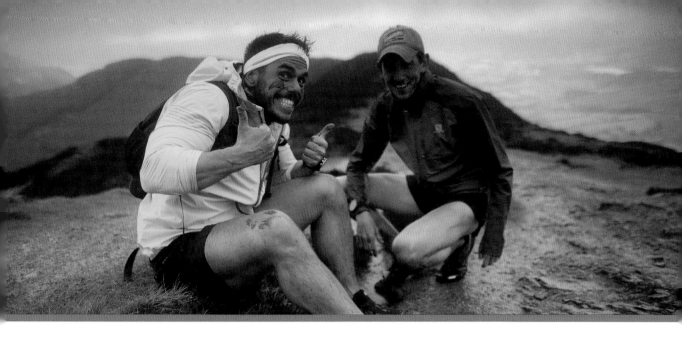

it's produced some of the greatest runners you've never heard of.

All because it's completely, utterly and defiantly unique and isolated to the Lake District.

Tracing its origins back to community fairs and games in the 19th century, fell racing took place alongside other sports such as wrestling and hammer throwing. It was one of many ways for communities of shepherds and agricultural labourers to compare speed, strength and stamina, and for individuals to gain local pride and notoriety. In fact, to this day this still remains the motive for many.

Superhuman feats of endurance are merely reported on in club newsletters, records are kept contained within Lake District folklore and some truly incredible runners will remain unknown, unreported and soon forgotten.

Understand this and you understand James Appleton.

This is because although a supremely talented runner, he is also an award-winning photographer, incredibly modest and much preferring being behind the camera.

Basically James – like all fell runners – runs for the love of the sport and the thrill of local competition and camaraderie. Global stardom, money and sponsorship were all foregone for personal pride, cake at the finish line and (at the very most) a picture in *Fellrunner* magazine and a trophy presented at the local pub.

This is fell running in its purest form. All delivered with a sizeable serving of eccentricity, resilience and grit. Muscle-bound ankles, wild facial hair and a feral appearance are optional but preferred. But to truly absorb the culture, James tells me I need to double-knot my shoe-laces, pack the shortest shorts I can find and head to Keswick to experience it at first hand. So that's what I did during the most gruelling 10 km I've ever run.

RUN 10 KM | UPHILL, DOWNHILL, FAST AND SLOW

'Run often. Run long. But never outrun your joy of running.'

JULIE ISPHORDING, Olympic Long-Distance Runner

It is 1pm on 21 April 2015, outside a coffee shop in Keswick.

James and I were grabbing a coffee and a toasted cheese panini before deciding on the best route to take for my maiden fell-running voyage. The weather had been kind too and although the sun was shining, there was a light breeze that would be very welcome mid-run. These were great running conditions, I thought, taking a bite of my panini.

Minutes later we were joined by one of James' training partners. Best described as a legend of the Lake District, it seems everyone knew the name Rupert Bonington. Son of the decorated British mountaineer Sir Chris Bonington, he grew up in a place called Nether Row, 15 miles over the fells from where we were sitting, and started running at the age of 10 up a fell called High Pike that he'd do with his dad when he was training for expeditions.

Later moving to Keswick at 23, he's now 46, which means he has been running across, up and down these fells for years and there is no running route he hasn't conquered. Needless to say, I immediately liked Rupert, who was now on the phone, clearing his plans for the day and joining us for a run.

Our running club was now three strong and our chat turned from toasted sandwiches to the fells as Rupert and James spoke in a language I could barely understand. But I did learn a few things that day:

It's never too hot or too cold to go for a run; actually, the wilder the better!

A 'fell' is a hill or stretch of high moorland, especially in northern England.

A 'crag' is a rugged cliff or rock face.

A 'bog' is an area of wet muddy ground that is too soft to support a heavy body.

'Scree' is a mass of small, loose stones that cover a slope on a mountain.

My level of running experience was embarrassing in comparison to theirs.

How embarrassing? Allow me to explain with some calculations I wrote on my panini napkin. In a year, Rupert's GPS watch informed us, he will run 1600 miles, with around 122,000 metres (400,000 ft) ascent, with an average 76-metre (250-ft) ascent per mile. To put that into perspective, that means he runs more than five marathons every month and climbs more than the height of Everest every month.

This doesn't even take into account the terrain. See, my mileage was often clocked on the immaculate synthetic rubber running track of Loughborough University, which the bones and ligaments in my feet loved. But James and Rupert's feet were made of something different. They each had feet that were forged over bogs, crags and scree.

In short, it would be a miracle if I finished the day with tendons intact.

But I was determined to return to Keswick town centre successful, even if I was sore. So I asked the waitress to reserve some freshly baked scones and locally sourced ice cream for my triumphant return.

Baptism of fire and fells

My first fell-running experience can only be described as brutally beautiful.

This is because after 68 minutes, 10 km and 600 metres (2000 ft) of ascent I was standing on a mountain top, but had been entirely humbled by the process of getting here. As I collapsed onto a patch of moss growing on a stone, James and Rupert were passionately proud of their 'back garden' and insisted I get to my feet and take in the view.

I'm glad they did. Yes, this was the hardest 10 km I've ever run. But it was also the most scenic.

'Welcome to the Lake District,' James said, smiling.

With my mouth wide open, what I saw was best described as a picturesque patchwork of lakes, valleys, woodlands and fells. I counted 20 different shades of green and could immediately see why this landscape had inspired every English poet and painter to pass through during the late 18th century.

In that moment my legs and lungs no longer hurt. My senses were entirely satisfied. So there we stood in silence. Not a word needed to be spoken. Instead, I relived the last 10 km in my head and was amazed how James and Rupert's technique had striking similarities to that of the San Bushmen. Gliding over every trail, gradient and terrain, their technique never faltering, their energy never wasted. Which is why I felt compelled to break the silence and speculatively ask, 'How long before I'm jumping fells in a single bound?'

'Thirty days.' James' immediate and definitive response surprised me.

'What? So, I just train in the fells for 30 days and BOOM! I graduate?' I asked.

He laughed and then explained how the giant U-shaped valleys of the Lake District were the greatest training aid ever created. Also, the rough grass, rocky paths, sheer vertical hillside tracks and fast-paced descents that tax your quads and confidence will be the best training partners I've ever had.

So, for the next 30 days, that's what I did, learning everything I could about the Lake District and the secrets the fell runners keep in their calves.

LEARN TO RUN UPHILL

'Hills never get easier, you get stronger.'
GREG LEMOND, Three-time Tour de France winner

Days later I was 20 minutes into my first hill-running session.

My knees are complaining. My legs are burning. My lungs are crying out for oxygen. This is because James and Rupert failed to mention that 'hill sprints' hosted in the Lake District mean something completely different to the rest of the world. They're longer, steeper and will test every bone in your feet and muscle fibre in your legs.

Basically, fell runners don't abide by the same rules as the rest of the running community.

Sweating and breathing more than any human in the history of fell running, I found Rupert running alongside me delivering small snippets of advice and encouragement as he effortlessly leapt up the cliff face.

'Imagine you're being pulled up the hill by a rope attached to the top of your chest. Keep your chin up and this will encourage you to open your chest, which will help your breathing and also encourage a strong running technique from the hips up, stopping you from collapsing your shoulders and slouching, which impacts on how smoothly you can run,' he said as he exaggerated his tip-tap running style that effortlessly glides up the hill.

'The increase in hip movement with running incline allows for the production of the power necessary to lift the body.'
JOURNAL OF EXPERIMENTAL BIOLOGY[8]

I nodded… Very appreciative… Unable to speak!

'Take small steps and forefoot strike to use the elasticity in your calves,' he said, pointing to James who was now 100 metres ahead of us and bounding over any rock, hill or river that came his way. Again, a nod was all I could manage.

'But what happens when I find it far too steep to run?' I tentatively asked given that virtually all of this fell was steep!

'That's when we get to power walk, hands pushing down on your lower thighs like pistons, maximising the power of your arms and shoulders combined with your legs,' Rupert says, giving me a quick demonstration.

What seemed like an eternity later I joined James and Rupert at the top. Gasping for air, I pointed at my calves and quads and gestured they were shot to pieces. With my message communicated I then fell onto a small, soft mound that perfectly protruded from the ground like a mud-based pillow that my hamstrings sunk into.

'That's no mud you're sat in,' James said, trying not to laugh.

'I did wonder why it was so warm,' I replied. Far too tired to care (or move) I asked out of curiosity: 'Sheep shit or cow crap?' James leant forward to give his verdict. 'You, my friend, are currently soothing your legs in sheep shit.'

'That now makes sense,' I said as I laid back, relaxed and made peace with my current predicament. As I did he then told me something that gave my lactic-ridden, shit-coated legs hope. 'Although I wasn't lying in animal excrement, where you're lying was me in 2013.'

'Uphill running requires greater muscular activity compared to level running and downhill running.'
SPORTS MEDICINE, 2017[9]

'It was the Spartan World Championships, and part of the course was up and down ski slopes. I basically got owned by the hills, since they use the terrain itself as an obstacle. This is why I decided to leave London and move up here, because you cannot train to be a good uphill runner without uphill running. It works completely different muscle groups.'

'During uphill running, the muscles most activated were the adductors (hips and thighs), biceps femoris (back of the legs), gluteal group, gastrocnemius (calves) and vastus group (quadriceps). Compared with horizontal running, uphill running required considerably greater muscle activation.'
JOURNAL OF APPLIED PHYSIOLOGY[10]

'How much uphill running?' I managed to ask now some oxygen had returned to my lungs.

'Around 5000 ft [1524 metres] of climbing a week,' was his prescription. 'I remember the first month I ran up here my quads (front of the legs) were in agony. They were just on fire during every run. But it was after 30 days that my hamstrings kind of woke up and said, "Oh we'll help you out" and then going uphill it felt like I had these diesel engines in the back of my legs.'

'After this extreme mountain ultra-marathon, the subjects modified only their uphill-running patterns for a more economical step mechanics.'
EUROPEAN JOURNAL OF APPLIED PHYSIOLOGY[11]

If my hamstrings could talk they would definitely not be saying, 'We'll help out.' They were probably saying, 'Why are we sat in shit?'

But I trusted James and the lessons contained among the rocks and bracken. So I stood up, stretched and prepared for another harsh lesson in running downhill descents.

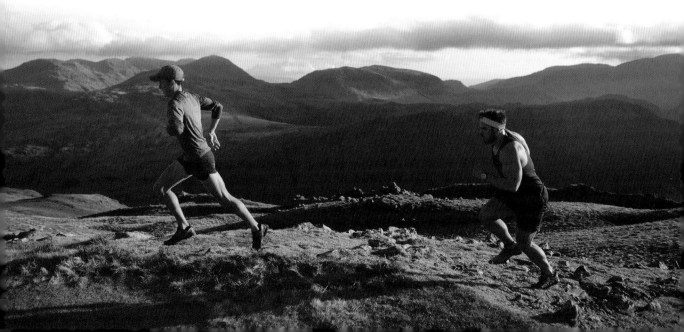

LEARN TO RUN DOWNHILL

What goes up, must come down. Which is why now, stood on a mountain top, Rupert tells me you can't become a good fell runner unless you master the art of downhill running. James nods and says it's a skill he's had to develop since moving to the Lakes.

'I'm better now than I was,' James admits. 'But following the local guys around here, they will put minutes between me and them during a race when running downhill. Going uphill I'm fitter and can beat them, but downhill they are another league. They've just been doing it years.'

'Incorporating downhill locomotion (running) in the training programmes of ultra-trailers may help to improve performance-related physiological and biomechanical parameters.'
JOURNAL OF SPORTS SCIENCE[12]

This didn't fill me with confidence as I looked down my steeply descending induction. 'Any tips and tricks?' I asked, desperate for any help anyone could offer.

Rupert responded, 'There are different schools of thought when it comes to running downhill. Ultimately, they both share one common theme: confidence. You have to have confidence in that in many instances the faster you go the less likely it is you'll slip or fall as in reality the faster you are moving the less time your feet have on the ground and thus slip.'

This sounded completely counter-intuitive, but then most of fell running is. So I listened intently and took mental notes and I ensured the double-knot on my trainers was tight.

'Whether you decide to go for the fast feet approach or large bounding steps you must try and commit. Keep your chin up so you're looking ahead, lean forward, relax and allow the momentum of the hill to power you. Also try and keep your ankles loose and foot placement as gentle as possible and attempt to midfoot strike since this will (again) allow your momentum to propel you down the hill.'

I won't lie, at this point I have gone from tentative to terrified, but it gets worse.

'Also, don't heel strike because it will hammer your quads and slow you down. That's unless you're on steeper ground. But I mean steep ground, where the gradient is enough to slide down on your bum. Then you do need to heel strike, but you keep your ankles and knees soft, lean forward and let yourself go. You can either quickly lift your knees to encourage fast feet or take the dramatic leaping/bounding motion which gets you down quickly but may result in a few speedy tumbles!'

'Wait, what?' My laces were now the least of my worries. 'Can we back up a minute? You're telling me this isn't considered steep?' I said now looking down the scariest descent I have ever come across.

'Also, let me get this right. Your measure of "steep" is when you no longer run but have to slide on your bum to get down? Is that right? Also, what's a "speedy tumble" and what's the fell running definition of a "few"?'

They both just laughed. 'Just remember, don't brake too much and commit.' And with that they took off. Without any time to consider my options, I began running too. Trying my best to mimic their footsteps, commit and leave my foot off the brake as they'd instructed.

With each step my life was flashing before my eyes.

I didn't know if I was committing or just falling uncontrollably, but whatever I was doing my quads were not a fan. As I left giant holes among the fells it was clear my ankles were far from loose and my footsteps were far from gentle. In contrast, James and Rupert were barely leaving a single footprint.

My 'elephant feet' from Namibia had returned and I was losing at this thing called fell running.

'Downhill running induces severe lower limb tissue damage.'
EUROPEAN JOURNAL OF APPLIED PHYSIOLOGY[13]

'Run soft, smooth and with speed,' they both shouted back up the hill. I couldn't shout back.

I was too preoccupied with stopping my ankles from snapping on the uneven rocks that weren't completely dry even though the morning mist had cleared. Each step I took became a trade-off between reducing the risk of falling and reducing the energy spent from braking.

'Metabolic cost increases during downhill running at steep angles.'
JOURNAL OF BIOMECHANICS[14]

Finally, it wasn't soft, smooth or quick, but I thankfully reached the bottom.

My legs were in pieces. I would rather survive a squat session with Andy Bolton than do another downhill run with Appleton and Bonington. I could literally feel the tiny muscle fibres tearing in my legs with every step.

'You were going too slow,' James said. He wasn't being rude; this was fact. 'Running can exert a load of as much as three times your bodyweight on a single leg as it comes into contact with the ground. When running downhill this is amplified since you're battling gravity. People don't understand just how fatiguing a mechanism braking can be.'

'During downhill running the role of eccentric work of the "anti-gravity" muscles is increased.'
BRITISH JOURNAL OF SPORTS MEDICINE[15]

My baptism of fire and fells was complete… but my training had just begun.

LEARN TO RUN SMARTER

Days later and I was thankfully back at sea level.

But after my hill-based initiation my legs were sore. Not just a little either, I mean unholy amounts of (delayed onset) muscle soreness as I hobbled through the cobbled streets of Keswick to meet James and Rupert. Watching me limp as they sat eating tuna toast melts they couldn't help but laugh.

I looked like Bambi (drunk) on ice.

Delayed onset of muscle soreness (DOMS) is a common response to exercise involving significant eccentric loading. Symptoms of DOMS vary widely and may include reduced force-generating capacity, significant alterations in muscle and connective tissue health, alteration of neuromuscular function and changes in mechanical performance.'[16]

'My legs are killing,' I said, pulling up a chair and ordering two more tuna toast melts.

'Also, my feet are blistered, I keep leaving holes in the Keswick countryside because I can't descend properly and I must have set a record for the most amount of "speedy tumbles" ever performed on a single fell.'

'I counted 17 in total between Steel Fell and Helm Crag,' James said, still smiling.

For those not familiar with the Lake District, Steel Fell and Helm Crag are two incredibly steep and incredibly iconic fells overlooking the stunning landscape of Grasmere. The views from both are absolutely stunning (I'm told), but of course I wouldn't know because I spent most of my time there tumbling down the sides of them.

But jokes aside, James and Rupert knew I was a walking, talking Exhaustion Phase waiting to happen and so said something that was music to my ears (and quads). 'Don't worry! For the rest of the week 80% of our training will be slow and only 20% fast.' I didn't know what they meant at the time, but I liked those percentages.

The 80/20 polarised training concept

To understand the concept of 80/20 polarised training you have to understand your anaerobic threshold.

This is the point when you're running at an intensity and speed that means your body cannot maintain its intake of oxygen. This results in excess lactic acid accumulating in the body (that burning sensation you get in your legs during a steep hill sprint), which in turn makes it difficult for the body to produce the energy required to continue running at that intensity and speed.

It sounds complicated but (again) it's not. Your anaerobic threshold is one of the main reasons you can't sprint an entire marathon.

It's that simple. In contrast, running at an intensity and speed below your anaerobic threshold means excess lactic acid does not accumulate in the body, you're able to supply enough oxygen to the muscles and therefore able to produce the energy required to continue running at that intensity and speed.

If you're running at a speed that you can maintain for a marathon, then that pace is below your anaerobic threshold.

Now there's technology that can accurately test your anaerobic threshold, and I regularly have mine tested at Loughborough University or at the ASICS Running Lab, but one of the easiest ways that James taught me was that if you can run and talk comfortably at the same time, you're probably running below your anaerobic threshold. But if you're running at a speed that means you're unable to speak in complete sentences, you're probably running above your anaerobic threshold.

Using the 80/20 polarised training concept:

- You spend 80% of your time running slow and below your anaerobic threshold to train movement mechanics, consistency and volume.
- You spend 20% of your time running fast and above your anaerobic threshold to train intensity.

LEARN TO RUN SLOW

Long, slow distance running simply involves running at a slow pace over long distances.

It's basically continuous running at a speed that's comfortable. This method helps runners improve aerobic metabolic capacity in the leg muscles (supplying them with oxygen) and develops the basic physical strength required to complete 10 km, 20 km or a marathon.

It also gives you plenty of time to learn to run, and because today I was running through the (flat) streets of Keswick way below my anaerobic threshold, it meant I could actually talk as James and Rupert launched into a full, scientific critique of my technique. To my surprise, everything they described was everything I had witnessed years before on the plains of Africa. Mile after mile they would shout the following cues:

'Relax the arms'

Increasing speed tends to stiffen a runner's arm swing. This can be avoided by removing tension from the shoulders and visualising a relaxed swinging style that starts from the elbows.

'Move at the hips'

An efficient running style makes use of the whole body, for example by using the large muscles around the hip joint that are close to the body's centre of mass, to enable a relaxed swinging of the legs. Swinging the legs upwards (as if straddling something) will enable runners to use their hip muscles. In addition, avoiding a mental image of pushing off will reduce the load on smaller muscles such as the calves.

'Land close to your body'

Landing your foot in a position far from the body should be avoided because it increases the leg's braking force. Aim to return the swing leg in a smooth, relaxed motion while ensuring your foot lands close to the body.

'High waist position'

An urge to push the leg off from the ground causes some runners to overflex the knees, resulting in a slumped lower back and waist and causing the legs to trail behind. When landing, be careful not to flex the knee too much. You should also aim to land lightly on the ground with the waist in a high position. This will ensure an efficient push-off. Everything practised during your slow-paced runs is based on the work of Dr Arthur Steindler. If you remember from the World's Longest Rope Climb (Chapter 5), his work defines your 'kinetic chain' as 'a combination of several successively arranged joints constituting a complex motor unit'. Put simply: how well all your joints and movements work together during certain movements.

LEARN TO RUN FAST

Sprint. Rest. Repeat.

This training method involves repeating a series of fast-paced and slow-paced running intervals, all to improve the body's ability to remove excess lactic acid (that burning sensation you get when halfway up a hill run). While many runners vary the speeds of their fast running, it is important to maintain a slow recovery jogging speed, and the next sprint interval should start before a runner's heart rate drops too far.

Why? Because this type of training improves both aerobic and anaerobic fitness.

In basic terms what this means is any activity (like running a marathon) can be classed as anaerobic and aerobic. Aerobic means 'with oxygen' since this relates to all activities that require us to breathe to complete them. Examples are 800-metre, 5-km or 10-km runs: trying to run these distances without oxygen is impossible.

Anaerobic exercise relates to those shorter, quicker activities that don't need as much oxygen, like a 100-metre sprint, which can be done without (heavy) breathing. Now running a marathon – and endurance generally – needs both aerobic and anaerobic fitness, which is why researchers wanted to test the 'effects of moderate-intensity endurance and high-intensity intermittent training on aerobic fitness and anaerobic fitness'. What did they find?

Basically, contrary to popular belief, they found 'That moderate-intensity aerobic training that improves aerobic fitness does not change anaerobic capacity and that adequate high-intensity intermittent training may improve both anaerobic and aerobic energy supplying systems significantly.'[17] Put simply, a leisurely 5-km run will improve your aerobic fitness, but may not be best suited to enhance your anaerobic fitness. But an interval-based workout – trying to complete ten 100-metre sprints with 40 seconds of rest in between – could potentially improve both.

MASTERING 'FASTER (ELEPHANT) FEET'

After 30 days of running up, down and around the fells I had graduated.

Completing my eight-year-long endurance-based pilgrimage that started by an elephant waterhole, I was desperate to see if I had cured my 'elephant feet'. So I laced up my trainers and headed to the sports laboratory to find out.

What did I find and conclude? In summary, the Ju-Wasi tribe, James and Rupert were among the greatest running partners I've ever had. Their technique was impeccable and their stamina undeniable. But after eight years I concluded that running is a skill that's incredibly personal and this idea of perfect 'textbook technique' doesn't exist. Yes, everyone can make refinements to gain more efficiency and speed (I know I made lots), but even three of the world's greatest athletes – with cabinets full to the brim with trophies – had their faults.

Paula Radcliffe is the current women's world record holder in the marathon. Her time of 2 hours 15 minutes and 25 seconds is incredible and is largely why she is a three-time winner of the London Marathon (2002, 2003, 2005) and three-time winner of the New York Marathon (2004, 2007, 2008).

She represented Great Britain at the Olympics four times consecutively and is considered by many to be the greatest female long-distance runner of modern times. But what's amazing is that all this was achieved despite many 'experts' claiming her head bobs around like it's independent from her body and she runs like she has a 'hiccup' in her stride.

Haile Gebrselassie is an Ethiopian running legend. He won two Olympic gold medals over 10,000 metres and four World Championship titles in the event. He won the Berlin Marathon four times consecutively and also had three straight wins at the Dubai Marathon. Further to this, he won four world titles indoors and was the 2001 World Half Marathon Champion.

And he did all this despite running with a 'crooked' left arm. This is because as a child growing up on a farm, he used to run 10 km to school every morning, and the same back every evening, which led to his distinctive running posture, with his left arm crooked as if still holding his school books.

Emil Zatopek is considered to be the greatest runner of the 20th century. Best known for winning three gold medals at the 1952 Summer Olympics in Helsinki, he took gold in the 5000 metres and 10,000 metres, but his final medal came when he decided at the last minute to compete in the first marathon of his life. Nicknamed the 'Czech Locomotive', in 1954 he became the first runner to break the 29-minute barrier in the 10,000 metres and three years earlier (1951) had broken the hour for running 20 km.

However, his running style was famously unsightly. Possibly due to his military background and years running in army boots, he ran like someone had shot him in both legs and his head bounced around uncontrollably.

Ross Edgley is the world's worst San Bushman and fell runner. Standing 178 cm (5 ft 10 in) and (sometimes) weighing over 100 kg (220 lb) , sports science (and logic) would say it would be impossible for him to take his moobs and 'elephant feet' around a marathon, never mind a triathlon with a tree. Believed to be too heavy and too clumsy.

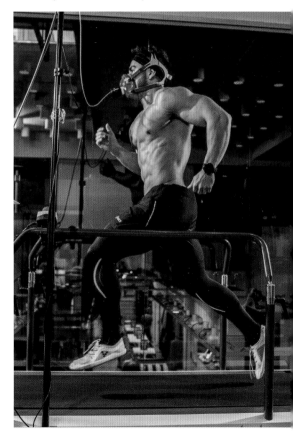

My body angle is good leaning forward, forefoot striking to absorb impact and carry on forward motion. (Semi) good range of motion at the hip (but could be better; as you'll notice my driving leg is not moving back beyond the middle of my body). Also moving in a slightly vertical motion (again caused by a lower range of motion at the hip), which is forcing my upper body to rotate more, my elbow to raise and essentially means I don't move forward as efficiently as possible (slightly wasted energy). In summary, I wouldn't ever class myself as a good runner and after eight years I was no closer to finding a definitive blueprint for endurance-based sporting success. But:

- Knowing my limitations and being conscious of my movement (and elephant feet) is a huge advantage.
- Learning to run efficiently can be just as rewarding as running fast.
- Exploring the intricacies of endurance is fascinating and something I continue to do.

YOUR 20-WEEK MARATHON GUIDE

Training notes

This 20-week marathon training guide puts all the theory into practice.

Remember, based on research from the Department of Sport, Health and Exercise Science at the University of Hull there is no universally agreed consensus on the best way to train for endurance sports (see page 255). But the programme is designed using all the principles described from Africa to the Lake District to get a relative beginner over the finish line of a marathon, in 20 weeks, in under five hours. The keys to this programme are:

- All units are listed in kilometres.
- The hardest and most intense training period is between weeks 12 and 17.
- Numbers that are in brackets indicate the run should be done at a pace higher than your anaerobic threshold pace.
- Numbers in red indicate you should run at race pace.
- The final long-distance run should be done two weeks prior to the race.
- Two days before the race, jog 2–3 km and increase speed over 1 km to simulate the race and stimulate the legs.

WEEK		MON	TUES	WED	THUR	FRI	SAT	SUN	DISTANCE PER WEEK (KM)
1	30-minute run (walk if necessary to acclimatise the body to the distance).	10			10		10		N/A
2	Jog at a slow and comfortable pace.		3	3	3		3		12
3			3	3	3		5		14
4	Run above your anaerobic threshold pace once per week.		5		5		5		15
5			5	5	5		5		20
6	Run faster than your anaerobic threshold pace twice a week. Perform a long-distance run on Sat/Sun that is slower than your anaerobic threshold pace.		(5)		(5)		7		17
7			(5)		(5)		10		20
8			(7)		(7)		10		24
9			(7)		(7)		12		26
10			(7)		(7)		15		29
11			(7)		(5)		15		27
12	Run faster than your anaerobic threshold pace once a week. Perform a long-distance run on Sat/Sun that is slower than your anaerobic threshold pace. On the other days, jog at a slow and comfortable pace.	5	(10)				20		35
13		5	(10)				25		40
14		5	(10)				15		30
15		5	(10)			5	25		45
16		5	(10)				15		30
17		5	(10)			5	30		50
18	Run at race pace, but be sure to avoid the Exhaustion Phase.		5	10			15		30
19		7		5			5		17
20		5		3		(1)	RACE		9

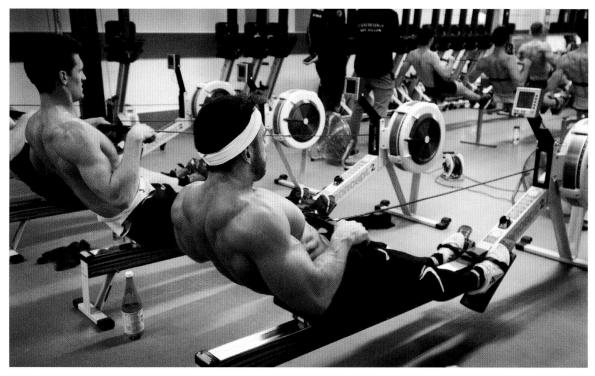

Becoming the strangest-shaped rower in the history of the Cambridge Rowing Club

HOW TO BUILD MUSCLE WITH CARDIO

MESSING ABOUT IN BOATS

'Anyone who has not rowed in a really close boat race cannot comprehend the level of pain.'

DAN TOPOLSKI, True Blue: The Oxford Boat Race Mutiny

It's 11 March 2015 and I find myself immersed in one of the world's oldest sporting rivalries.

An age-old rowing event of such global notoriety it's known simply as 'The Boat Race'. An annual event where the dark blue boat of Oxford University meets the light blue boat of Cambridge on the historic banks of the River Thames to race side-by-side across 4 miles and 374 yards (6.779 km) from Putney to Mortlake.

Why? Because 'tradition'.

See, many years ago, two friends from Harrow School – Charles Wordsworth (nephew of the poet William Wordsworth), of Christ Church College, Oxford, and Charles Merrivale of St John's, Cambridge – decided to set up a challenge. On 10 February 1829 a meeting of the Cambridge University Boat Club requested Mr Snow of St John's to write immediately to Mr Staniforth of Christ Church stating 'That the University of Cambridge hereby challenges the University of Oxford to row a match at or near London, each in an eight-oared boat during the ensuing Easter vacation.' Over 100 years later the rivalry is as fierce as ever.

THE CAMBRIDGE BOATHOUSE

The time is 6:45am and I arrive early at the entrance of the Cambridge Boathouse.

It was always a privilege to train here just weeks away from the race. There's an excitement and anticipation in the air that's hard to explain. Every minute is planned with military precision. Essentially, if it won't help win The Boat Race, it doesn't have a place at the boathouse.

This is why, no matter where I am in the world, every year I will always gratefully accept an invitation from Head Coach Steve Trapmore to join the ranks for a training session and each time leave having found leg strength and lung capacity I never knew I had. Basically, I don't just come to become a better rower, I come to become a better athlete.

'Rowing, particularly sculling, inflicts on the individual in every race a level of pain associated with few other sports. There was certainly pain in football during a head-on collision, pain in other sports on the occasion of a serious injury. That was more the threat of pain; in rowing there was the absolute guarantee of it every time.'
DAVID HALBERSTAM, The Amateurs

Walking through the doors, I feel I should bow as if entering a temple. It feels elite, smells historic and looks prestigious.

I entered the gym on the bottom floor through the giant, folding stable doors. It has around 30 indoor rowing machines hanging from every available wall space while oars and other equipment are hung from the huge, exposed wooden beams that stretch across the ceiling. Also it's coated in a strange, thick turquoise paint that I'm later told makes mopping up the buckets of sweat easier.

To the side of the larger hall is a small weights room. The equipment is made from hardened steel and feels industrially antique, like the barbells and leather medicine balls were made for the first ever Cambridge team, but were created to be so durable they've accidentally become usable rowing relics.

Upstairs is completely different. Performance and function are replaced with grandeur and heritage, with plaques, crests and Boat Race collectables proudly placed on every wall. It's impossible for any athlete not to be inspired by it. The motivation you get from standing there is far more potent than any caffeinated pre-workout.

But my appreciation is cut short. In that moment I hear Steve's voice echoing from the hall downstairs. Game time! Walking down the stairs to join the ranks, I was about to uncover the training secrets kept under lock and key at the Cambridge Boathouse.

The false start

The warm-up was efficient and my introduction to the team brief. This was not a social trip and I didn't want any preferential treatment, despite the fact I could possibly lay claim to being the smallest attendee of a Cambridge Boathouse indoor rowing session. At 178 cm (5 ft 10 in) I was over a foot smaller than the tallest member of the team (a 211-cm/6-ft 11-in giant from Harvard).

But despite my lack of limb length I was made to feel so welcome, seamlessly slotting into the ranks as the runt of the rowing litter.

'How we feeling?' Steve asked, greeting me with the giant things he calls hands.

'Still awaiting a growth spurt, but overall good,' I replied. Steve laughed and assured me I'd be fine.

This was typical of him though. Nothing seemed to faze him. Partly because when it came to rowing he'd done it all. Starting at the age of 15, by 17 he was in the Great Britain Junior Team. As he grew, so did his medal collection, and as a senior he won a gold, silver and bronze medal at the World Championships, later adding Olympic Gold at coxed eights at the 2000 Summer Olympics in Sydney. Essentially, rowing coaches don't come more qualified than Steve.

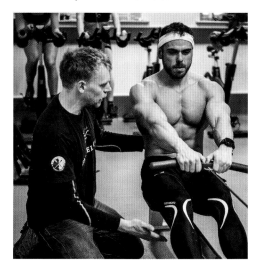

Which is why when he tells me to take an indoor rower off the wall, that's exactly what I do. Placing it in formation with the rest of the team, I was told to sit next to Luke (the captain). His form was impeccable and I'm told it would help me 'keep in sync' with the team, almost like learning to row through osmosis.

'Ready! 3, 2, 1...' The session begun.

Out of the corner of my eye I tried to watch Luke. His form was smooth and relaxed, yet powerful and precise. It was like watching my running mentors: not an ounce of energy was wasted. In comparison, my technique was disjointed, forced and I was far too dependent on my biceps that were rapidly filling with lactic acid.

Although I said I didn't want any preferential treatment, the coach in Steve couldn't help but come to my aid. 'How honest do you want me to be?' he asked, laughing.

Red-faced and riddled with lactic acid throughout my body, I decided my ego couldn't hurt much more than my arms right now so asked him to be brutally honest.

'You're not using your most powerful muscles in your legs. You're trying too hard to pull with your arms, which is completely inefficient. Think of it like a deadlift into a row, rather than a bicep curl.'

He then proceeded to cradle me like a small child as I sat on the rower. Moving my legs, arms and back in a motion that slightly resembled the rest of the team's. Although it must have looked so odd, I didn't care. With each row it got easier and easier. Eventually, Steve released me like a proud dad watching his son ride a bike for the first time. I was away. As I looked to him for approval, he nodded.

I was now (kind of) rowing.

THE PERFECT ROW

So what does a biomechanically efficient row look like? Well, according to the *National Strength and Conditioning Association Journal*, 'The stroke is a coordinated muscle action that requires repetitive, maximum, yet smooth application of force', which can be achieved by 'breaking the stroke up into the following sequence':[18]

The Catch: 'Be sure to relax the muscles of the spine. This will increase flexibility in the core, which in turn allows you to reach as far forward as possible during "the catch" phase of the row.'

The Leg Drive: 'Like in most sports, the power of your legs should not be underestimated in rowing. They represent a key part of your kinetic chain, which is why each stroke should start with a powerful "leg drive".'

The Body Drive: 'Only once the legs are fully extended, continue the movement's momentum and drive with the entire body. All the time ensuring you hinge at the hip and fully extend the back.'

The Arm Drive: 'This final phase should only be completed when all other parts of the stroke are efficiently executed. As you finish the "body drive", complete the movement with an arm drive. The biceps (and arms) are a very small muscle group in this kinetic chain, which is why each stroke should finish with an "arm drive". Too many people begin the movement with this, which is biomechanically inefficient, and you'll fatigue very quickly.'

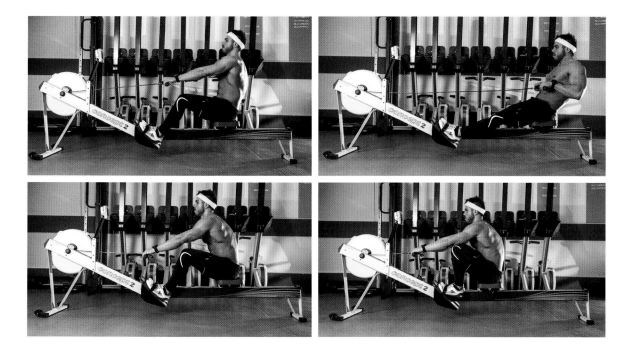

Strength and stamina

We rowed for 60 minutes in total, during which time my breathing started to regulate, my arms no longer hurt and the larger muscles in my legs started to (thankfully) take most of the strain. I was (semi) in sync with the test of the team and by the time the session ended I felt that as well as being the smallest rower in Cambridge Boathouse history, I was also the most improved.

But despite this sense of personal achievement I was under no illusion: my rowing metrics were far below that of an elite Boat Race competitor. Looking at Luke's screen, every one of his strokes was longer, stronger and more powerful than mine. In that moment the large legs, wide backs, huge lungs and low body fat of every boathouse inhabitant made sense.

This is because when looking at the physiological makeup of a rower, sports scientists claim: 'Elite oarsmen and oarswomen possess large body dimensions and show outstanding aerobic and anaerobic qualities.' They added that rowers also 'exhibit excellent strength and power when compared with other elite athletes'.[19]

As for the low body fat, the study notes they burn calories like a furnace: 'The caloric expenditure of rowing estimated from a 6-minute rowing ergometer exercise was calculated at 36 kcal/min, one of the highest energy costs so far reported for any predominantly aerobic-type sport.'

Why was this so important? Because contrary to what many believe, rowers are living proof that strength and stamina can co-exist.

HOW DOES CARDIO 'BURN' MUSCLE?

First, it must be noted that under certain conditions cardio can 'burn' muscle.

We covered this with Robert Hickson's theory on Concurrent Training in Chapter 7 (see page 190) and there are thousands of studies that support this idea. Each study describes the conditions under which strength and stamina training do not exist optimally together.

'During the last several decades many researchers have reported an interference effect on muscle strength development when strength and endurance were trained concurrently. The majority of these studies found that the magnitude of increase in maximum strength was higher in the group that performed only strength training compared with the concurrent training group, commonly referred to as the "interference phenomenon".'[20]

But the purpose of this chapter is to describe other conditions, offer another perspective, show that cardio and strength training shouldn't be completely feared when done together.

So where does this fear of cardio and muscle loss actually come from? Well, there is the view that to bulk up you need to consume more calories than you use and any form of cardio will burn those precious calories and therefore your muscles. But personally (and from those World Champions in strength sports) I've found this to be a very, very simple view of the human body.

This is because (again) we are not calorie-controlled machines. It's not as simple as counting calories in and out and then watching the muscle grow or shrink in relation to this. As we'll discover, there are thousands more processes within the human body that have an influence on this (capillary density being just one we will discuss).

While this is a whole other article in itself, it's enough to know that if you're meeting your macronutrient needs (protein, carbs and fats) with a nutrient-dense diet with sufficient calories (it's important to note 'sufficient' and not excessive like so many people believe), you won't simply waste away by going for a jog a few times a week.

Next, it's often been quoted in strength and conditioning journals that cardio will cause the body to develop slow-twitch muscle fibres. These are better for endurance training and less prone to fatigue but they're also smaller in size than fast-twitch muscle fibres that are needed for strength, speed and power.

This identified difference is often accompanied by a misleading picture of a lean and light Kenyan Olympic long-distance runner standing next to a sprinter to illustrate this point. But you have to understand this type of muscle adaptation only occurs after months – if not years – of endurance training. As proven by scientists from Ohio University in Athens, who discovered that after a lifetime of training, long-distance runners had a higher proportion of slow-twitch muscle fibres compared to their strength athlete counterparts.[21]

But these were athletes (powerlifters and distance runners) who were conditioned over years. If you're a beginner and new to training, almost any form of training can improve strength and stamina. So don't get caught up in specifics and just enjoy training.

'Results indicate combined training can induce substantial concurrent and compatible increases in VO2 peak (lung capacity) and strength performance.'
MEDICINE AND SCIENCE IN SPORTS AND EXERCISE[22]

Performing 40 minutes of cardio a few days a week with your strength training will not suddenly transform your physique into that of a Kenyan long-distance runner.

Lastly, there is the argument that cardio will reduce your testosterone levels. Obviously it's a hormone of particular importance for strength athletes, but scientists from the University of Carolina, USA, were quick to point out that this dip in testosterone only occurred after 'Chronic exposure to prolonged endurance training'. Performing 30–45 minutes of cardio is certainly not considered 'chronic exposure' so don't feel you'll wake up feeling weak as a kitten with low testosterone following a brief stint on the cross-trainer.[23]

'These results suggest that strength gains can be maintained with resistance training once or twice a week while focusing on improving aerobic endurance performance without compromising the latter.'
CANADIAN JOURNAL OF APPLIED PHYSIOLOGY[24]

So, to come back to the original question that haunts strength athletes: Under what conditions can strength and stamina exist in harmony? The answer (supported by Swedish scientists) is: rowing, cycling, Strongman and many more…

ROW AND RUN YOUR MUSCLES BIGGER?

Traditionally, bulking up consisted of mountains of food and heavy weights.

Cardio – or anything that sent your heart rate above 100 beats per minute – was avoided in fear that it would plunge your muscles into a catabolic state and 'eat away' at your hard-earned muscle. But it is research like that published by the Department of Health Sciences at Mid Sweden University in Östersund (and rowers around the world) that seems to contradict this well-established rule of gym folklore.

'In the quest to maximize average propulsive stroke impulses over 2000-m racing, testing and training of various strength parameters have been incorporated into the physical conditioning plans of rowers.'[25]

But Swedish researchers not only exorcised the myth, they proved cardio could actually 'elicit greater muscle hypertrophy than resistance exercise alone'. What this means is combining cardio with weight training could actually increase muscle size.[26]

To test this theory, the Swedish study took 10 healthy men between the ages of 25 and 30 and subjected them to five weeks of unilateral knee extensor exercises. One leg was trained in a manner similar to most conventional strength training routines: completing 4 sets of 7 repetitions at 75–80% of their one-rep max. The other leg was subjected to exactly the same strength routine, coupled with a 45-minute cycle during each session.

After five weeks, researchers used an MRI scan (magnetic resonance imaging) and muscle biopsies to determine any changes in the cross-sectional area and volume of the leg muscles. Specifically, the vastus lateralis (muscle located on the side of the leg) and the quadriceps femoris (muscle found at the front of the leg) were analysed.

What did they find?

The leg subjected to both cardio and strength training was noticeably bigger than the leg that performed strength training alone. Results revealed the vastus lateralis had increased in size by 17% in the cardio-strength trained leg compared to 9% in the strength-trained leg. Furthermore, the volume of the quadriceps femoris had increased by 14% in the cardio-strength trained leg compared to 8% in the strength-trained leg.

'These results provide novel insight into human muscle adaptations… and offer the very first genomic basis explaining how aerobic exercise may augment (improve), rather than compromise, muscle growth induced by resistance exercise.'
AMERICAN JOURNAL OF PHYSIOLOGY[27]

So where did this gym-based wizardry come from?

Hard to say, but it's widely known that performing any form of cardiovascular training dramatically improves your capillary density. Capillaries are the small blood vessels that network through the muscles, and by increasing their density you also increase your own ability to supply the working muscles with blood, oxygen and nutrients during training.

This is one of the most overlooked aspects of strength training as power-based athletes arguably place too much emphasis on shifting iron at the expense of looking after their capillaries. However, using the sport of Strongman as an example (a sport that contains some of the world's largest and strongest athletes), it could be argued that most past champions were well aware of this fact.

Five-time World's Strongest Man Mariusz Pudzianowski was famously a boxer before taking up the sport of Strongman and notably incorporated intense skipping sessions into his training before most weights sessions. Also, despite weighing 150 kg (330 lb)

Strongman legend Geoff Capes had a pretty impressive 200-metre sprint time, clocking 23.7 seconds. Equally, three-time world's strongest man Bill Kazmaier was a huge advocate of cardio training and heavily incorporated it into his training throughout his career.

But let's put evidence aside for the moment.

It seems research could also support this idea of caring for your capillaries. That's because a study published in *The Journal of Applied Physiology* set out to monitor the adaptive changes in the muscles that occur during intensive endurance-based training. Scientists took seven athletes and had them complete a 24-week training programme that was heavily cardio based. After 24 weeks, muscle biopsies were taken and it was found that athletes displayed 'an increased capillary supply of all muscle fibre types'. [28] They concluded that this would improve the efficiency of the entire cardio-respiratory system.

For strength athletes, this would also mean faster recovery rates between sets and therefore an ability to increase work capacity, which as we know from Chapter 7 could be invaluable. But most notably, a well-designed cardiovascular routine has been shown to work very well in conjunction with German Volume Training (GVT) to increase muscle mass.

Often referred to as the 'tens sets method', this is one of the oldest and most effective forms of training that involves completing 10 sets of 10 repetitions. Believed to have originated in Germany in the 1970s, it was made popular by Germany's weight-lifting coach Rolf Feser, who advocated its use to weightlifters who wanted to move up a weight class during the off-season.

Canadian weightlifter Jacques Demers – silver medallist in the Los Angeles Olympics – also famously used this training protocol and credited it for the renowned size of his thighs.

Now the entire programme works on the premise that you subject the muscles to an extensive volume of repeated efforts on a single exercise. The muscles are then forced to adapt and grow as the body is loaded above its habitual level (what it's accustomed to). Typically, it involves choosing a large compound movement such as the squat, bench or deadlift and using a weight that's roughly 60% of your one-rep max (or a weight you could perform 20 repetitions with). You then perform 10 sets of 10 repetitions, with 60–90 seconds of rest in between.

As a muscle-building training protocol it's believed very few workouts are supported by as many experts as German Volume Training. But it's clear to see how cardio and an improved capillary density can help you in those final sets. Even the strongest of athletes would struggle without any endurance capability, and as a result, would be unable to complete the workload recommended by GVT training to increase muscle mass.

But the strength/stamina benefits don't stop there.

CAN YOU CYCLE YOURSELF STRONGER?

If you want to be a good cyclist... get on your bike. But, if you want to be a great cyclist... get on your bike and in the weights room. No, seriously!

'Adding strength training to usual endurance training improved determinants of cycling performance as well as performance in well-trained cyclists.'
EUROPEAN JOURNAL OF APPLIED PHYSIOLOGY[29]

After the 2016 Rio Olympics, British Cycling had dominated three successive Olympiads. Outside the Games, cycling was still dominated by British teams.

Team Sky – a British professional cycling team that competes in the UCI World Tour – is based at the National Cycling Centre in Manchester, England, and is managed by British Cycling's former performance director Dave Brailsford. It was widely reported that their initial aim in 2010 was to 'create the first British winner of the Tour de France within five years'.

This changed... Though they later cut back to just aiming to 'win the Tour de France within five years', Sky achieved their initial goal within just three years when Bradley Wiggins won the 2012 Tour de France, becoming the first British winner in its history.

How? Through hard work, technological innovation, an insane endurance-based work ethic and an understanding of how strength training improves stamina, say English Institute of Sport coaches Scott Pearson and Joe Hewitt: 'Strength work will make you faster on the bike, but it will also deliver a host of other benefits. It will slow and even reverse the loss of muscle mass, facilitate weight control, improve bone health, which is an issue even for Grand Tour riders.' They add: 'By being more robust and resilient, you will be less likely to injure, which means more time out on your bike.'[30]

An idea supported by the *Scandinavian Journal of Medicine and Science in Sport* in 2010: 'It is concluded that strength training can lead to enhanced long-term (longer than 30 minutes) and short-term (less than 15 minutes) endurance capacity in highly trained top-level endurance athletes'.[31]

And 2011: 'In conclusion, adding strength training to usual endurance training improves leg strength and 5-minute all-out performance following 185 minutes of cycling in well-trained cyclists.'[32]

Where does this cycling strength-stamina wizardry come from?

MORE MUSCLE FIBRES

Remember, sports science teaches us that there are two types of muscle fibres.

These are Type I fibres and Type II fibres, which can be further subdivided into Type IIa and Type IIb. Type I fibres (more commonly known as 'slow-twitch' muscle fibres) are great for endurance are needed to get through all stages of the Tour de France. They are much more resistant to fatigue.

Type II muscle fibres are more commonly known as 'fast-twitch' muscle fibres and these are needed to power up the hills during a steep ascent since they have a faster contractile speed. How do you build more of these for cycling? Yes, strength training: 'Concurrent strength/endurance training in young elite competitive cyclists led to an improved 45-minute time-trial endurance capacity that was accompanied by an increased proportion of Type IIa muscle fibre.'[33]

Better muscle movement

Remember, if you move better you move further.

This I discovered on the planes of Africa and the fells of the Lake District, but it seems strength training can help you on your next cycle too.

'Adding heavy strength training improved cycling performance, increased fractional utilization of VO2 max (lung capacity) and improved cycling economy (movement and efficiency).'[34]

THE 1300-REPETITION ROWING WORKOUT

Presenting the 1300-repetition workout forged under the roof of the Cambridge Boathouse. Created to develop this concept of enduring strength, it's a workout that's become renowned at the club. Performed from start to finish with absolutely no rest, the large, full-body, compound movements performed with a high number of repetitions closely mimic the physical race demands.

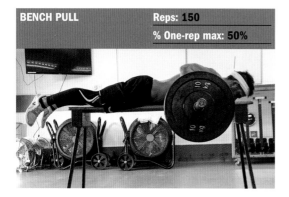

BENCH PULL   Reps: 150
% One-rep max: 50%

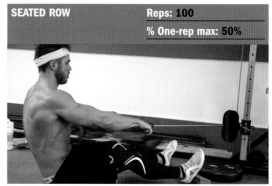

SEATED ROW   Reps: 100
% One-rep max: 50%

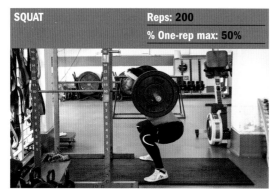

SQUAT   Reps: 200
% One-rep max: 50%

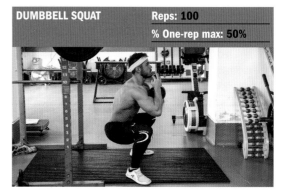

DUMBBELL SQUAT   Reps: 100
% One-rep max: 50%

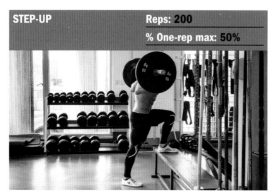

STEP-UP   Reps: 200
% One-rep max: 50%

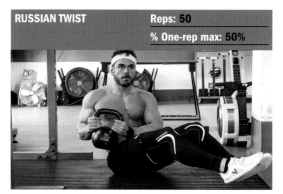

RUSSIAN TWIST   Reps: 50
% One-rep max: 50%

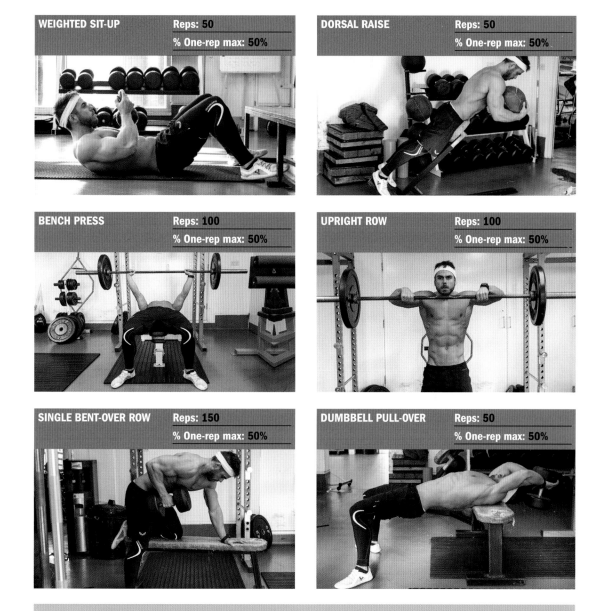

| WEIGHTED SIT-UP | Reps: 50 |
| | % One-rep max: 50% |

| DORSAL RAISE | Reps: 50 |
| | % One-rep max: 50% |

| BENCH PRESS | Reps: 100 |
| | % One-rep max: 50% |

| UPRIGHT ROW | Reps: 100 |
| | % One-rep max: 50% |

| SINGLE BENT-OVER ROW | Reps: 150 |
| | % One-rep max: 50% |

| DUMBBELL PULL-OVER | Reps: 50 |
| | % One-rep max: 50% |

TOTAL REPS: 1300

'Think of aerobics plus weightlifting minus the music or camaraderie. Combine unalloyed endurance with straightforward strength and demand poise, timing, and practiced form as well. Think of pure pain: that's the ergometer.'

BARRY STRAUSS, Rowing Against the Current

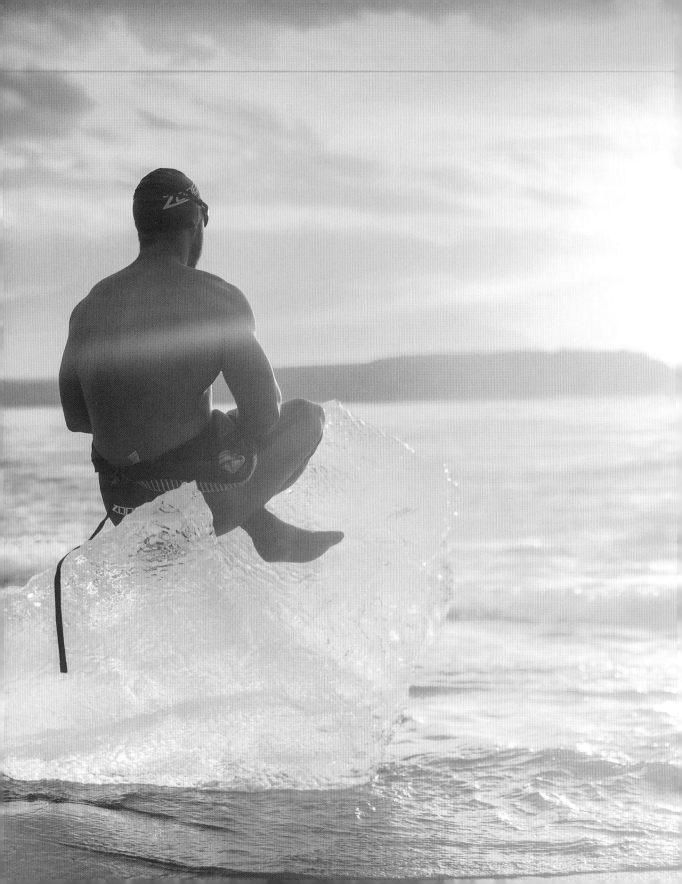

"A HUMAN BEING NEEDS A FRAMEWORK OF VALUES, A PHILOSOPHY OF LIFE TO LIVE BY AND UNDERSTAND BY, IN ABOUT THE SAME SENSE HE NEEDS SUNLIGHT, CALCIUM OR LOVE."

ABRAHAM MASLOW: Hierarchy of Human Needs

PART IV:
YOUR BEGINNING

THE WORLD'S TOUGHEST PILGRIMAGE |
Japan

TACKLING THE OKUGAKE

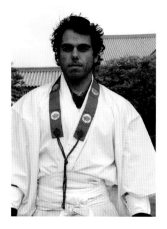

11 March 2008 and I'm on Mount Sanjogatake in Japan.

I've joined a team of trainee Yamabushi warrior priests as they embark on an annual endurance-based pilgrimage of self-discipline and enlightenment called an Okugake. But there's a slight problem. With no means of communicating with my new hosts I'm a little clueless as to what the month ahead entails.

Yet again the words 'creek' and 'without a paddle' come to mind.

But the occasional nod of approval from the Yamabushi leads me to believe I am doing OK. So here I am, five days in and halfway up a mountain wearing the world's most uncomfortable pair of sandals, a dressing gown and what can only be described as a giant nappy.

What had I learnt?

Well, this is far from the official description of an Okugake, since it's basically as random as it is hard to explain. But as a series of spiritual tasks it's like a month-long church sermon mixed with extreme sports.

My morning routine began with a 4am wake-up call. This was then followed by as much green tea as I could drink and lots of meditating. Once high on tea leaves and sufficiently cleansed, I'd then embark on a 20-km hike that finished with a test of faith – called the Nishino Nozoki – where I was hung off a cliff by a rope tied around my ankles and asked a series of questions.

Again hard to explain, but imagine a bungee jump and quiz rolled into one.

Historically, this was used to filter out any spies who were trying to infiltrate the monastery. If you hesitated or couldn't answer the question it was obvious you weren't a monk and you were promptly dropped off the cliff and out of monk school. Thankfully, I survived the Nishino Nozoki – and subsequent rope burns – and was granted entry into a neighbouring monastery.

Upon arrival lunch was served, more green tea was poured and we chanted ancient mantras for dessert. But I should point out that these morning festivities were merely a warm-up. After lunch the training would be taken up a notch.

It was time to find some ice-cold waterfalls, then meditate under them.

Spiritual enlightenment is COLD!

It's Day 7 of the Okugake and we're hopping from one monastery to the next.

The terrain up here is brutal.

The rocks are jagged, the air is thin and the ever-unstable footing tests both the durability of your ankles and the limits of your patience. But 18 km into that day's hike – and as altitude gripped my lungs with 1524 metres (5000 ft) of elevation – we are joined by the Chief Yamabushi Monk Miyagi-San.

Standing 168 cm (5 ft 6 in) tall and weighing close to 90 kg, he is far more nimble than his stature suggests and his short legs have yet to find a cliff face they couldn't conquer. It's almost soothing watching him scale the mountain as his facial expression changes from inner peace to mild amusement.

But the main reason I was so glad to see Miyagi-San was because he spoke a little English. Not a lot, but enough for me to break the seven days of silence I've just endured and to find out a little more about the sacred pilgrimage I now find myself a quarter of the way through.

I'm especially keen to know more about my impending date with an ice-cold waterfall.

But moments later no explanation is needed. Beneath a 10-metre waterfall the water crashes into the rocks below with such force it's created a 20-metre wide pool.

'This won't be pleasant will it?' I ask as I take off my robe.

Miyagi-San sees the concern on my face but, almost too honest for his own good, simply laughs and shakes his head. Without a moment's hesitation he strips down to his nappy. Rubs his belly and plunges himself into the water and under the waterfall. Then – still with a stoic smile – he immediately enters a trance-like state and begins meditating.

Not wanting to miss a moment's spiritual enlightenment, I follow, but my entry into the water is less graceful.

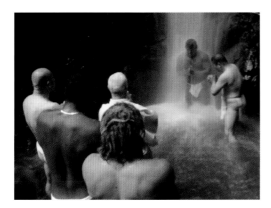

Jumping in at the deepest point, I lose both my breath and my underwear.

The force of the waterfall had hit my shoulders, rushed down my back and ripped the nappy (I'd forgotten to tighten it) clean off. Gasping for air, I didn't want to ask for help, so under the confused gaze of the Yamabushi warrior priests I was now naked in their sacred pool, searching for my underwear and self-respect.

On my third attempt – with my white butt cheeks bobbing on the surface – I found it caught on a rock.

Unhooking the cotton, and with what little dignity I had left, I put it on, apologised to all the Yamabushi in attendance and then joined Miyagi-San to meditate under the waterfall.

It was cold and it was painful. Each droplet of water came crashing down onto your head and it felt like you were getting hit by a giant fist made of ice, over and over again. After my wardrobe malfunction it was only my ego that hurt. Now it was my head, neck and shoulders.

Thirty minutes passed. My first waterfall meditation was complete. We then hiked to another monastery 20 km away. But during this time I came to a realisation.

Not through hours of meditation and not when searching for my underwear at the bottom of a pool. It was because during that day's hike I couldn't explain the concept of my dissertation to Miyagi-San. For whatever reason, he couldn't understand this idea of putting your own health completely in the hands of someone else.

Whether that's a personal trainer or a magazine, to fully surrender control of your fitness and food to someone else seemed so strange to him.

'You are your own best expert,' he told me. Then just like that, it was like my personal Okugake was complete.

'Every human being is the author of his own health or disease.'
BUDDHA

DON'T OUTSOURCE YOUR HEALTH

'There are many things you can outsource, but your health should not be one of them. Own your food and fitness with conviction.'
ROSS EDGLEY

Japan was like a month of enlightenment for me.

Fitness is now shrouded in rules and restrictions. There are too many training plans, too many diets and (above all else) too many self-proclaimed experts. We're basically being left to find our way blindly through a fitness-based minefield set inside a maze of misinformed advice.

'Spoon feeding in the long run teaches us nothing but the shape of the spoon.'
E.M. FORSTER

The solution? Take control of your food and fitness. Stop completely outsourcing it.

It's an idea I've obsessed over since Japan. It's also an idea that's been present throughout history and embraced by some of the greatest minds ever to live, from Jiddu Krishnamurti to Isaac Asimov. Even Steve Jobs, one of the greatest entrepreneurial geniuses of the 21st century, was forever quick to point out:

'Everything around you that you call life was made up by people that were no smarter than you.'

STEVE JOBS

Expanding on this, it was the Nobel Prize-winning German novelist Hermann Hesse who said we should 'look for perfection of ourselves'. This was a quote from his award-winning novel *The Glass Bead Game*, which embodies this idea of 'self-empowerment' and 'true wisdom':

'The doctrine you desire, absolute, perfect dogma that alone provides wisdom, does not exist. Nor should you long for a perfect doctrine, my friend. Rather, you should long for the perfection of yourself.'

HERMANN HESSE

Many leading psychologists agree too.

Take the work of Anders Ericsson, who's recognised as one of the world's leading theoretical and experimental researchers on expertise.[1] He believed there are no experts, only well-practised individuals, claiming: 'The term expert is used to describe highly experienced professionals. When experts exhibit their superior performance in public their behavior looks so effortless and natural that we are tempted to attribute it to special talents.'

But, wait for it, he adds: 'When scientists began measuring the experts' supposedly superior powers with psychometric tests, no general superiority was found.[2] Not even IQ.[3] Differences between experts and less proficient individuals nearly always reflect attributes acquired by the experts during their lengthy training.'

Basically, they had just been training more and learning longer. That's it.

Applying this to food and fitness it's therefore safe to say that 'experts' and authors – myself included – are not mentally more advanced than you. In reality, they're just a little more practised in that field.

Stop looking to them for answers!

Instead, become your own expert. It's amazing what you can achieve once you do.

Just look at the super-athletes spawned from the days of the Soviet Union. Yes, granted many argue that chemical concoctions and anabolic aids had a role to play. But one factor that cannot be ignored is the psychology of the USSR sportsmen and women.

Pioneered by Avksenty Tcezarevich Puni – one of the fathers of Russian sport psychology – the Russian approach expected athletes to understand the basic physiological and psychological processes taking place in the body during training.[4] Puni called it 'boevaya gotovnost', and it means a self-empowered readiness to fight.

It's a very different approach to following bullet points in glossy magazines.

'I cannot teach anybody anything, I can only make them think.'

SOCRATES

Going back even further, the great 19th-century strongman Eugen Sandow also stressed the importance of self-education. Born in Germany in 1867, he is considered the 'father of modern bodybuilding' and, long before Puni and Soviet sporting success, his book entitled *Strength: How to Obtain It* stressed the need to understand and study fitness first.

'You must learn to exercise your mind. This first of all lessons in physical training is of the utmost importance. Exercise without using the mind in conjunction is of no use. It is the brain that develops the muscles. Let me strongly advise every student to study well the anatomical chart.' It was the perfect fusion of self-empowerment and fitness, but it's an approach time forgot.

'The body, in fact, like a child, wants to be educated, and only through a series of exercises can this education be given.'

EUGEN SANDOW

THE BOOK'S BUSHIDO

PRINCIPLES FOR FITNESS

'If you don't have solid beliefs, you cannot build a stable life. Beliefs are like the foundation of a building, and they are the foundation to build your life upon.'

ALFRED A. MONTAPERT

Japan will always be a very special place for me.

I learnt so many things from my time there. The ice-cold meditation techniques I still practise to this day and have since combined with Wim Hof's methods; an understanding of food completely different to anywhere else I've ever been; and, of course, the lifelong friends I made in the monastery.

But one of the most important things I took from Japan was a code of conduct that I borrowed from the philosophy of the Samurai. If you're not familiar with them, basically they're this badass ancient military nobility. Feared and revered throughout the world, they lived their lives by eight virtues they called the Bushido. Translated, this means 'the way of the warrior' and I remember at the time thinking this sounded like a pretty good idea.

That's why this book now has its very own 'Bushido'. A set of principles that I hope remain with you long after you've finished reading the book. They're not concrete rules and are far from foolproof, so please feel free to pick and choose which ones you want and add your own. But in my experience adopting even a few can bring about positive and meaningful changes to your food, fitness and life.

Just like a badass Samurai.

'If you don't change your beliefs, your life will be like this forever. Is that good news?'
WILLIAM SOMERSET MAUGHAM

Principle 1: Be Balanced

Life is for living and many of us aren't.

Yes, to be so unfit[5] you can't enjoy a barefoot run on a sun-soaked beach is a crime.[6] But to diet so strictly you never know the joy a rack of chocolate balsamic-glazed pork ribs can bring is also a sin.[7] Find your happy and healthy medium.

Principle 2: Learn From the Past

Biologically speaking we've remained relatively unchanged for 200,000 years. Granted, in science's continual effort to understand fitness, fat and food we have made some amazing discoveries to expand our understanding of the human body. In no way am I trying to belittle that. But as a whole, we've long been aware of core principles that shape our food and fitness.

Learn the basics from the past and you won't go far wrong.

Principle 3: Keep it Simple

Too often 'experts' make training and nutrition more complicated that it needs to be. Albert Einstein said it best when he said, 'If you can't explain it to a six-year-old you don't understand it well enough.' In short, make food and fitness as complicated as it needs to be, not as complicated as it can be.

Principle 4: Question Everything

Question everything and anything.

This includes the contents of this book. Just because I wrote it, don't consider it gospel. The famous Greek philosopher Socrates once said 'The only thing I know for certain is I know nothing.' He was a clever man, so it's safe to say me, you and others probably aren't all-knowing and all-seeing.

On that note, I always say we humans are restricted by our five senses. We know there's light we can't see and sounds we can't hear, but we know they exist. So, let's not be so arrogant as to think we know, see and hear everything. We don't, can't and may never do.

Principle 5: Always Pursue Happiness

A happy life stems from food, water and sleep.[8]

Contrary to many 'advanced' self-help guidebooks and a session on a psychiatrist's couch, I know. But taking inspiration from the world of psychology – and Maslow's hierarchy of human needs – it's clear to see that if we better organise our fridges and gym routines, we better organise our happiness.

Principle 6: Embrace Individuality

We are all biologically unique.

No body is the same, no limb is identical and no hormonal response to training is equal. The relatively new field of nutrigenomics – the study of how our genes interact with our food – teaches us our diet is no different either. For these exact reasons, there is no perfect workout or diet plan! This is why the *National Strength and Conditioning Journal* stated in 1991:

'Is there a single, perfect workout? A workout with the best weight training, plyometric, flexibility and endurance exercises? A workout with the precise number of sets and repetitions? A workout that tells the athlete exactly how much weight to use? The answer is "No".'[9]

The very idea of the 'perfect' workout that's broadcasted to the masses defies the Law of Biological Individuality. All contradictory to the advice found in glossy magazines, I know. It's also a little scary for some who find comfort in law and order. But the human body simply doesn't work like that. Therefore, with every training or meal plan always ask, 'Does this suit my individual biology?'

Principle 7: You're Your Best Expert

No one knows your body better than you.

How come? Well as we've discovered we are all biologically different. No response to training or food is ever the same from person to person, so how can any 'guru' write a diet or training programme for you? Yes, they can guide you, and I know many great coaches and personal trainers who do. But you have the potential to be your own best expert.

So take control of your fitness, or at the very least play a large role in it.

Principle 8: Live Beyond Books

I'm a writer, so of course love books.

But I also acknowledge they have their limitations. That's because they teach us what we already know, but not what remains to be found. That's why in many ways creativity and imagination are more powerful. Books can serve as the fuse to light the fire of discovery. To quote Albert Einstein, 'Imagination is more important than knowledge. For knowledge is limited to all we now know and understand, while imagination embraces the entire world, and all there ever will be to know and understand.'

Principle 9: Never Stop Exploring

This is just a book, not a bible.

Do not let your study of the body and thirst for knowledge stop within these pages. The study of fitness and food is evolving at an exponential rate, and our exploration of each should too.

LIST OF WORKOUTS AND RECIPES

WORKOUTS

RECIPES

NOTES

FOREWORD

1. Freire, Paulo (2007) *Pedagogy of the Oppressed*. New York: Continuum.
2. Greene, Robert (2021) *Mastery*. London: Profile Books.

THE BEGINNING

1. Verkhoshansky, Yuri and Mel Siff (2009) *Supertraining*. Supertraining Institute.
2. Baechle, T.R. and R.W. Earle (eds) (2000) *Essentials of Strength and Conditioning*. Champaign, IL: Human Kinetics.
3. American College of Sports Medicine (2006) *ACSM's guidelines for exercise testing and prescription*. Baltimore: Lippinncott, Willians and Wilkins.
4. Edgley, Ross (2007) 'An analysis of the Editorial Policy of selected Commercial Health and Fitness Publications and an examination of the extent to which they promote "Body Dissatisfaction", Disempowerment and Dependence.'
5. Kiely, John (2012) 'Periodization Paradigms in the 21st Century: Evidence-Led or Tradition-Driven?' *International Journal of Sports Physiology and Performance*, 7, 242–250.
6. '10 Facts About Obesity.' The World Health Organization, February 2014. Retrieved from http://www.who.int/features/factfiles/obesity/en/.
7. Lucan, S.C. and Di Nicolantonio (2015) 'How calorie-focused thinking about obesity and related diseases may mislead and harm public health. An alternative.' *Public Health Nutrition*, 18(4), 571–81.

CHAPTER 1

1. Wathen, Dan and Thomas Baechle (2008) *Periodization: Essentials of Strength Training and Conditioning*, Third Edition. Human Kinetics and NSCA.

CHAPTER 2

1. Walleczek, J. (ed.) (2000) *Self-Organized Biological Dynamics and Nonlinear Control: Toward Understanding Complexity, Chaos and Emergent Function in Living Systems*. Cambridge: Cambridge University Press.
2. Selye, Hans (1936) 'A syndrome produced by diverce nocuous agents.' *Nature*, Volume 138.
3. Rippetoe, Mark and Andy Barker (2014) *Practical Programming for Strength Training*, Third Edition. The Aasgaard Company.
4. Carlile, F. (1961) 'The athlete and adaptation to stress.' *Track Tech*, 156–8.

5. Todd, J.S., J.P. Shurley and T.C. Todd (2012) 'Thomas L. DeLorme and the science of progressive resistance exercise.' *Journal of Strength and Conditioning Research*, 11, 2913–23.
6. Verkhoshansky, Natalia (2012) 'General Adaptation Syndrome and its applications in sport training.' Verkhoshansky Special Strength Training Methodology.

CHAPTER 3

1. Epstein, Y., J. Rosenblum, R. Burstein and M.N. Sawka (1988) 'External load can alter the energy cost of prolonged exercise.' *European Journal of Applied Physiology and Occupational Physiology*, Volume 57, Issue 2, 243–7.
2. Toussaint, H.M. and A.P. Hollander (1994) 'Energetics of competitive swimming. Implications for training programmes.' *Sports Medicine*, 18(6), 384–405.
3. Tarnanen, Sami P., Jari J. Ylinen, MD, PhD, Kirsti M. Siekkinen, PT, Esko A. Mälkiä, PhD, Hannu J. Kautiainen, BA and Arja H. Häkkinen, PhD (2008) 'Effect of Isometric Upper-Extremity Exercises on the Activation of Core Stabilizing Muscles.' *Archives of Physical Medicine and Rehabilitation*, 89(3), 513–21.
4. Duc, S., W. Bertucci and F. Grappe (2008) 'Muscular activity during uphill cycling: Effect of slope, posture, hand grip position and constrained bicycle lateral sways.' *Journal of Electromyography and Kinesiology* 18(1), 116–27.
5. Harman, Everett, Ki-Hoon Han and Peter Frykman (2001) 'Load-Speed Interaction Effects on the Biomechanics of Backpack Load Carriage.' Army Research, Institute of Environmental Medicine, Natick, MA: Defense Technical Information Center.

CHAPTER 4

1. Shephard, R.J. (2010) 'Development of the discipline of exercise immunology.' *Exercise Immunology Review* 16, 194–222, 2010.
2. Walsh, N.P. et al (2011) 'Position Statement Part one: Immune function and exercise.' *Exercise Immunology Review*, 17, 6–63.
3. Castell, L.M (2002) 'Exercise-Induced Immunodepression in Endurance Athletes and Nutritional Intervention with Carbohydrate, Protein and Fat—What Is Possible, What Is Not?' *Nutrition*, 18(5), 371–5.
4. Chamorro-Viña, Carolina, Maria Fernandez-del-Valle and Anna M. Tacón (2013) 'Excessive Exercise and Immunity: The J-Shaped Curve.' *The Active Female*, 357–72.

5. Shephard, R.J. (2010) 'The history of exercise immunology.' In C. Tipton (ed.) *The history of exercise physiology*. Champaign, IL: Human Kinetics.
6. Shephard, R.J. (1997) *Physical activity, training and the immune response*. Carmel, IN: Cooper Publishing Group.
7. Brenner, I.K., P.N. Shek and R.J. Shephard (1994) 'Infection in athletes.' *Sports Medicine* 17, 86–107.
8. Oliver, S.J., S.J. Laing, S. Wilson, J.L. Bilzon, R. Walters and N.P. Walsh (2007) 'Salivary immunoglobulin A response at rest and after exercise following a 48 h period of fluid and/or energy restriction.' *British Journal of Nutrition*, 97, 1109–16.
9. Nieman, D.C., S.L. Nehlsen-Cannarella, P.A. Markoff, A.J. Balk-Lamberton, H. Yang, D.B. Chritton, J.W. Lee and K. Arabatzis (1990) 'The effects of moderate exercise training on natural killer cells and acute upper respiratory tract infections.' *International Journal of Sports Medicine*, 11, 467–73.
10. 'Immune function and Exercise': Loughborough University Institutional Repository.
11. Kox, Matthijs, Lucas T. van Eijk, Jelle Zwaag, Joanne van den Wildenberg, Fred C.G.J. Sweep, Johannes G. van der Hoeven and Peter Pickkersa (2014) 'Voluntary activation of the sympathetic nervous system and attenuation of the innate immune response in humans.' *Proceedings of the National Academy of Sciences of the United States of America*, 2014 May 20, 111 (20), 7379–84.
12. Ibid.
13. Janský, L., D. Pospíšilová, S. Honzová, B. Uličný, P. Šrámek, V. Zeman and J. Kamínková (1996) 'Immune system of cold-exposed and cold-adapted humans.' *European Journal of Applied Physiology and Occupational Physiology*, Volume 72, Issue 5, 445–50.

CHAPTER 5

1. Wathen, Dan and Thomas Baechle (2008) *Periodization: Essentials of Strength Training and Conditioning*, Third Edition. Human Kinetics and NSCA.
2. Hardman, A.E. and A. Hudson (1994) 'Brisk walking and serum lipid and lipoprotein variables in previously sedentary women--effect of 12 weeks of regular brisk walking followed by 12 weeks of detraining.' *British Journal of Sports Medicine*, 28, 261–6.

3. Stensel, D.J., K. Brooke-Wavell, A.E. Hardman, P.R.M. Jones and N.G. Norgan (1994) 'The influence of a 1-year programme of brisk walking on endurance fitness and body composition in previously sedentary men aged 42–59 years.' *European Journal of Applied Physiology and Occupational Physiology*, Volume 68, Issue 6, 531–7.

4. Midgley, A.W., L.R McNaughton and A.M. Jones (2007) 'Training to enhance the physiological determinants of long-distance running performance: can valid recommendations be given to runners and coaches based on current scientific knowledge?' *Sports Medicine*, 37(10), 857–80.

5. Koukoubis, T.D., L.W. Cooper, R.R. Glisson, A.V. Seaber and J.A. Feagin Jr (1995) 'An electromyographic study of knee muscles during climbing.' *Knee Surgery, Sports Traumatology, Arthroscopy*, 3(2), 121–4.

6. Rooks, Michael D. (2012) 'Rock Climbing Injuries.' *Sports Medicine*, 23(4), 261–270.

7. Deuster, Patricia. A. (1997) *The Navy Seal Physical Fitness Guide.* Department of Military and Emergency Medicine Uniformed Services University of Health Sciences.

8. Harman, Everett A., David J. Gutekunst, Peter N. Frykman, Bradley C. Nindl, Joseph A. Alemany, Robert P. Mello, and Marilyn A. Sharp (2008) 'Effects of Two Different Eight-Week Training Programs on Military Physical Performance.' *Journal of Strength and Conditioning Research*, 22, (2), 524–34.

9. Caine, Dennis J., Keith Russell and Liesbeth Lim (2013) 'Handbook of Sports Medicine and Science: Gymnastics.' *Olympic Handbook of Sports Medicine*, 2013.

10. Schwanbeck, Shane, Philip D. Chilibeck and Gordon Binsted (2009) 'A Comparison of Free Weight Squat to Smith Machine Squat Using Electromyography.' *Journal of Strength and Conditioning Research*, 23(9), 2588–91.

11. Behm, D.G., A.M. Leonard, W.B. Young, W.A. Bonsey and S.N. MacKinnon (2005) 'Trunk muscle electromyographic activity with unstable and unilateral exercises.' *Journal of Strength and Conditioning*, 19(1), 193–201.

12. Snarr, R.L. and M.R. Esco (2013) 'Electromyographic Comparison of Traditional and Suspension Push-Ups.' *Journal of Human Kinetics*, 39, 75–83.

13. Snarr, R.L., M.R. Esco, E.V. Witte, C.T. Jenkins and R.M. Brannan (2013) 'Electromyographic activity of rectus abdominis during a suspension push-up compared to traditional exercises.' *Journal of Exercise Physiology*, 16(3), 1–8.

14. Hubbard, Daniel (2010) 'Is Unstable Surface Training Advisable for Healthy Adults?' *Strength & Conditioning Journal*, 32, 64–66.

15. Flint, M. Marilyn and Janet Gudgell (2013) 'Electromyographic Study of Abdominal Muscular Activity during Exercise.' *Research Quarterly, American Association for Health, Physical Education and Recreation*, 36(1).

16. Tarnanen, Sami P. et al (2008) 'Effect of Isometric Upper-Extremity Exercises on the Activation of Core Stabilizing Muscles.' *Archives of Physical Medicine and Rehabilitation*, 89(3) , 513–21.

17. Gutin, B. and S. Lipetz (1971) 'An Electromyographic Investigation of the Rectus Abdominis in Abdominal Exercises.' *Research Quarterly, American Association for Health, Physical Education and Recreation*, 42(3).

18. Vogt, M. and H.H. Hoppeler (1985) 'Eccentric exercise: mechanisms and effects when used as training regime or training adjunct.' *Journal of Applied Physiology*, 116(11), 1446–54.

CHAPTER 6

1. Alhassan, S.,S. Kim, A. Bersamin, A.C. King and C.D. Gardner (2008) 'Dietary adherence and weight loss success among overweight women: results from the A to Z weight loss study.' *International Journal of Obesity*, 32(6), 985–91.

2. Stewart, T.M., D.A. Williamson and M.A. White (2002) 'Rigid vs. flexible dieting: association with eating disorder symptoms in nonobese women.' *Appetite*, 38(1), 39–44.

3. Hargove, James L. (2007) 'Does the history of food energy units suggest a solution to "Calorie confusion"?' *Nutrition Journal*, 6, 44.

4. Beecher, G.R., K.K. Stewart, J.M. Holden, J.M. Harnly and W.R. Wolf (2009) 'Legacy of Wilbur O. Atwater: human nutrition research expansion at the USDA–-interagency development of food composition research.' *The Journal of Nutrition*, 139(1), 178–84.

5. Schoeller, D.A. (2009) 'The energy balance equation: looking back and looking forward are two very different views.' *Nutrition Reviews*, 67(5), 249–54.

6. Hall, Kevin D. (2008) 'What is the Required Energy Deficit per unit Weight Loss?' *International Journal of Obesity*, 32(3), 573–6.

7. Elliot et al (1989) 'Sustained depression of the resting metabolic rate after massive weight loss.' *American Journal of Clinical Nutrition*, 49(1), 93–6.

8. Cavallo, E., F. Armellini, M. Zamboni, R. Vicentini, M.P. Milani and O. Bosello (1990) 'Resting metabolic rate, body composition and thyroid hormones. Short term effects of very low calorie diet.' *Hormone and Metabolic Research*, 22(12), 632–5.

9. Polivy, Janet (1996) 'Psychological Consequences of Food Restriction.' *Nutrition Research Newsletter*. FindArticles.com, 2012.

10. Saris, W.H. (2001) 'Very-low-calorie diets and sustained weight loss.' *Obesity Review*, 9(4), 295–301.

11. Wadden, T.A., A.J. Stunkard, S.C. Day, R.A. Gould and C.J. Rubin (1987) 'Less food, less hunger: reports of appetite and symptoms in a controlled study of a protein-sparing modified fast.' *International Journal of Obesity*, 11(3), 239–49.

12. Wadden, T.A., A.J. Stunkard, K.D. Brownell and S.C. Day (1985) 'A comparison of two very-low-calorie diets: protein-sparing-modified fast versus protein-formula-liquid diet.' *American Journal of Clinical Nutrition*, 41(3), 533–9.

13. Astrup, A. and S. Rossner (2001) 'Lessons from obesity management programmes: greater initial weight loss improves long-term maintenance.' *Obesity Reviews*, 1(1), 17–19.

14. Rodriguez, N.R., N.M. Di Marco, and S. Langley (2009) 'American College of Sports Medicine position stand. Nutrition and athletic performance.' *Medicine and Science in Sport and Exercise*, 41(3), 709–31.

15. Economos, C.D., S.S. Bortz and M.E. Nelson (1993) 'Nutritional practices of elite athletes. Practical recommendations.' *Sports Medicine*, 16(6), 381–99.

16. Zalesin, K.C., B.A. Franklin and M.A. Lillystone (2010) 'Differential loss of fat and lean mass in the morbidly obese after bariatric surgery.' *Metabolic Syndrome and Related Disorders*, 8(1), 15–20.

17. Martin, C.K., S.K. Das, L. Lindblad et al (2011) 'Effect of calorie restriction on the free-living physical activity levels of nonobese humans: results of three randomized trials.' *Journal of Applied Physiology*, 110(4), 956–63.

18. Withers, R.T., C.J. Noell, N.O. Whittingham, B.E. Chatterton, C.G. Schultz and J.P. Keeves (1997) 'Body composition changes in elite male bodybuilders during preparation for competition.' *Australian Journal of Science and Medicine in Sport*, 29(1), 11–16.

19. van der Ploeg, G.E., A.G. Brooks, R.T. Withers, J. Dollman, F. Leaney and B.E. Chatterton (2001) 'Body composition changes in female bodybuilders during preparation for competition.' *European Journal of Clinical Nutrition*, 55(4), 268–77.

20. Muller, M.J. and A. Bosy-Westphal (2013) 'Adaptive thermogenesis with weight loss in humans.' *Obesity*, 21(2), 218–28.

21. Dulloo, A.G., J. Jacquet, J-P. Montani and Y. Schutz (2012) 'Adaptive thermogenesis in human body weight regulation: more of a concept than a measurable entity?' *Obesity Review*, 13(2), 105–21.

22. Manninen, A.H. (2004) 'Is a calorie really a calorie? Metabolic advantage of low-carbohydrate diets.' *Journal of the International Society of Nutrition*, 1(2), 21–6.

23. Lucan, S.C. and Di Nicolantonio (2015) 'How calorie-focused thinking about obesity and related diseases may mislead and harm public health. An alternative.' *Public Health Nutrition*, 18(4), 571–81.

24. Hill J.O., J.C. Peters, D. Yang, T. Sharp, M. Kaler, N.N. Abumrad and H.L. Greene (1989) 'Thermogenesis in humans during overfeeding with medium-chain triglycerides.' *Metabolism*, 38(7), 641–8.

25. St-Onge, M.P. and P.J. Jones (2002) 'Physiological effects of medium-chain triglycerides: potential agents in the prevention of obesity.' *The Journal of Nutrition*, 132(3), 329–32.

26. Feinman, Richard D. and Eugene J. Fine (2004) '"A calorie is a calorie" violates the second law of thermodynamics.' *Nutrition Journal*, 3, 9.

27. Vandewater, Kristin and Zata Vickers (1996) 'Higher-protein foods produce greater sensory-specific satiety.' *Physiology & Behaviour*, 59(3), 579–83.

28. Johnston, C.S., C.S. Day and P.D. Swan (2002) 'Postprandial thermogenesis is increased 100% on a high-protein, low-fat diet versus a high-carbohydrate, low-fat diet in healthy, young women.' *Journal of American College Nutrition*, 21(1), 55–61.

29. Cordain, Lauren et al (2005) 'Origins and evolution of the Western diet: health implications for the 21st century'. *American Journal of Clinical Nutrition*, 81(2), 341–54.

30. Tarnopolsky, M.A., J.D. MacDougall and S.A. Atkinson (1988) 'Influence of protein intake and training status on nitrogen balance and lean body mass.' *Journal of Applied Physiology*, (64)1, 187–93.

31. Chandra, R.K. (1997) 'Nutrition and the immune system: an introduction.' *American Journal of Clinical Nutrition*, 66(2), 460–3.

32. Schoeller, D.A. and A.C. Buchholz (2005) 'Energetics of obesity and weight control: does diet composition matter?' *Journal of the American Dietetic Association*, 105(5 Suppl 1), 24–8.

33. Paddon-Jones, Douglas, Eric Westman, Richard D. Mattes, Robert R. Wolfe, Arne Astrup and Margriet Westererp-Plantenga (2008) 'Protein, weight management, and satiety.' *Journal of the American Dietetic Association*, 87(5), 1558–61.

34. Kim, J.E., L.E. O'Connor, L.P. Sands, M.B. Slebodnik and W.W. Campbell (2016) 'Effects of dietary protein intake on body composition changes after weight loss in older adults: a systematic review and meta-analysis.' *Nutrition Reviews* 74(3), 210–24.

35. Williams, C., J. Brewer and M. Walker (1992) 'The effect of a high carbohydrate diet on running performance during a 30-km treadmill time trial.' *European Journal of Applied Physiology and Occupational Physiology*, 65(1), 18–24.

36. Balsom, P.D., G.C. Gaitanos, K. Söderlund and B. Ekblom (1999) 'High-intensity exercise and muscle glycogen availability in humans.' *Acta Physioligca Scandinavia*, 165(4), 337–45.

37. Burke, L.M., G.R. Cox, N.K. Cummings and B. Desbrow (2001) 'Guidelines for daily carbohydrate intake: do athletes achieve them?' *Sports Medicine*, 31(4), 267–99.

38. Ibid.

39. Gifford, K.D. (2002) 'Dietary fats, eating guides, and public policy: history, critique, and recommendations.' *The American Journal of Medicine*, 30, 11.

40. Ibid.

41. Lambert, Estelle V., David P. Speechly, Steven C. Dennis and Timothy D. Noakes (1994) 'Enhanced endurance in trained cyclists during moderate intensity exercise following 2 weeks adaptation to a high fat diet.' *European Journal of Applied Physiology and Occupational Physiology*, 69(4), 287–93.

42. R.C. Brown (2002) 'Nutrition for optimal performance during exercise: carbohydrate and fat.' *Current Sports Medicine Reports*, 1(4), 222–9.

43. Davis, Richard C. (September 1984) 'Arctic Profiles: Frederick Schwatka (1849-1892)'. *Arctic*, 37(3), 302.

44. Pivovarova, Olga, et al (2014) 'Changes of Dietary Fat and Carbohydrate Content Alter Central and Peripheral Clock in Humans.' *The Journal of Clinical Endocrinology & Metabolism*, 100(6).

45. Stephen H. Boutcher (2011) 'High-Intensity Intermittent Exercise and Fat Loss.' *Journal of Obesity*, 2011: 868305.

46. King, Abby C. and Diane L. Tribble (1991) 'The Role of Exercise in Weight Regulation in Nonathletes.' *Sports Medicine*, 11(5), 331–49.

47. Tremblay, A., J.A. Simoneau and C.Bouchard (1994) 'Impact of exercise intensity on body fatness and skeletal muscle metabolism.' *Metabolism*, 43(7), 814–8.

48. Treuth, M.S. et al (1994) 'Effects of strength training on total and regional body composition in older men.' *Journal of Applied Physiology*, 77(2), 614-62.

49. Melby, C., C. Scholl, G. Edwards and R. Bullough (1993) 'Effect of acute resistance exercise on postexercise energy expenditure and resting metabolic rate.' *Journal of Applied Physiology*, 75(4), 1847-53.

50. Ballor, D.L., V.L .Katch, M.D. Becque and C.R. Marks (1988) 'Resistance weight training during caloric restriction enhances lean body weight maintenance.' *American Journal of Clinical Nutrition*, 47(1), 19–25.

51. Scala, Dwight, Jim McMillan, Danny Blessing, Ralph Rozenek and Mike Stone (1987) 'Metabolic Cost of a Preparatory Phase of Training in Weight Lifting: A Practical Observation.' *Journal of Strength & Conditioning Research*, 1(3).

52. Bruce, C.R. et al (2006) 'Endurance Training in Obese Humans Improves Glucose Tolerance and Mitochondrial Fatty Acid Oxidation and Alters Muscle Lipid Content.' *American Journal of Physiology: Endocrinology and Metabolism*, 291, E99–E107.

53. Grassi, Davide, Cristina Lippi, Stefano Necozione, Giovambattista Desideri and Claudio Ferri (2005) 'Short-term administration of dark chocolate is followed by a significant increase in insulin sensitivity and a decrease in blood pressure in healthy persons.' *American Journal of Clinical Nutrition*, 81(3), 611–614.

54. Halsted, C.H. (1980) 'Alcoholism and malnutrition. Introduction to the symposium.' *American Journal of Clinical Nutrition*, 33(12), 2705–8.

55. Schutz, Y. (2000) 'Role of substrate utilization and thermogenesis on body-weight control with particular reference to alcohol.' *The Proceedings of the Nutrition Society*, 59(4), 511–7.

56. Apovian, Caroline M. (2004) 'Sugar-Sweetened Soft Drinks, Obesity, and Type 2 Diabetes.' *The Journal of American Medical Association*, 292(8), 978–9.

57. Arima, H. et al (2002) 'Alcohol reduces insulin-hypertension relationship in a general population: the Hisayama study.' *The Journal of Clinical Epidemiology*, 55(9), 863–9.

58. Frémont, Lucie (2000) 'Biological effects of resveratrol.' *Life Sciences*, 66(8), 663–73.

59. Spiegel, Karine, Esra Tasali, Plamen Penev and Eve Van Cauter (2004) 'Brief Communication: Sleep Curtailment in Healthy Young Men Is Associated with Decreased Leptin Levels, Elevated Ghrelin Levels, and Increased Hunger and Appetite.' *Annals of Internal Medicine*, (11), 846–50.

60. Davidson, J.R., H. Moldofsky and F.A. Lue (1991) 'Growth hormone and cortisol secretion in relation to sleep and wakefulness.' *Journal of Psychiatry and Neuroscience*, 16(2), 96–102.

61. Born, J., T. Lange, K. Hansen, M. Mölle and H.L. Fehm (1997) 'Effects of sleep and circadian rhythm on human circulating immune cells.' *The Journal of Immunology*, 158 (9), 4454–64.

62. Signore, A.P., F. Zhang, Z. Weng, Y. Gao and J. Chen (2008) 'Leptin neuroprotection in the CNS: mechanisms and therapeutic potentials.' *Journal of Neurochemistry*, 106(5), 1977–90.

63. (2004) 'Summaries for patients. Sleep duration and levels of hormones that influence hunger.' *Annals of Internal Medicine*, 141(11), 152.

64. Nedeltcheva, Arlet V., Jennifer M. Kilkus, Jacqueline Imperial, Dale A. Schoeller and Plamen D. Penev (2010) 'Insufficient sleep undermines dietary efforts to reduce adiposity.' *Annals of Internal Medicine*, 153(7), 435–41.

65. Harris, James Arthur and Francis Gano Benedict (1919) *A Biometric Study Of Basal Metabolism In Man*. Carnegie Institution of Washington.

66. Alhassan, S., S. Kim, A. Bersamin, A.C. King, and C.D. Gardner (2008) 'Dietary adherence and weight loss success among overweight women: results from the A to Z weight loss study.' *International Journal of Obesity*, 32(6), 985–91.

67. Burke, L.M., G.R. Cox, N.K. Cummings and B. Desbrow (2001) 'Guidelines for daily carbohydrate intake: do athletes achieve them?' *Sports Medicine*, 31(4), 267–99.

68. Schoeller, D.A. and A.C. Buchholz (2005) 'Energetics of obesity and weight control: does diet composition matter?' *The Journal of the American Dietetic Association*, 105(5 Suppl 1), S24–8.

69. Lambert, Estelle V., David P. Speechly, Steven C. Dennis, Timothy D. Noakes (1994) 'Enhanced endurance in trained cyclists during moderate intensity exercise following 2 weeks adaptation to a high fat diet.' *European Journal of Applied Physiology and Occupational Physiology*, 69(4), 287–93.

70. Brand, J.C., P.L. Nicholson, A.W. Thorburn and A.S. Truswell (1985) 'Food processing and the glycemic index.' *The American Journal of Clinical Nutrition*, 42(6), 1192–6.

71. Macari, M., M.J. Dauncey and D.L. Ingram (1983) 'Changes in food intake in response to alterations in the ambient temperature: modifications by previous thermal and nutritional experience.' *European Journal of Physiology*, 396(3), 231–7.

72. Burke, L.M., G.R. Cox, N.K. Cummings and B. Desbrow (2001) 'Guidelines for daily carbohydrate intake: do athletes achieve them?' *Sports Medicine*, 31(4), 267–99.

73. Schoeller, D.A. and A.C. Buchholz (2005) 'Energetics of obesity and weight control: does diet composition matter?' *The Journal of the American Dietetic Association*, 105(5 Suppl 1), S24–8.

74. Lambert, Estelle V., David P. Speechly, Steven C. Dennis, name? Timothy and D. Noakes (1994) 'Enhanced endurance in trained cyclists during moderate intensity exercise following 2 weeks adaptation to a high fat diet.' *European Journal of Applied Physiology and Occupational Physiology*, 69(4), 287–93.

CHAPTER 7

1. Tucker, R. and M. Collins (2012) 'What makes champions? A review of the relative contribution of genes and training to sporting success.' *British Journal of Sports Medicine*, 46(8), 555–61.

2. Baar, Keith (2014) 'Using Molecular Biology to Maximize Concurrent Training.' *Sports Medicine*, 44(Suppl 2), 117–25.

3. Hickson, Robert C. (1980) 'Interference of strength development by simultaneously training for strength and endurance.' *European Journal of Applied Physiology and Occupational Physiology*, 45(2–3), 255–63.

4. Zatsiorsky, Vladimir M. (1995) *Science and Practice of Strength Training*. Champaign, IL: Human Kinetics Publishers.

5. Winwood, P.W., P.A., Hume, J.B. Cronin and J.W. Keogh (2014) 'Retrospective injury epidemiology of strongman athletes.' *Journal of Strength and Conditoning*, 28(1), 28–42.

6. Siewe, J. et al (2014) 'Injuries and overuse syndromes in competitive and elite bodybuilding.' *International Journal of Sports Medicine*, 35(11), 943–8.

7. Keogh, J., P.A. Hume and S. Pearson (2006) 'Retrospective injury epidemiology of one hundred one competitive Oceania power lifters: the effects of age, body mass, competitive standard, and gender.' *Journal of Strength and Conditioning Research*, 20(3), 672–81.

8. Raske, A. and R. Norlin (2002) 'Injury incidence and prevalence among elite weight and power lifters.' *American Journal of Sports Medicine*, 30(2), 248–56.

9. Calhoon, G. and A.C. Fry (1999) 'Injury rates and profiles of elite competitive weightlifters.' *Journal of Athletic Training*, 34(3), 232–8.

10. Haykowsky, Mark J., D. Warburton and E.R. Darren (1999) 'Pain and Injury Associated with Powerlifting Training in Visually Impaired Athletes.' *Journal of Visual Impairment & Blindness*, 93(4), 236–41.

11. Brown E.W., and R.G. Kimball (1983) 'Medical history associated with adolescent powerlifting.' *Pediatrics*, 72(5), 636–44.

12. Hak, P.T., E. Hodzovic and B. Hickey (2013) 'The nature and prevalence of injury during CrossFit training.' *Journal of Strength and Conditioning Research*.

13. Brechue, W.F. and T. Abe (2002) 'The role of FFM accumulation and skeletal muscle architecture in powerlifting performance.' *European Journal of Applied Physiology*, 86(4), 327–36.

14. Lovera, M. and J. Keogh (2015) 'Anthropometric profile of powerlifters: differences as a function of bodyweight class and competitive success.' *The Journal of Sports Medicine and Physical Fitness*, 55(5), 478–87.

15. Kaminski, T.W., C.V. Wabbersen and R.M. Murphy (1998) 'Concentric versus enhanced eccentric hamstring strength training: clinical implications.' *Journal of Athletic Training*, 33(3), 216–21.

16. Vogt, Michael and Hans H. Hoppeler (2014) 'Eccentric exercise: mechanisms and effects when used as training regime or training adjunct.' *Journal of Applied Physiology*, 116(11), 1446–54.

17. Wernbom, M., J. Augustsson and R. Thomeé (2007) 'The influence of frequency, intensity, volume and mode of strength training on whole muscle cross-sectional area in humans.' *Sports Medicine*, 37(3), 225–64.

18. Burd, Nicholas A. et al (2012) 'Muscle time under tension during resistance exercise stimulates differential muscle protein sub-fractional synthetic responses in men.' *The Journal of Physiology*, 590(2), 351–62.

19. Jenkins, Nathaniel D.M. and Ty Palmer (2012) 'Implement Training for Concentric-Based Muscle Actions.' *Strength and Conditioning Journal*, 34(2), 1–7.

20. Housh, D.J., T.J. Housh, J.P. Weir, L.L. Weir, T.K. Evetovich and P.E. Donlin (1998) 'Effects of unilateral concentric-only dynamic constant external resistance training on quadriceps femoris cross-sectional area.' *Journal of Strength & Conditioning Research*.

21. Evetovich, T.K., T.J. Housh, D.J. Housh, G.O. Johnson, D.B. Smith and K.T. Ebersole (2001) 'The effect of concentric isokinetic strength training of the quadriceps femoris on electromyography and muscle strength in the trained and untrained limb.' *Journal of Strength and Conditioning*, 15(4), 439–45.

22. Kaidar-Person, O, B. Person, S. Szomstein and R.J. Rosenthal (2008). 'Nutritional deficiencies in morbidly obese patients: a new form of malnutrition? Part A: vitamins.' *Obesity Surgery*, 18(7), 870–6.

23. Fuhrman, J. and D.M. Ferreri (2010) 'Fueling the vegetarian (vegan) athlete.' *Current Sports Medicine Reports*, 9(4), 233–41.

24. Knez, Wade L. and Jonathan M. Peake (2010) 'The Prevalence of Vitamin Supplementation in Ultraendurance Triathletes.' *International Journal of Sport Nutrition and Exercise Metabolism*, 20(6).

25. Applegate, E.A. (1991) 'Nutritional considerations for ultra-endurance performance.' *International Journal of Sports Nutrition*, 1(2), 118–26.

26. Leveritt, M. and P.J. Abernethy (1999) 'Effects of Carbohydrate Restriction on Strength Performance.' *Journal of Strength & Conditioning Research*.

27. Cribb, P.J. and A. Hayes (2006) 'Effects of supplement timing and resistance exercise on skeletal muscle hypertrophy.' *Medicine and Science in Sports Exercise*, 38(11), 1918–25.

28. Esmarck, B. et al (2001) 'Timing of postexercise protein intake is important for muscle hypertrophy with resistance training in elderly humans.' *The Journal of Physiology*, 535(1), 301–11.

29. Jentjens, R. and A. Jeukendrup (2003) 'Determinants of post-exercise glycogen synthesis during short-term recovery.' *Sports Medicine*, 33(2), 117–44.

CHAPTER 8

1. Yessis, M. (1972) 'Kinesiological Research in the Soviet Union.' *Journal of Health, Physical Education, Recreation*, 43(1), 93–8.

2. Santello, M. (2005) 'Review of Motor Control Mechanisms Underlying Impact Absorption from Falls.' *Gait & Posture*, 21(1), 85–94.

3. Verkhoshansky, Yuri V. and V.V. Lazarev (1989) 'Principles of planning speed and strength/speed endurance training in sports.' *National Strength and Conditioning Journal*, 11(2), 58–61.

4. Markovic, G. and P. Mikulic (2010) 'Neuro-musculoskeletal and performance adaptations to lower-extremity plyometric training.' *Sports Medicine*, 40(10), 859-95.

5. Rouis, M., E. Attiogbé, H. Vandewalle, H. Jaafar, T. D. Noakes and T. Driss (2014) 'Relationship between vertical jump and maximal power output of legs and arms: Effects of ethnicity and sport.' *Scandinavian Journal of Medicine & Science in Sports*, 25(2), 197–207.

6. Zehr, E. Paul and Digby G. Sale (1994) 'Ballistic Movement: Muscle Activation and Neuromuscular Adaptation.' *Canadian Journal of Applied Physiology*, 19(4), 363–78.

7. Mangine, Gerald T. et al (2008) 'The Effects of Combined Ballistic and Heavy Resistance Training on Maximal Lower- and Upper-Body Strength in Recreationally Trained Men.' *Journal of Strength & Conditioning Research*, 22(1), 132–9.

8. Zehr, E.P. and D.G. Sale (1994) 'Ballistic movement: muscle activation and neuromuscular adaptation.' *Canadian Journal of Applied Physiology*, 19(4), 363–78.

9. Anderson, C.E., G.A. Sforzo and J.A. Sigg (2008) 'The effects of combining elastic and free weight resistance on strength and power in athletes.' *The Journal of Strength & Conditioning Research*, 22(2), 567–74.

10. Ibid.

11. Ghigiarelli, J.J., E.F. Nagle, F.L. Gross, R.J. Robertson, J.J. Irrgang and T. Myslinski (2009) 'The effects of a 7-week heavy elastic band and weight chain program on upper-body strength and upper-body power in a sample of division 1-AA football players.' *Journal of Strength and Conditioning Research*, 23(3), 756–64.

12. Treiber, F.A. et al (1998) 'Effects of Theraband and lightweight dumbbell training on shoulder rotation torque and serve performance in college tennis players.' *American Journal of Sports Medicine*, 26(4), 510–15.

13. Page, P.A., J. Lamberth, B. Abadie, R. Boling, R. Collins and R. Linton (1993) 'Posterior Rotator Cuff Strengthening Using Theraband® in a Functional Diagonal Pattern in Collegiate Baseball Pitchers.' *Journal of Athletic Training*, 28(4), 346–54.

14. Stevenson M.W., J.M. Warpeha, C.C. Dietz, R.M. Giveans and A.G. Erdman (2010) 'Acute effects of elastic bands during the free-weight barbell back squat exercise on velocity, power, and force production.' *Journal of Strength & Conditioning Research*, 24(11), 2944–54.

15. Hatfield, Fred (1989) *Power: A scientific approach*. McGraw-Hill.

16. Fry, A.C. (2012) 'The role of resistance intensity on muscle fibre adaptations.' *Sports Medicine*, 34(10), 663–79.

17. Fry, C. (2004) 'The role of resistance exercise intensity on muscle fibre adaptations.' *Sports Medicine*, 10, 663–79.

18. Crewther, B.T., T. Heke and J.W. Keogh (2011) 'The effects of training volume and competition on the salivary cortisol concentrations of Olympic weightlifters.' *Journal of Strength & Conditioning Research*, 25(1), 10-15.

19. Storey, A. and H.K. Smith (2012) 'Unique aspects of competitive weightlifting: performance, training and physiology.' *Sports Medicine*, 42(9), 769–90.

20. Crewther, B.T., T. Heke and J.W. Keogh (2011) 'The effects of training volume and competition on the salivary cortisol concentrations of Olympic weightlifters.' *Journal of Strength & Conditioning Research*, 25(1), 10–15.

21. Mujika, I., S. Padilla, D. Pyne, T. Busso (2004) 'Physiological changes associated with pre-event taper in athletes.' *Sports Medicine*, 34(13), 891–927.

CHAPTER 9

1. Midgley, A.W., L.R. McNaughton and A.M. Jones (2007) 'Training to enhance the physiological determinants of long-distance running performance: can valid recommendations be given to runners and coaches based on current scientific knowledge?' *Sports Medicine*, 37(10), 857–80.

2. Applegate, E. (1989) 'Nutritional concerns of the ultra-endurance triathlete.' *Medicine and Science in Sports and Exercise*, 21 (5 Suppl), S205-8.

3. Nielsen, Rasmus, Joshua M. Akey, Mattias Jakobsson, Jonathan K. Pritchard, Sarah Tishkoff and Eske Willerslev (2017) 'Tracing the peopling of the world through genomics.' *Nature* 541, 302–10.

4. Daoud, A.I., G.J. Geissler, F. Wang, J. Saretsky, Y.A. Daoud and D.E. Lieberman (2012) 'Foot strike and injury rates in endurance runners: a retrospective study.' *Medicine and Science in Sport and Exercise*, 44(7),1325–34.

5. Applegate, E. (1989) 'Nutritional concerns of the ultra-endurance triathlete.' *Medicine and Science in Sports and Exercise*, 21(5 Suppl), S205–8.

6. Eckel, R.H. et al (2006) 'Carbohydrate balance predicts weight and fat gain in adults.' *American Journal of Clinical Nutrition*, 83(4), 803–8.

7. Porter, Ruth and Julie Whelan (2008) 'Human Muscle Fatigue: Physiological Mechanisms.' Ciba Foundation Symposium 82, 2008.

8. Roberts, Thomas J. and Richard A. Belliveau (2005) 'Sources of mechanical power for uphill running in humans.' *Journal of Experimental Biology*, 208, 1963–1970.

9. Vernillo, G., M. Giandolini, W.B. Edwards, J. Morin, P Samozino, N. Horvais and G.Y. Millet (2017) 'Biomechanics and Physiology of Uphill and Downhill Running.' *Sports Medicine*, 47(4), 615–29.

10. Sloniger, Mark A., Kirk J. Cureton, Barry M. Prior and Ellen M. Evans (1997) 'Lower extremity muscle activation during horizontal and uphill running.' *Journal of Applied Physiology*, 83(6), 2073–9.

11. Vernillo, G., A. Savoldelli, A. Zignoli, P. Trabucchi, B. Pellegrini, G.P. Millet and F. Schena (2014) 'Influence of the world's most challenging mountain ultra-marathon on energy cost and running mechanics.' *European Journal of Applied Physiology*, 114(5), 929–39.

12. Vernillo, G., A. Savoldelli, A. Zignoli, S. Skafidas, A. Fornasiero, A. La Torre, L. Bortolan, B. Pellegrini and F. Schena (2015) 'Energy cost and kinematics of level, uphill and downhill running: fatigue-induced changes after a mountain ultramarathon.' *Journal of Sports Science*, 33(19), 1998–2000.

13. Giandolini, M., G. Vernillo, P. Samozino, N. Horvais, W.B. Edwards, J.B. Morin and G.Y. Millet GY (2016) 'Fatigue associated with prolonged graded running.' *European Journal of Applied Physiology*, 116(10), 1859–73.

14. Jinger, S. Gottschall and Rodger Kram (2005) 'Ground reaction forces during downhill and uphill running.' *Journal of Biomechanics*, 38(3), 445–52.

15. Eston, R.G., J. Mickleborough and V. Baltzopoulos (1995) 'Eccentric activation and muscle damage: biomechanical and physiological considerations during downhill running.' *British Journal of Sports Medicine*, 29, 89–94.

16. Braun, William A. and Darren J. Dutto (2003) 'The effects of a single bout of downhill running and ensuing delayed onset of muscle soreness on running economy performed 48 h later.' *European Journal of Applied Physiology*, 90(1), 29–34.

17. Tabata, I., K. Nishimura, M. Kouzaki, Y. Hirai, F. Ogita, M. Miyachi and K. Yamamoto (1996) 'Effects of moderate-intensity endurance and high-intensity intermittent training on anaerobic capacity and VO2max.' *Medicine and Science in Sport and Exercise*, 28(10), 1327-30.

18. Mazzone, Thomas M.D. (1988) 'Kinesiology of the rowing stroke.' *National Strength & Conditioning Association Journal*, 10(2), 4–13.

19. Hagerman, Fredrick C. (1984) 'Applied Physiology of Rowing.' *Sports Medicine*, 1(4), 303–26.

20. García-Pallarés, Jesús and Mikel Izquierdo (2011) 'Strategies to Optimize Concurrent Training of Strength and Aerobic Fitness for Rowing and Canoeing.' *Sports Medicine*, 41(4), 329–43.

21. Prince, Frederick P, Robert S. Hikida and Fredrick C. Hagerman (1976) 'Human muscle fiber types in power lifters, distance runners and untrained subjects.' *Pflügers Archive*, 363(1), 19–26.

22. McCarthy, J.P., J.C. Agre, B.K. Graf, M.A. Pozniak and A.C. Vailas (1995) 'Compatibility of adaptive responses with combining strength and endurance training.' *Medicine and Science in Sport and Exercise*, 27(3), 429–36.

23. Hackney, Anthony C. (1989) 'Endurance Training and Testosterone Levels.' *Sports Medicine*, 8(2), 117–127.

24. Bell, G.J., D.G. Syrotuik, K. Attwood and H.A. Quinney (1993) 'Maintenance of Strength Gains While Performing Endurance Training in Oarswomen.' *Canadian Journal of Applied Physiology*, 18(1), 104–115.

25. Lawton, T.W., J.B. Cronin and M.R. McGuigan (2011) 'Strength testing and training of rowers: a review.' *Sports Medicine*, 41(5), 413–32.

26. Lundburg, Tommy R., Rodrigo Fornandez Gonzalo, Thomas Gustafsson and Per A. Tesch (2012) 'Aerobic exercise does not compromise muscle hypertrophy response to short-term resistance training.' *Journal of Applied Physiology*, 114(1), 81–89.

27. Lundberg, T.R., R. Fernandez-Gonzalo, P.A. Tesch, E. Rullman and T. Gustafsson (2016) 'Aerobic exercise augments muscle transcriptome profile of resistance exercise.' *American Journal of Physiology*, 310(11), R1279–87.

28. Ingjer, F. (1979) 'Effects of endurance training on muscle fibre ATP-ase activity, capillary supply and mitochondrial content in man.' *The Journal of Physiology*, 294, 419–32.

29. Rønnestad, B.R., E.A. Hansen and T. Raastad (2010) 'Effect of heavy strength training on thigh muscle cross-sectional area, performance determinants, and performance in well-trained cyclists.' *European Journal of Applied Physiology*, 108(5), 965–75.

30. www.britishcycling.org.uk/knowledge/bike-kit/article/izn20160113-Ask-the-experts-how-to-Beginner-strength-exercises-for-cyclists-0; www.britishcycling.org.uk/knowledge/bike-kit/set-up/article/20161103-Do-I-need-a-professional-bike-fit-0

32. Aagaard, P. and J.L. Andersen (2010) 'Effects of strength training on endurance capacity in top-level endurance athletes.' *Scandinavian Journal of Medicine and Science in Sport*, 20(Suppl 2), 39–47.

32. Rønnestad, B.R., E.A. Hansen and T. Raastad (2011) 'Strength training improves 5-min all-out performance following 185 min of cycling.' *Scandinavian Journal of Medicine and Science in Sport*, 21(2), 250–9.

33. Vikmoen, O., S. Ellefsen, Ø. Trøen, I. Hollan, M. Hanestadhaugen, T. Raastad and B.R. Rønnestad (2016) 'Strength training improves cycling performance, fractional utilization of VO2max & cycling economy in female cyclists.' *Scandinavian Journal of Medicine and Science in Sport*, 26(4), 384–96.

34. Ibid.

CHAPTER 10

1. Ericsson, K. Anders, Ralf T. Krampe and Clemens Tesch-Romer (1993) 'The Role of Deliberate Practice in the Acquisition of Expert Performance.' *Psychological Review*, 100(3), 363–406.

2. Taylor, I.A. (1975) 'A retrospective view of creativity investigation.' In I.A. Taylor and J.W. Getzels, (eds) *Perspectives in creativity*. Chicago, IL: Aldine Publishing Co, 1–36.

3. Doll, J., and U. Mayr (1987) 'Intelligenz und Schachleistung - eine Untersuchung an Schachexperten. [Intelligence and achievement in chess - a study of chess masters].' *Psychologische Beiträge*, 29, 270–89.

4. Stambulova, Natalia B., Craig A. Wrisberg and Tatiana V. Ryba (2006) 'A Tale of Two Traditions in Applied Sport Psychology: The Heyday of Soviet Sport and Wake-Up Calls for North America.' *Journal of Applied Sport Psychology,* 18(3).

5. 'Worldwide obesity has doubled since 1980.' The World Health Organization, February 2014: www.who.int/gho/ncd/risk_factors/obesity_text/en/

6. 'Physical inactivity is the fourth leading risk factor for global mortality.' The World Health Organization, February 2014: www.who.int/mediacentre/factsheets/fs385/en/

7. Stewart, T.M., D.A. Williamson and M.A. White (2002) 'Rigid vs. flexible dieting: association with eating disorder symptoms in nonobese women.' *Appetite*, 38(1), 39–44.

8. McNaughton, S.A., D. Crawford, K. Ball and J. Salmon (2012) 'Understanding determinants of nutrition, physical activity and quality of life among older adults: the Wellbeing, Eating and Exercise for a Long Life (WELL) study.' *Health Quality of Life Outcomes*, 10, 109.

9. Curtis.T. 'Strength Training Modalities: The Perfect Workout?' *National Strength & Conditioning Association Journal*, 13(6), 83–5.

INDEX

ACKNOWLEDGEMENTS

The title of *The World's Fittest Book* is a bold one. But it's not a reference to me or my achievements. Instead it's a tribute to the Olympians, World Champions, decorated Royal Marines and food-based geniuses who contributed so generously to the knowledge within it. Each one shared my vision to create something that would educate and empower millions and without them there would be no book. Which is why I will forever be indebted to every person you've come to learn about.

The book was only made possible by the incredible people I feel privileged to have met, trained and travelled with. It's essentially a by-product of the expertise they selflessly donated, and that expertise begins with the immensely talented team of photographers who captured every image you see here. To James Appleton, Simon Howard, Harvey Gibson, Chris Bailey and Richard Hunter, thank you so much for following me over mountains, through lakes and into gyms all over the world with your cameras to bring this book to life.

My family and friends have helped me plot, plan and often complete each and every adventure I've embarked on. They typically begin with an idea hatched over a Sunday roast dinner and end with my family on a support boat battling seasickness and 6-ft waves halfway across the Caribbean sea as I swim with a tree attached to my trunks (as odd as it sounds). This sort of selfless commitment epitomises just how lucky I am to have these people in my life.

To Mark, Nick, Karl, Laura and the team at THE PROTEIN WORKS™, I don't think there's any other brand in the world where competing in a triathlon with a tree on your back or running a marathon pulling a car is actually encouraged as part of a job. For helping every one of my crazy adventures with unbridled support (and an endless supply of protein brownies) I want to say one huge thank you.

Finally, to the amazing publishing team at Little, Brown. Without them this entire book would only exist as scribbles in my travel diary and as a 10-year-old document saved on my laptop. But because Adam Strange had the monk-like patience to sit through over 200,000 words of my fitness and food musings, Alex Cooper had the endurance to trek around the country with me visiting gyms, and Stephanie, Duncan, Abby, Sian, Alison and the entire team didn't mind taking conference calls with me sitting on a spin bike or on the side of a pool during a 30-km swim... my dream of publishing my book became a reality.

ABOUT THE AUTHOR

Ross Edgley is an athlete, adventurer and author whose decade-long career spans every area of sport, fitness and nutrition imaginable. He's set world records around the globe and has been called 'The World's Most Travelled Fitness Expert' (*GQ*, 2016). Ross was listed in the World's 50 Top Fittest Men in 2016 by Askmen.com after he...

- Ran a marathon pulling a 1.4-tonne car (dubbed 'The World's Strongest Marathon' by the media).
- Climbed 8848 metres, the height of Everest, up a rope ('The World's Longest Rope Climb').
- Ran 1000 miles barefoot in a month carrying a 50-kg backpack.
- Completed an Olympic-distance triathlon carrying a 100-lb tree.
- Ran 31 marathons in 31 days on a treadmill in his kitchen, trialling different recipes.
- Swam over 100 km across the Caribbean Sea pulling a 100-lb tree.
- Swam non-stop for 48 hours at the Commando Training Centre for the Royal Marines.

Founder of 2017's most downloaded training app (Primal 9) with Menshealth.com, co-founder of Europe's most innovative sports nutrition brand (THE PROTEIN WORKS™) and proud alumnus of Loughborough University's world-renowned School of Sport and Exercise Science, Ross has an 'aversion to the average' and, through his work, wants to teach millions that the human body is far more powerful than we are often led to believe.

'Fitness is a journey everyone should start, but no one should finish.'

ROSS EDGLEY